D1692269

Atlas *of* Emergency Procedures

ATLAS *of* EMERGENCY PROCEDURES

EDITED BY

Peter Rosen, M.D.
Residency Director Emeritus
Director of Education
Department of Emergency Medicine
University of California San Diego Medical Center
San Diego, California

Theodore C. Chan, M.D.
Assistant Clinical Professor of Medicine
Associate Medical Director
Department of Emergency Medicine
University of California San Diego Medical Center
San Diego, California

Gary M. Vilke, M.D.
Assistant Clinical Professor of Medicine
Director, Prehospital Services
Department of Emergency Medicine
University of California San Diego Medical Center
San Diego, California

George Sternbach, M.D.
Clinical Professor of Surgery
Attending Physician in Emergency Medicine
Stanford Medical Center
Stanford, California
Emergency Physician
Seton Medical Center
Daly City, California

ILLUSTRATED BY

Elizabeth Weadon Massari, CMI
Tim Hengst, CMI

Mosby
A Harcourt Health Sciences Company
St. Louis   London   Philadelphia   Sydney   Toronto

Mosby
A Harcourt Health Sciences Company

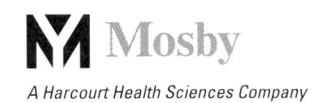

Publisher: Richard Lampert
Acquisitions Editor: Judith Fletcher
Managing Editor: Kathy Falk
Project Manager: Patricia Tannian
Designer: Liz Young

Copyright © 2001 by Mosby, Inc.

All rights reserved. No part of this publication may be reproduced or transmitted in any form or by any means, electronic or mechanical, including photocopy, recording, or any information storage and retrieval system, without permission in writing from the publisher.

NOTICE
Pharmacology is an ever-changing field. Standard safety precautions must be followed, but as new research and clinical experience broaden our knowledge, changes in treatment and drug therapy may become necessary or appropriate. Readers are advised to check the most current product information provided by the manufacturer of each drug to be administered to verify the recommended dose, the method and duration of administration, and contraindications. It is the responsibility of the licensed prescriber, relying on experience and knowledge of the patient, to determine dosages and the best treatment for each individual patient. Neither the publisher nor the editor assumes any liability for any injury and/or damage to persons or property arising from this publication.

Permission to photocopy or reproduce solely for internal or personal use is permitted for libraries or other users registered with the Copyright Clearance Center, provided that the base fee of $4.00 per chapter plus $.10 per page is paid directly to the Copyright Clearance Center, 222 Rosewood Drive, Danvers, Massachusetts 01923. This consent does not extend to other kinds of copying, such as copying for general distribution, for advertising or promotional purposes, for creating new collected works, or for resale.

Mosby, Inc.
A Harcourt Health Sciences Company
11830 Westline Industrial Drive
St. Louis, Missouri 63146

Printed in United States of America

Library of Congress Cataloging in Publication Data

Atlas of emergency procedures / edited by Peter Rosen . . . [et al.]; illustrated by Elizabeth Weadon Massari, Tim Hengst.
     p. ; cm.
  Includes bibliographical references and index.
  ISBN 0-8151-7402-0 (alk. paper)
  1. Emergency medicine—Atlases. 2. Surgical emergencies—Atlases.
I. Rosen, Peter, 1935-
  [DNLM: 1. Emergencies—Atlases. 2. Surgical Procedures, Operative—methods—Atlases. WO 517 A8792 2001]
  RC86.7.A854 2001
  616.02'5'0222—dc21
                                                      00-052538

01 02 03 04 05 TG/MV 9 8 7 6 5 4 3 2 1

Contributors

JAMES T. AMSTERDAM, D.M.D., M.D., M.M.M., F.A.C.E.P.
Head, Emergency Medicine Department
HealthPartners Regions Hospital
Professor of Clinical Emergency Medicine
University of Minnesota School of Medicine
Minneapolis, Minnesota

ERIK D. BARTON, M.D.
Associate Residency Director
Department of Emergency Medicine
Brigham and Women's Hospital
Boston, Massachusetts

KENNETH J. BRAMWELL, M.D.
Fellow, Pediatric Emergency Medicine
Primary Children's Medical Center
Salt Lake City, Utah

COLLEEN J. CAMPBELL, M.D.
Assistant Clinical Professor of Medicine
Department of Emergency Medicine
University of California San Diego Medical Center
San Diego, California

THEODORE C. CHAN, M.D.
Assistant Clinical Professor of Medicine
Associate Medical Director
Department of Emergency Medicine
University of California San Diego Medical Center
San Diego, California

JOSEPH E. CLINTON, M.D.
Chief of Service
Department of Emergency Medicine
Hennepin County Medical Center
Professor of Clinical Emergency Medicine
University of Minnesota School of Medicine
Minneapolis, Minnesota

DANIEL F. DANZL, M.D.
Professor and Chair
Department of Emergency Medicine
University of Louisville School of Medicine
Louisville, Kentucky

DANIEL P. DAVIS, M.D.
Assistant Clinical Professor
Department of Emergency Medicine
University of California San Diego Medical Center
San Diego, California

JAMES DUCHARME, M.D.
Professor
Department of Emergency Medicine
Dalhousie University
Clinical Director
Department of Emergency Medicine
Atlantic Health Sciences Corporation
Saint John, New Brunswick
Canada

KIM M. FELDHAUS, M.D.
Attending Physician
Department of Emergency Medicine
Denver Health Medical Center
Denver, Colorado

MARY ANNE FUCHS, M.D.
Assistant Clinical Professor
Department of Emergency Medicine
University of California San Diego Medical Center
San Diego, California

PHILLIP M. HARTER, M.D.
Assistant Professor of Surgery
Division of Emergency Medicine
Stanford University
Stanford, California

KENNETH C. JACKIMCZYK, M.D.
Associate Chairman
Department of Emergency Medicine
Maricopa Medical Center
Phoenix, Arizona

PASCAL S.C. JUANG, M.D.
Chief Resident
Harvard Affiliated Emergency Medicine Residency
Brigham and Women's Hospital and
Massachusetts General Hospital
Clinical Fellow in Medicine
Harvard Medical School
Boston, Massachusetts

SAMUEL M. KEIM, M.D.
Associate Professor and Residency Director
Department of Emergency Medicine
University of Arizona Health Sciences Center
Tucson, Arizona

JOHN L. KENDALL, M.D.
Department of Emergency Medicine
Denver Health Medical Center
Denver, Colorado

JAMES P. KILLEEN, M.D.
Assistant Clinical Professor of Medicine
Department of Emergency Medicine/Hyperbaric Medicine
University of California San Diego Medical Center
San Diego, California

MARK I. LANGDORF, M.D., M.H.P.E.
Associate Professor of Clinical Emergency Medicine
Chief and Residency Director
Division of Emergency Medicine
Medical Director, UC Irvine Medical Center
Department of Emergency Medicine
Irvine, California

JAMES L. LARSON, Jr., M.D.
Assistant Professor and Assistant Residency Director
Department of Emergency Medicine
University of North Carolina Chapel Hill
School of Medicine
Chapel Hill, North Carolina

STEVEN LARSON, M.D.
Assistant Professor
Department of Emergency Medicine
Hospital of the University of Pennsylvania
Philadelphia, Pennsylvania

SIDNEY I. LEE, M.D., F.A.C.E.P.
Chairman
Department of Primary Care
Kapiolani Medical Center
Honolulu, Hawaii

VINCENT J. MARKOVCHICK, M.D.
Director
Emergency Medicine
Denver Health
Denver, Colorado

JOHN MARX, M.D.
Chair
Department of Emergency Medicine
Carolinas Medical Center
Charlotte, North Carolina
Clinical Professor of Emergency Medicine
University of North Carolina School of Medicine
Chapel Hill, North Carolina

HARVEY W. MEISLIN, M.D.
Professor and Chief
Department of Emergency Medicine
University of Arizona Health Sciences Center
Tuscon, Arizona

LESLIE W. MILNE, M.D.
Assistant Clinical Instructor
Department of Emergency Medicine
Massachusetts General Hospital
Boston, Massachusetts

MICHAEL F. MURPHY, M.D.
Associate Professor
Departments of Emergency Medicine and Anesthesiology
Dalhousie University
Halifax, Nova Scotia, Canada

GARY J. ORDOG, M.D., F.A.C.E.P.
Department of Emergency Medicine
Mayo/Newhall Memorial/UCLA Hospital
Santa Clarita, California

CHRISTOPHER F. RICHARDS, M.D.
Assistant Professor
Department of Emergency Medicine
Oregon Health Sciences University
Portland, Oregon

GHAZALA Q. SHARIEFF, M.D.
Assistant Clinical Professor of Medicine and Pediatrics
University of California San Diego
Director of Pediatric Emergency Medicine
Palomar-Pomerado Health System
San Diego, California

BARRY C. SIMON, M.D.
Chairman and Program Director
Department of Emergency Medicine
Alameda County Medical Center
Oakland, California

REBECCA SMITH-COGGINS, M.D.
Associate Professor of Surgery/Emergency Medicine
Emergency Medicine Residency Director
Stanford University School of Medicine
Stanford, California

GEORGE STERNBACH, M.D.
Clinical Professor of Surgery
Attending Physician in Emergency Medicine
Stanford Medical Center
Stanford, California
Emergency Physician
Seton Medical Center
Daly City, California

MATTHEW DAVID SZTAJNKRYCER, M.D., Ph.D.
Assistant Professor
Department of Emergency Medicine
University of Cincinnati
Cincinnati, Ohio

N. NOUNOU TALEGHANI, M.D.
Attending Physician
Division of Emergency Medicine
Stanford University Hospital
Stanford, California

JAMES H. TRUONG, M.D.
Department of Emergency Medicine
University of California Irvine Medical Center
Orange, California

GARY M. VILKE, M.D.
Assistant Clinical Professor of Medicine
Director, Prehospital Services
Department of Emergency Medicine
University of California San Diego Medical Center
San Diego, California

RON M. WALLS, M.D.
Associate Professor of Medicine (Emergency Medicine)
Harvard Medical School
Chairman
Department of Emergency Medicine
Brigham and Women's Hospital
Boston, Massachusetts

EDWARD A. WALTON, M.D.
Clinical Assistant Professor
Departments of Emergency Medicine and Pediatrics
University of Michigan
Ann Arbor, Michigan

MICHAEL B. WOLFE, M.D.
Attending Emergency Physician
Community Hospital of Los Gatos
Los Gatos, California

DONALD DEMETRIUS ZUKIN, M.D.
Attending Physician
Department of Emergency Medicine
Children's Hospital Oakland
Oakland, California
Clinical Assistant Professor
Department of Pediatrics
University of California San Francisco
San Francisco, California

PREFACE

Emergency medicine encompasses a wide spectrum of conditions that involve the acute distortions of normal physiology. For both the less serious and the most critical problems, emergency physicians must frequently perform invasive technical procedures. They must possess a complete armamentarium of technical skills, the knowledge of when to use them, the willingness to modify techniques in the face of difficulty, and the aggressiveness to perform a major technical invasion when a less invasive route has failed. Medical education, even at the advanced level of residency training, has tended to ignore the putatively easy technical tasks in favor of a concentration on cognitive knowledge.

Atlases have traditionally been illustrated texts that depict the performance of surgical procedures. We believe that a comparable volume is appropriate to delineate the procedures performed in the emergency department and the prehospital care arena. A number of books describe emergency procedures, but none offers a visual display of the techniques being described. The purpose of the *Atlas of Emergency Procedures* is to provide that very kind of guide.

Although the publication of surgical atlases is an established tradition, the purpose of an atlas is often misunderstood. The text contained in an atlas must be concise rather than comprehensive, and although references may be cited, an atlas is not meant to provide an all-inclusive bibliography. The function of the *Atlas of Emergency Procedures* is to give the clinician an illustrated guide to the completion of both basic and advanced techniques required in emergency practice. It is meant to complement rather than replace a textbook of emergency medicine. The *Atlas of Emergency Procedures* is intended not only for the student and resident physician in training, but also as a reference for the physician in clinical practice who performs both simple and difficult invasive procedures. In addition, many emergency medical technicians, paramedics, and flight nurses perform these procedures and could use this atlas as a learning and reference resource.

Eminent teachers of emergency medicine who are also in active practice have written the procedures in the *Atlas of Emergency Procedures*. A brief discussion of indications, contraindications, and complications and their management is included for each procedure. The technical steps of each procedure are depicted in detailed drawings done from the perspective of the emergency physician. In every case we have selected a methodology that stems from an active emergency medicine practice, but recognizing that any given problem has multiple technical solutions, we have attempted to give some acceptable variations in the discussions that follow each procedure description. In discussions of the most difficult and complex procedures the contributors share their own experience and technical tricks.

The goal of the *Atlas of Emergency Procedures* is to provide readers with a constant source of education for the procedures demanded in emergency medicine. Our intent is not that the atlas will replace bedside teaching or practice, but rather that it will supplement them. Technical tasks are visual and spatial, and we hope that this atlas will enhance the visual orientation that will enable successful technical performance.

Peter Rosen
Theodore C. Chan
Gary M. Vilke
George Sternbach

Contents

CHAPTER 1 AIRWAY, 1

Assisted mask ventilation, 2
DANIEL F. DANZL

Endotracheal intubation, 4
   Standard endotracheal intubation, 4
   DANIEL F. DANZL

   Fiberoptic intubation, 8
   MICHAEL F. MURPHY

   Retrograde intubation, 10
   JAMES P. KILLEEN

   Digital intubation, 12
   JAMES P. KILLEEN

   Endotracheal intubation using a lighted stylet, 14
   JAMES P. KILLEEN

   Nasotracheal intubation, 16
   DANIEL F. DANZL

   Pediatric endotracheal intubation, 18
   GHAZALA Q. SHARIEFF

Tracheal suctioning, 20
DANIEL F. DANZL

Needle cricothyrotomy, 22
KENNETH J. BRAMWELL

Cricothyrotomy, 24
RON M. WALLS

CHAPTER 2 THORAX, 31

External defibrillation, 32
JAMES H. TRUONG, MARK I. LANGDORF

Intercostal nerve block, 34
ERIK D. BARTON

Thoracentesis, 36
ERIK D. BARTON

Needle thoracostomy, 38
MICHAEL B. WOLFE AND REBECCA SMITH-COGGINS

Tube thoracostomy, 40
KIM M. FELDHAUS

Thoracotomy, 46
KENNETH C. JACKIMCZYK AND GARY J. ORDOG

Open cardiac massage, 50
KENNETH C. JACKIMCZYK

Cardiorrhaphy, 54
GARY J. ORDOG

Internal defibrillation, 56
KENNETH C. JACKIMCZYK

Aortic cross clamping, 58
GARY J. ORDOG

CHAPTER 3 CARDIOVASCULAR SYSTEM, 61

Radial artery cannulation, 62
JOHN L. KENDALL

Pericardiocentesis, 66
VINCENT J. MARKOVCHICK

Peripheral venous access, 68
   Peripheral venipuncture, 68
   CHRISTOPHER F. RICHARDS

Central venous access, 74
   General approach to central venous access (Seldinger guidewire technique), 74
   PHILLIP M. HARTER AND SIDNEY I. LEE

   Subclavian central venous access, 78
   MATTHEW DAVID SZTAJNKRYCER

   Internal jugular central venous access, 82
   JOSEPH E. CLINTON

   Femoral central venous access, 86
   DONALD DEMETRIUS ZUKIN

Alternative venous access, 90
   Greater saphenous venous cutdown, 90
   GEORGE STERNBACH

Saphenofemoral venous cutdown, 94
GEORGE STERNBACH

Upper extremity venous cutdown, 96
GEORGE STERNBACH

Intraosseous infusion, 98
EDWARD A. WALTON

Umbilical venous catheter, 100
EDWARD A. WALTON

CHAPTER 4 ABDOMEN, 103

Nasogastric intubation, 104
JOHN MARX

Semiopen diagnostic peritoneal lavage, 108
JOHN MARX

Paracentesis, 112
THEODORE C. CHAN

Anoscopy, 114
STEVEN LARSON

Excision of thrombosed external hemorrhoid, 116
STEVEN LARSON

Pilonidal abscess drainage, 118
STEVEN LARSON

Perianal abscess drainage, 120
STEVEN LARSON

CHAPTER 5 GENITOURINARY SYSTEM, 123

Urethral catheterization, 124
GARY M. VILKE

Cystostomy, 128
GARY M. VILKE

Bladder aspiration, 130
GARY M. VILKE

Dorsal slit in phimosis, 132
GARY M. VILKE

Manual paraphimosis reduction, 134
GARY M. VILKE

Zipper removal, 136
GARY M. VILKE

CHAPTER 6 OBSTETRICS AND GYNECOLOGY, 139

Culdocentesis, 140
COLLEEN J. CAMPBELL

Vaginal delivery, 142
COLLEEN J. CAMPBELL

Perimortem cesarean section, 146
COLLEEN J. CAMPBELL

Episiotomy and repair, 150
COLLEEN J. CAMPBELL

Incision and drainage of Bartholin's abscess, 152
COLLEEN J. CAMPBELL

CHAPTER 7 NERVOUS SYSTEM, 155

Lumbar puncture, 156
JAMES L. LARSON, JR.

Facial and oral blocks, 158
   Supraorbital nerve block, 158
   N. NOUNOU TALEGHANI AND GEORGE STERNBACH

   Infraorbital nerve block, 160
   N. NOUNOU TALEGHANI AND GEORGE STERNBACH

   Internal maxillary–superior alveolar nerve block, 162
   JAMES T. AMSTERDAM

   Mandibular and inferior alveolar nerve block, 164
   JAMES T. AMSTERDAM

   Mental nerve block, 166
   JAMES T. AMSTERDAM

Extremity blocks, 168
   Bier block, 168
   JAMES DUCHARME

   Wrist blocks, 170
   JAMES DUCHARME

   Digital nerve block, 174
   N. NOUNOU TALEGHANI AND GEORGE STERNBACH

   Foot blocks, 176
   N. NOUNOU TALEGHANI AND GEORGE STERNBACH

CHAPTER 8 EYE, 179

Corneal foreign body removal, 180
PASCAL S.C. JUANG

Eversion of the upper eyelid, 182
PASCAL S.C. JUANG

Contact lens removal, 184
PASCAL S.C. JUANG

Measurement of intraocular pressure–Schiøtz tonometry, 186
PASCAL S.C. JUANG

CHAPTER 9 EAR, NOSE, AND THROAT, 189

Anterior packing, 190
THEODORE C. CHAN

Posterior packing, 194
THEODORE C. CHAN

Septal hematoma drainage, 198
THEODORE C. CHAN

Auricular hematoma drainage, 200
THEODORE C. CHAN

Peritonsillar abscess drainage, 202
JAMES T. AMSTERDAM

Mandibular reduction, 204
JAMES T. AMSTERDAM

CHAPTER 10 SKIN AND SUBCUTANEOUS TISSUE, 207

Interrupted and running suture, 208
BARRY C. SIMON

Mattress suture, 210
BARRY C. SIMON

Intradermal (buried) suture, 212
BARRY C. SIMON

Scalp laceration repair, 214
BARRY C. SIMON

Corner stitch (half-buried horizontal mattress), 216
BARRY C. SIMON

Dog ear repair, 218
BARRY C. SIMON

V-Y closure, 220
BARRY C. SIMON

Abscess incision and drainage, 222
HARVEY W. MEISLIN AND SAMUEL M. KEIM

CHAPTER 11 EXTREMITIES, 227

Fascial compartment pressure measurement (anterior compartment, lower leg), 228
LESLIE W. MILNE

Arthrocentesis of the knee, 232
LESLIE W. MILNE

Arthrocentesis of the ankle, 234
LESLIE W. MILNE

Arthrocentesis of the metatarsophalangeal joint, 236
LESLIE W. MILNE

Aspiration of the shoulder, 238
LESLIE W. MILNE

Arthrocentesis of the elbow, 240
LESLIE W. MILNE

Arthrocentesis of the wrist, 242
LESLIE W. MILNE

Hand, 244

Felon drainage, 244
SAMUEL M. KEIM AND HARVEY W. MEISLIN

Paronychia drainage, 246
SAMUEL M. KEIM AND HARVEY W. MEISLIN

Ring removal, 248
SAMUEL M. KEIM AND HARVEY W. MEISLIN

Nail removal, 252
HARVEY W. MEISLIN AND SAMUEL M. KEIM

Fish hook removal, 254
HARVEY W. MEISLIN AND SAMUEL M. KEIM

CHAPTER 12 REDUCTION AND SPLINTING, 257

Dislocation reduction, 258

Closed reduction of anterior shoulder dislocations, 258
MARY ANNE FUCHS

Posterior elbow dislocation reduction with the puller technique, 262
MARY ANNE FUCHS

Radial head subluxation reduction by the flexion-supination method, 264
MARY ANNE FUCHS

Finger dislocations, 266
MARY ANNE FUCHS

Posterior hip reduction by the standard supine (Allis) method, 268
MARY ANNE FUCHS

Patellar dislocation reduction, 270
MARY ANNE FUCHS

Splinting, 272
DANIEL P. DAVIS

CHAPTER 1

AIRWAY

Assisted Mask Ventilation ■ DANIEL F. DANZL

Indications
- Patient with apnea or respiratory failure
- Before endotracheal intubation

Contraindications
- None

Equipment
- Bag-valve-mask (BVM) resuscitator (neonatal, pediatric, and adult sizes)
- Oxygen source and tubing
- Reservoir bag

Procedure

1. Check equipment, and make certain the BVM resuscitator has a reservoir bag.
2. If cervical spine injury is not suspected, move the patient's head into the sniffing position and place a small towel roll under the occiput to align the oropharyngolaryngeal axes.
3. Two-person technique:
   a. One person holds the mask to the patient's face by placing the thumb and index finger on each side of the mask to obtain a good seal *(A)*.
   b. Elevate the mandible with the remaining fingers to open the airway.
   c. The other person compresses the bag and delivers adequate tidal volumes of 10 to 15 cc/kg.
4. One-person technique:
   a. With one hand hold the mask to the patient's face by placing the thumb and index finger on top of the mask to obtain a good seal *(B)*.
   b. Elevate the mandible with the remaining fingers to open the airway.
   c. With the other hand compress the bag and deliver adequate tidal volumes of 10 to 15 cc/kg.

Complications

- Hypoventilation
- Hypoxemia
- Hypercarbia
- Pulmonary barotrauma
- Gastric insufflation
- Aspiration

Discussion

- The presence of facial fractures, oropharyngeal obstruction, cervical or temporomandibular arthritis, and facial hair can make the procedure difficult.
- If there is difficulty in ventilating the patient, make sure there is a good seal with the mask and the airway is clear. Adjusting the patient's head position and ensuring adequate mandible elevation with the fingers often improves mask ventilation. Insert a nasopharyngeal or oropharyngeal airway to improve airway patency if the patient is unconscious.
- An additional person can apply concurrent cricoid pressure to reduce gastric insufflation.
- If the reservoir bag does not reinflate, check for a system leak or a tubing disconnection.

References

Benhamou D et al: Nasal mask ventilation in acute respiratory failure: experience in elderly patients, *Chest* 102:912-917, 1992.

Carden E, Hughes T: Evaluation of manually operated self-inflating resuscitation bags, *Anesth Analg* 54:133-138, 1975.

Daya M, Mariani R, Fernandes C: Basic life support. In Dailey RH et al, eds: *The airway: emergency management*, St Louis, 1992, Mosby.

Pennock BE et al: Noninvasive nasal mask ventilation for acute respiratory failure: institution of a new therapeutic technology for routine use, *Chest* 105:441-444, 1994.

Stewart RD et al: Influence of mask design on bag-mask ventilation, *Ann Emerg Med* 14:403-406, 1985.

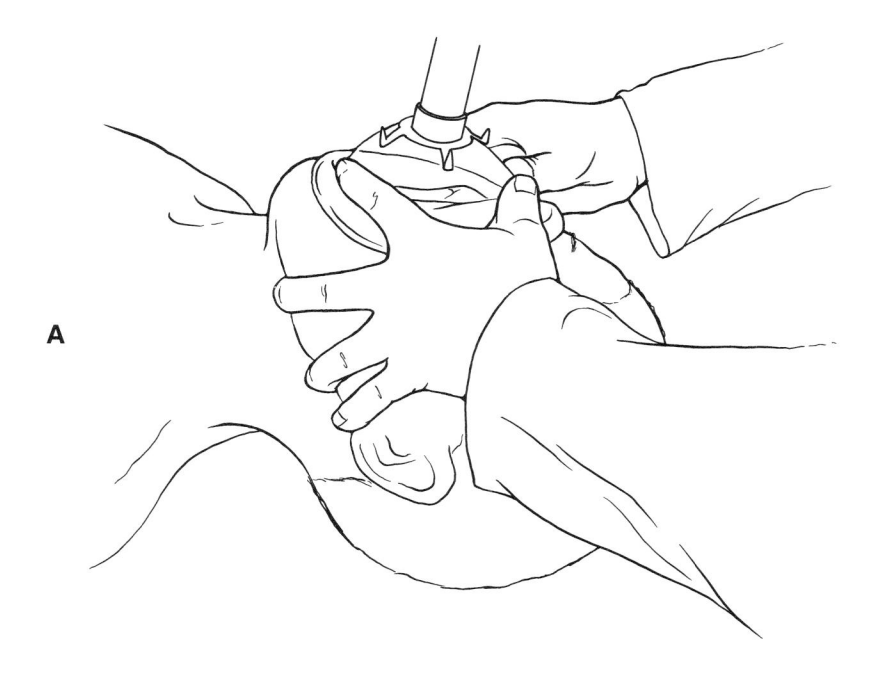

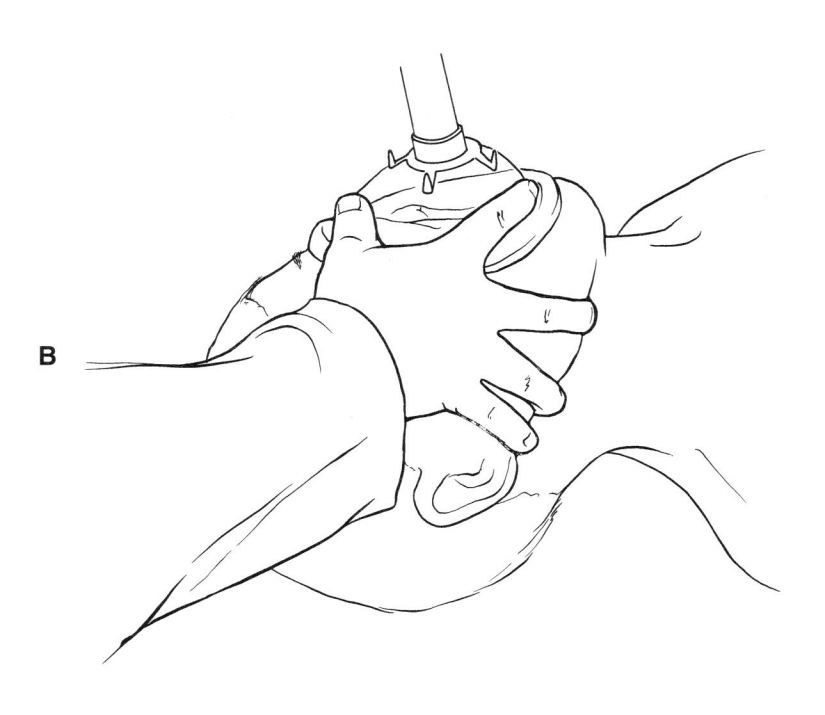

Airway

A

B

Endotracheal Intubation

Standard Endotracheal Intubation   Daniel F. Danzl

Indications
- Apnea
- Respiratory failure
- Inability to protect airway
- Altered level of consciousness
- Maintenance of patent airway

Contraindications
- Laryngotracheal injuries
- Maxillofacial trauma or deformities that prevent orotracheal intubation

Equipment
- Cardiac monitor and pulse oximeter
- Oxygen source
- Suction source and equipment
- Laryngoscope and blades
- Straight (Miller) blade sizes 2 and 3
- Curved (MacIntosh) blade sizes 3 and 4
- Endotracheal (ET) tubes (variety of sizes):
  - Average adult male: 8 to 8.5 mm internal diameter
  - Average adult female: 7.5 to 8 mm internal diameter
- Stylet
- 10-ml syringe
- Confirmation device (e.g., end-tidal CO_2 detector, esophageal intubation detector)
- Securing device (twill tape or other)

Procedure

1. Initiate continuous cardiac monitoring and pulse oximetry.
   a. Select the appropriate-size ET tube and insert the stylet.
2. Check the equipment, including ET tube cuff, laryngoscope light, and suction.
3. Evaluate the patient's airway anatomy: oral cavity size, neck mobility, teeth, mentum-cricoid distance, and dentures (which should be removed). Ease of laryngoscopy correlates with the ability to visualize the soft palate, uvula, and faucial pillars *(A)*.
4. If cervical spine injury is not suspected, position the patient in the sniffing position and place a towel roll under the occiput to align the oropharyngolaryngeal axes *(B)*.
5. Preoxygenate with 100% oxygen for 1 to 2 minutes, and suction the oral cavity as necessary.
6. With the operator at the head of the patient, adjust the height of the bed to a comfortable level for the operator.
7. Place the laryngoscope in the left hand and the ET tube in the right hand.
8. Insert the blade into the right corner of the patient's mouth.
   a. If using the straight blade, align the blade down the center of the tongue and directly lift the epiglottis with the tip of the blade *(C)*.
   b. If using the curved blade, sweep the tongue to the left side of the oropharynx, insert the blade tip into the vallecula, and indirectly lift the epiglottis off the larynx *(D)*.

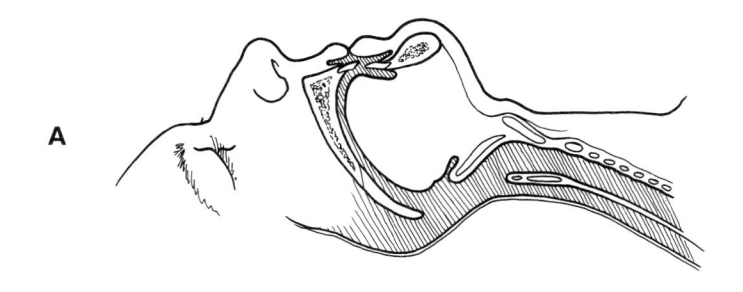

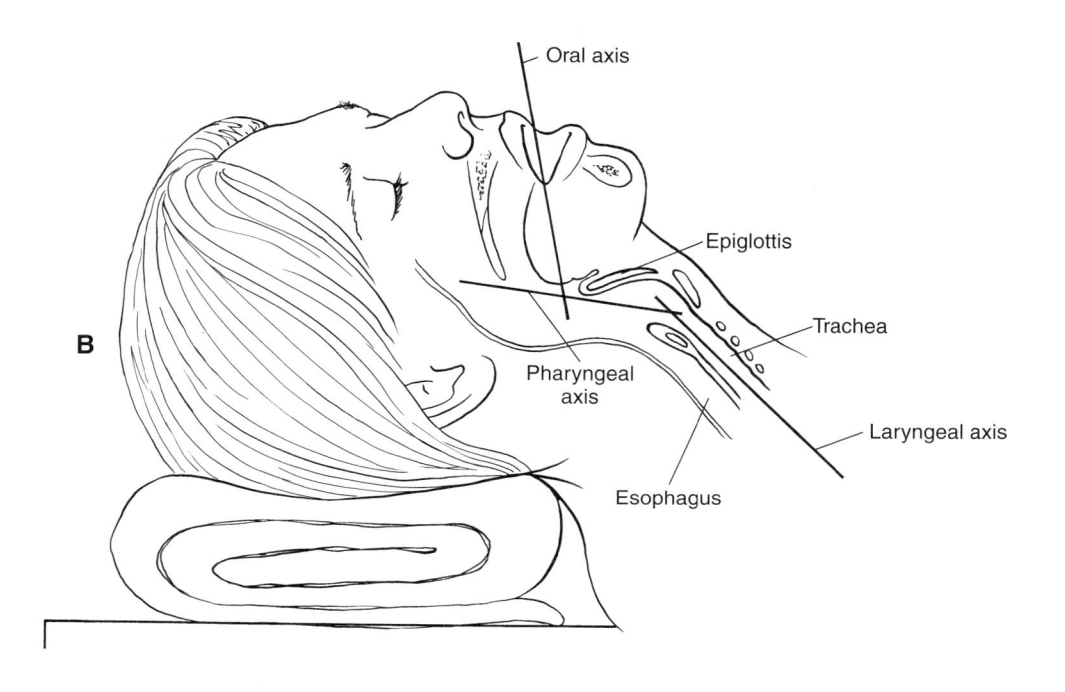

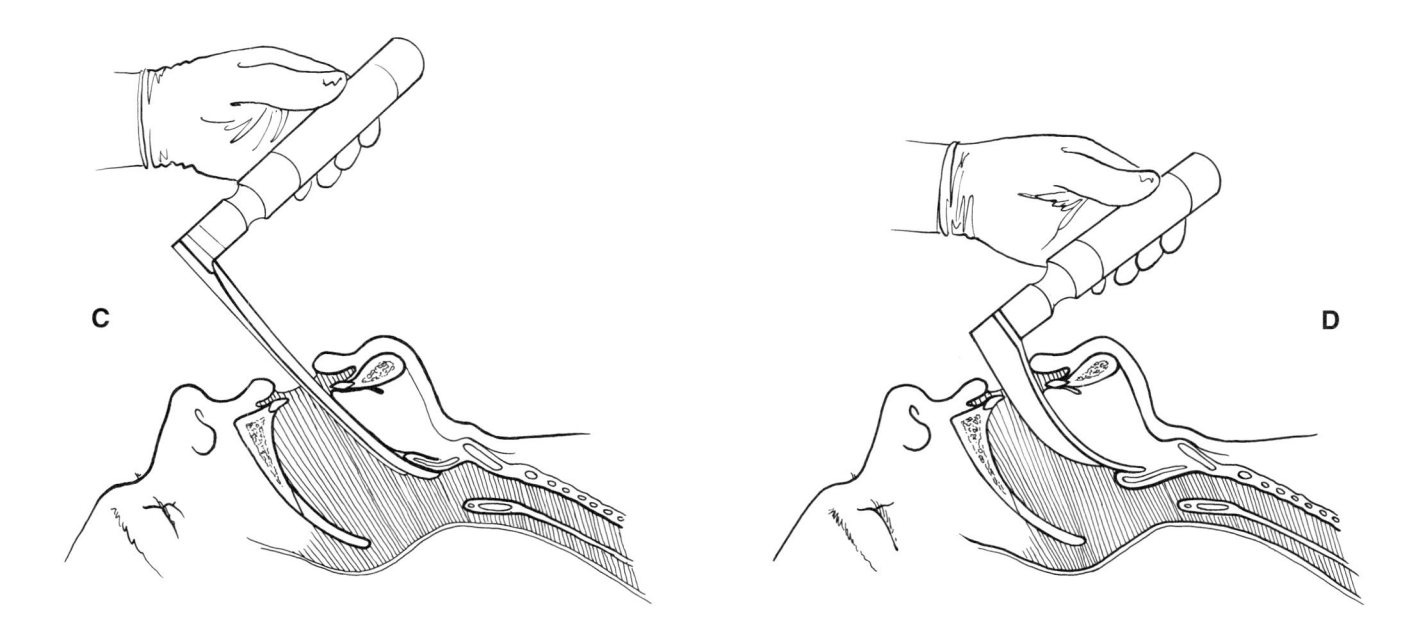

Airway

A

B
- Oral axis
- Epiglottis
- Trachea
- Pharyngeal axis
- Laryngeal axis
- Esophagus

C

D

9. Apply lifting force on the laryngoscope handle in the direction that it points, at a 90-degree angle to the blade. Do not torque the handle back because this might damage the teeth.
10. Directly visualize the vocal cords *(E)*, and insert the ET tube with the stylet into the trachea until the cuff passes through the cords *(F)*. The tube should not be passed unless the cords are visualized. The correct depth of insertion is approximately 23 cm from the corner of the mouth in men and 21 cm in women.
11. Carefully remove the stylet and inflate the cuff with 10 cc of air *(G)*.
12. Confirm tube placement by checking bilateral breath sounds and using other available methods *(H)*.
13. Secure the tube with available devices.

Complications

- Hypoxemia
- Hypercarbia
- Esophageal intubation
- Endobronchial intubation (most commonly right mainstem)
- Cardiac dysrhythmias
- Hypertension
- Elevated intracranial pressure
- Dental trauma
- Direct mucosal injury
- Arytenoid cartilage displacement
- Exacerbation of existing cervical spine injury

Discussion

- Medications, including sedatives and paralytic agents, are commonly used to facilitate intubation. Operators should be familiar with the appropriate uses, indications, contraindications, and complications of these medications.
- Selection of the laryngoscope blade is often based on personal preference. The wider curved blade is easier to use for the majority of intubations and is recommended particularly for operators with less experience. The narrower straight blade is useful for the patient with an anteriorly placed airway or large epiglottis. The operator should be familiar with the use of both blades.
- Bending the distal ET tube with stylet anteriorly before insertion can facilitate passage of the tube into the anterior larynx rather than the posterior esophagus.
- A chest radiograph is useful in confirming tube insertion depth, since the tip should be approximately 2 cm above the carina.
- ET intubation is commonly performed by paramedics in the field when patients are in cardiac arrest or have respiratory failure. Medications to facilitate intubation, particularly paralytic agents, are used in a number of prehospital settings. In these situations rescue airway techniques must be available.
- When an unconscious patient may have a cervical spine injury, in-line stabilization (not traction) during intubation is the rule.

Bibliography

Fernandez R et al: Endotracheal tube cuff pressure assessment: pitfalls of finger estimation and need for objective measurement, *Crit Care Med* 18:1423-1426, 1990.

Franklin C et al: Life-threatening hypotension associated with emergency intubation and the initiation of mechanical ventilation, *Am J Emerg Med* 12:425-428, 1994.

Jenkins WA et al: The syringe aspiration technique to verify endotracheal tube position, *Am J Emerg Med* 12:413-416, 1994.

Roberts JR et al: Proper depth of placement of oral endotracheal tubes in adults prior to radiographic confirmation, *Acad Emerg Med* 2:20-24, 1995.

Scannell G et al: Orotracheal intubation in trauma patients with cervical fractures, *Arch Surg* 128:903-906, 1993.

Airway

E

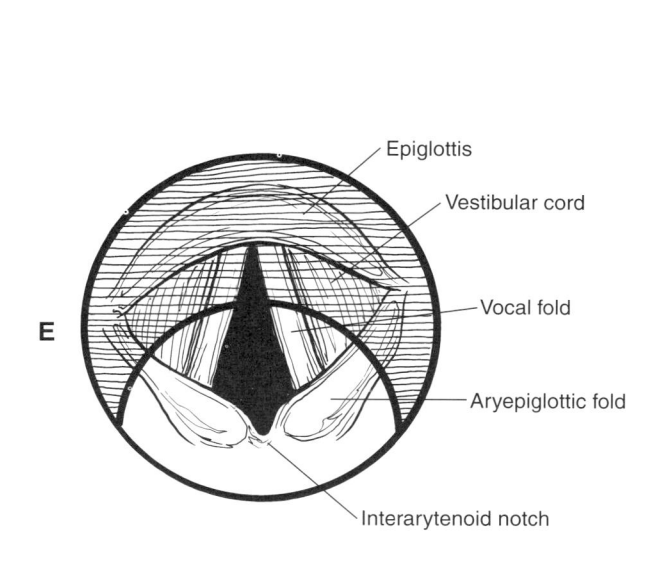

- Epiglottis
- Vestibular cord
- Vocal fold
- Aryepiglottic fold
- Interarytenoid notch

F

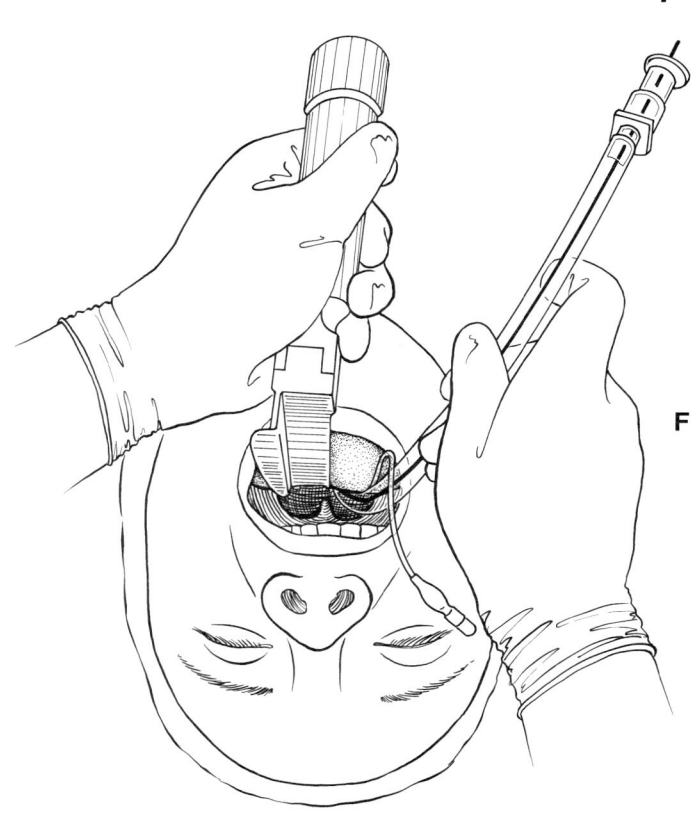

G

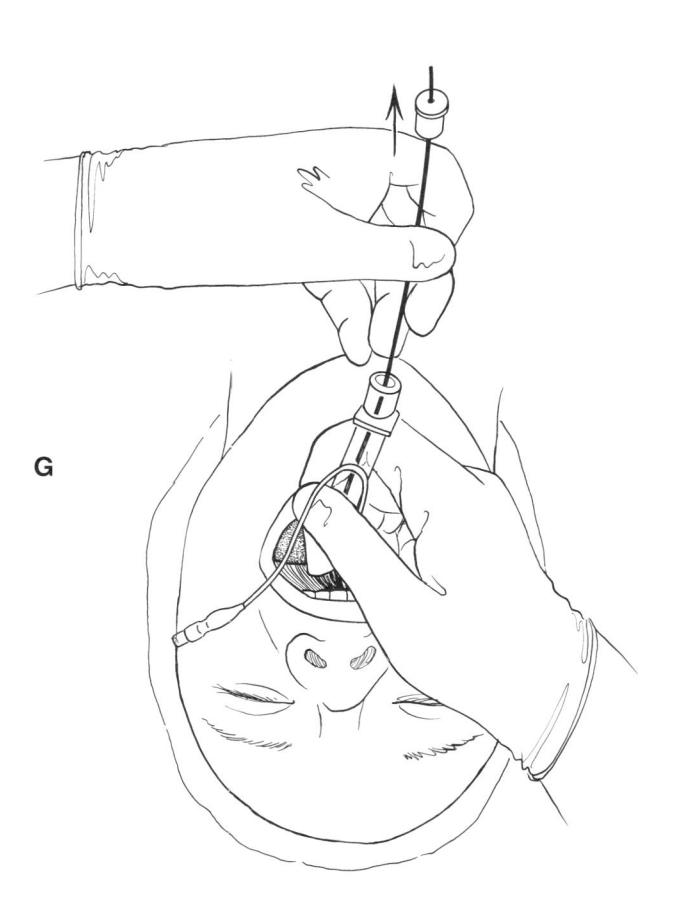

H

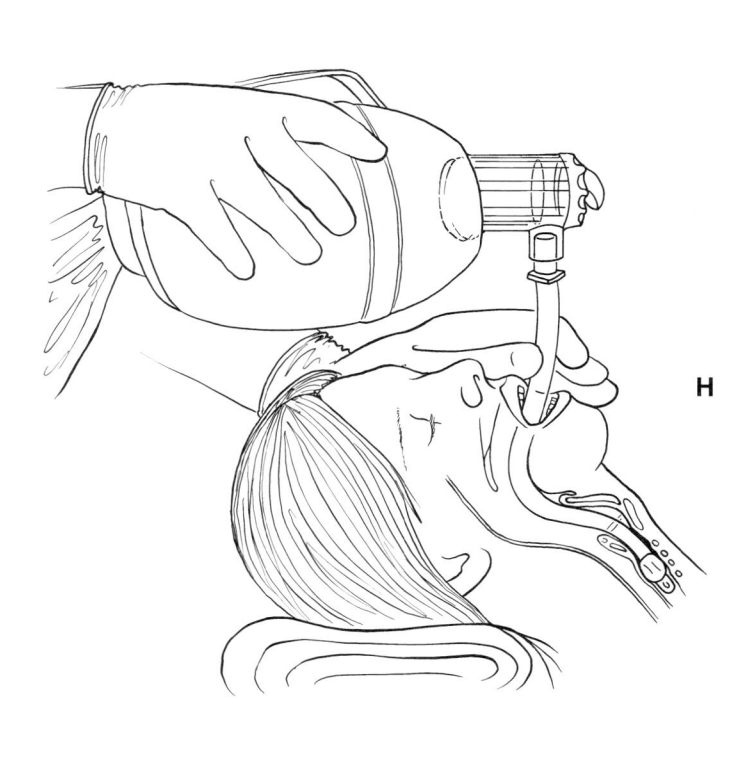

Fiberoptic Intubation   Michael F. Murphy

Indications
- Anticipated difficult intubation
- Cervical spine immobilization
- Failed intubation

Contraindications
- Excessive blood and secretions in upper airway
- Upper airway obstruction caused by foreign bodies or other lesions
- Patient's inability to maintain adequate oxygenation during the time required for fiberoptic intubation

Equipment
- Fiberoptic scope
- Endotracheal (ET) tube
- Suction equipment
- Oxygen source
- Bite block
- Topical anesthetic agent (e.g., benzocaine)
- Water-soluble lubricant
- Silicone liquid

Procedure

1. Initiate continuous cardiac monitoring and pulse oximetry.
2. Provide sedation as appropriate for the patient's relaxation.
3. Apply topical anesthetic to the oropharynx if the patient is awake or has a gag reflex.
4. Provide supplemental oxygen.
5. Lubricate the ET tube, and place it over the laryngoscope up to the handpiece.
6. Put a drop of silicone liquid on the tip of the scope to prevent fogging.
7. Put the bite block in for the oral route.
8. Stand up straight at the head of the bed, moving hands and arms, not the torso.
9. Stay in midline.
10. Hold the body of the scope in the dominant hand, using the thumb to toggle the tip control lever up and down *(A)*.
11. Use the nondominant hand to advance, withdraw, and manipulate the scope.
12. Maintain gentle tension between the hands to permit left and right rotation of the tip.
13. Use the little finger of the scope hand to feel the lower lip and keep the scope at midline.
14. Advance the tip over the tongue until the epiglottis comes into view at the top of the visual field.
15. As the tip is advanced, the white vocal cords are seen.
16. Advance the tip through the cords during inspiration, and advance it toward the carina.
17. Advance the ET tube over the scope into the airway.
18. Inflate the cuff with 10 cc of air.
19. Confirm tube placement by checking bilateral breath sounds and using other available methods.
20. Secure the tube with available devices.

Complications

- Hypoxemia
- Hypercarbia
- Esophageal intubation
- Endobronchial intubation (most commonly right mainstem)
- Cardiac dysrhythmias
- Hypertension
- Elevated intracranial pressure
- Dental trauma
- Direct mucosal injury

Discussion

- Operators should be familiar with the use of the fiberoptic scope. Appropriate sterilization techniques should have been performed.
- An antisialogogue, such as glycopyrrolate 0.01 mg/kg IM, may be useful in controlling secretions.
- If following the nasal route, apply vasoconstrictor agent inside the nose.
- Avoid touching the carina with the scope because this will induce coughing.
- Administration of 2 to 4 mg of 4% lidocaine through the working channel of the scope may be needed if the cords close or a cough reflex begins.
- A chest radiograph may be useful in confirming the depth of tube insertion. The tip should be approximately 2 cm above the carina.

Bibliography
Afilalo M et al: Fiberoptic intubation in the emergency department: a case series, *J Emerg Med* 1:387-391, 1993.
Delaney KA et al: Emergency flexible fiberoptic nasotracheal intubation: a report of 60 cases, *Ann Emerg Med* 17:919-926, 1988.
Messeter MD et al: Endotracheal intubation with the fiberoptic bronchoscope, *Anaesthesia* 35:294-298, 1980.
Mlinek EJ et al: Fiberoptic intubation in the emergency department, *Ann Emerg Med* 19:359-362, 1990.
Schafermeyer RW: Fiberoptic laryngoscopy in the emergency department, *Am J Emerg Med* 2:160-163, 1984.

A

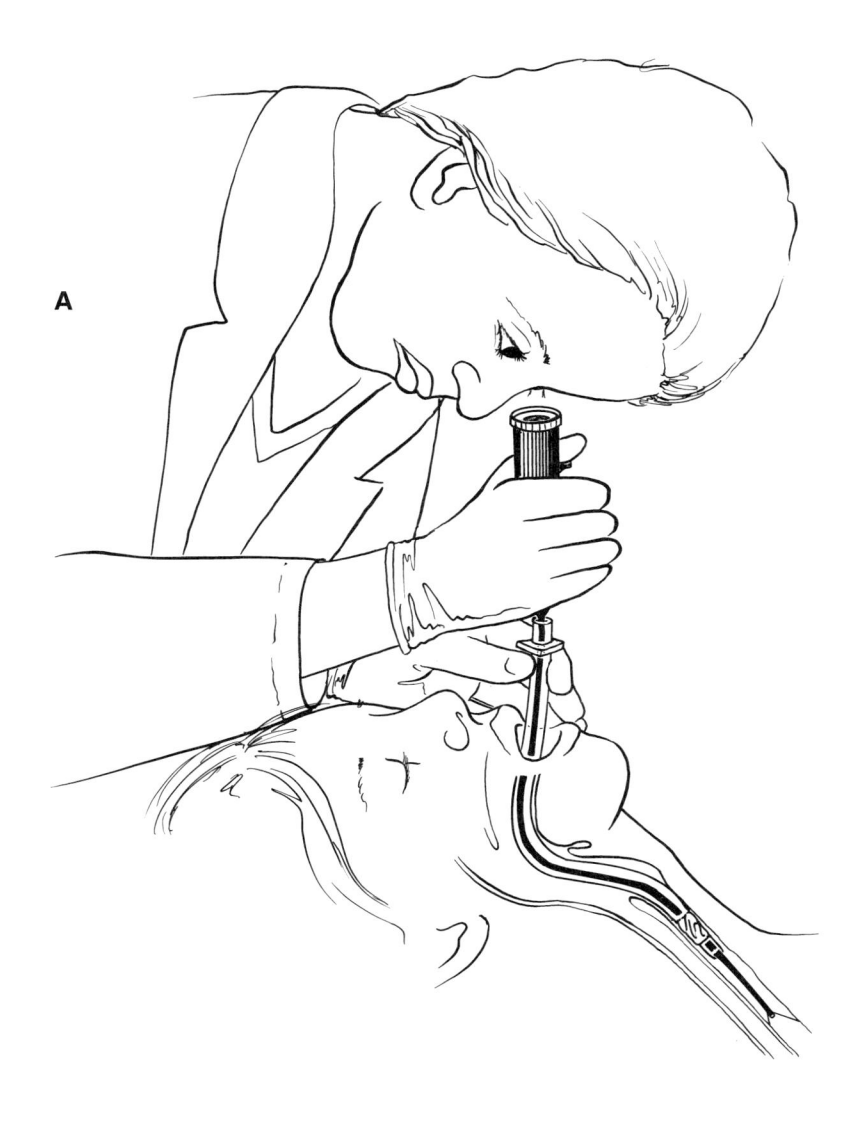

Retrograde Intubation   James P. Killeen

Indications
- Inability to visualize the vocal cords secondary to secretions, trauma, or infection
- Inability to achieve orotracheal intubation
- Difficult airway
- Cervical spinal injury
- Congenital abnormalities
- Anatomic distortion from injury, infection, surgery, trauma, or tumor

Contraindications
- Inability to open mouth for catheter retrieval
- Coagulation disorder
- Neck tumor
- Large thyroid
- Infection overlying cricothyroid membrane
- Obscure cricothyroid anatomy

Equipment
- Endotracheal tube
- Introducer needle
- Through-the-needle catheter or flexible-tip guidewire (approximately 70 cm)
- Small syringe
- Wire cutters
- Sterile gloves
- Betadine or antiseptic solution
- Or prepackaged kit including the above

Procedure
1. Prepare the anterior neck region in sterile fashion.
2. Stabilize the larynx using the thumb and middle finger of one hand.
3. Identify the thyroid cartilage (the only V-shaped cartilage in the neck) with the index finger, and move caudally to the small space just cephalad to the cricoid cartilage. This space overlies the cricothyroid membrane (CTM).
4. With the index finger as a guide, pierce the skin overlying the CTM with the syringe-needle unit.
5. Angle the needle 30° to 40° caudally to puncture the inferior aspect of the CTM, avoiding the superiorly placed cricothyroid arteries.
6. Use the free flow of air aspiration to confirm proper placement.
7. Remove the syringe of the syringe-needle unit, and angle the needle 30° to 40° cephalad *(A)*.
8. Feed the guidewire through the needle, and advance into the oropharynx or nasopharynx *(B, C)*.
9. Remove the needle.
10. Feed the guidewire through the endotracheal tube side hole (Murphy's eye) into the endotracheal tube lumen and out the proximal end *(D)*. This allows approximately 1 cm of tube to be below the vocal cords before removal of the guidewire.
11. Clamp the wire at the neck with a hemostat as the endotracheal tube is threaded over the guidewire into the trachea.
12. Exert a slight pressure onto the tube when it meets resistance.
13. Cut and then release the guidewire at the skin level, and pull it from the proximal end of the endotracheal tube to prevent contamination of the cervical soft tissues.
14. Advance the endotracheal tube, and confirm proper placement by auscultation, chest radiograph, or end-tidal CO_2 detector.

Complications
- Laryngospasm
- Soft tissue neck infections
- Subcutaneous emphysema
- Hemoptysis
- Submucosal hematoma
- Esophageal intubation
- Failure to obtain an airway

Bibliography
American Society of Anesthesiologists Task Force on Management of the Difficult Airway: Practice guidelines for management of the difficult airway, *Anesthesiology* 78(3):597-602, 1993.

Blosser SA, Stauffer JL: Intubation of critically ill patients, *Clin Chest Med* 17(3):355-378, 1996.

Butler FS, Cirillo AA: Retrograde tracheal intubation, *Anesth Analg Curr Res* 39:333-338, 1960.

McNamara RM: Retrograde intubation of the trachea, *Ann Emerg Med* 16(6):680-682, 1987.

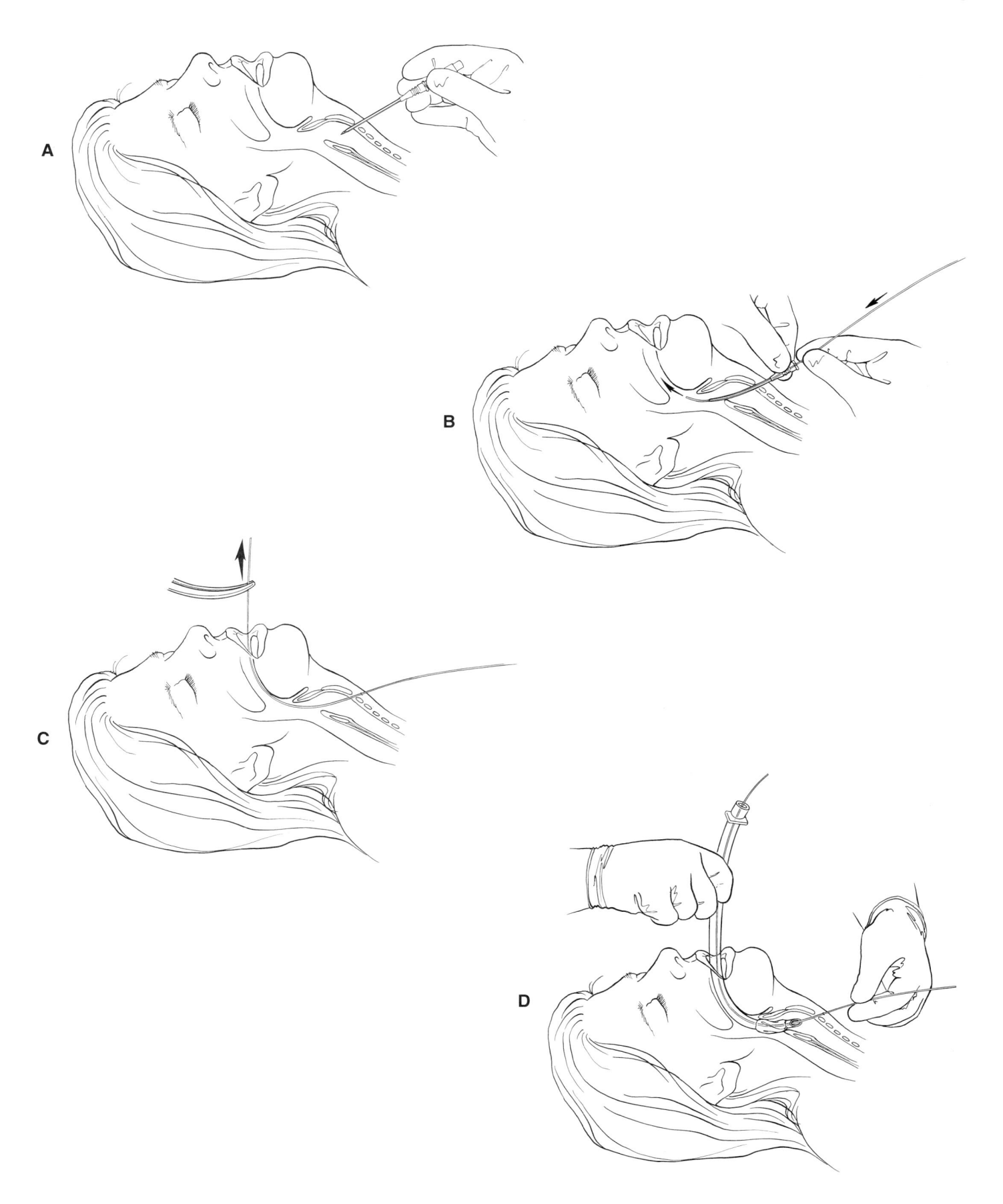

Airway

A

B

C

D

Digital Intubation JAMES P. KILLEEN

Indications
- Copious oral secretions
- Inability to directly visualize the epiglottis and vocal cords
- Confined spaces that do not allow direct visualization
- Severe head injury requiring immobilization of the cervical spine
- Anatomic anomalies
- Prolonged apnea

Contraindications
- Awake patient

Equipment
- Sterile gloves
- Endotracheal tube
- Bite block (optional)

Procedure
1. If right handed, stand on the left side of the patient, facing the patient, to perform this maneuver.
2. Place the index and middle fingers of the left hand onto the right side of the mouth, and extend toward the base of the tongue with the palmar surface of the fingers against the dorsal surface of the tongue.
3. Palpate the epiglottis and arytenoids with the left hand.
4. Pass the endotracheal tube along the dorsum of the left index and middle fingers by entering the mouth on the left side *(A)*.
5. Confirm tube placement using standard methods.

Complications
- Esophageal intubation
- Induction of emesis
- Trauma
- Hypoxia from multiple attempts
- Tissue dissection
- Mainstem bronchus intubation
- Bitten fingers (operator hazard)

Discussion
- A stylet can be used to form a hook or curve in the endotracheal tube to facilitate digital intubation.
- Biting injury to the operator can be prevented by use of a bite block, but digital intubation should be reserved for comatose patients.

Bibliography

Cook RT Jr, Polson DL: Use of BAAM with a digital intubation technique in a trauma patient, *Prehosp Disaster Med* 8:357-358, 1993.

Hardwick WC, Bluhm D: Digital intubation, *J Emerg Med* 1(4):317-320, 1984.

Stewart RD: Tactile orotracheal intubation, *Ann Emerg Med* 13(3):175-178, 1984.

Walls RM: Management of the difficult airway in the trauma patient, *Emerg Med Clin North Am* 16(1):45-61, 1998.

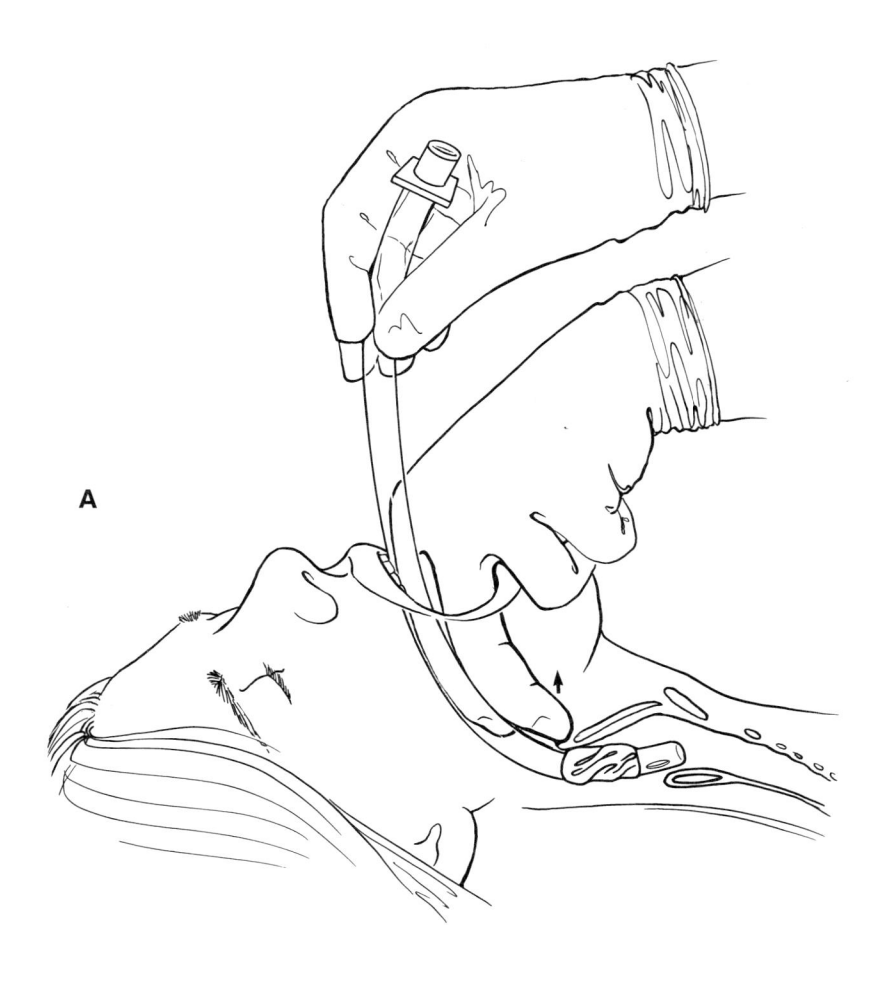

Airway

A

Endotracheal Intubation Using a Lighted Stylet   JAMES P. KILLEEN

Indications
- Difficult airway in which anatomy (temporomandibular or cervical spine immobility) or physiologic changes (secretions) hinder the ability to view the vocal cords

Contraindications
- Upper airway foreign body
- Neck tumor
- Retropharyngeal abscess
- Friable tissue along the oropharynx and larynx

Equipment
- Power source
- Lighted stylet setup, consisting of three movable parts: reusable handle, flexible wand with distal illuminating light, and stiff retractable stylet; the light is designed to focus forward and laterally in wide angles to illuminate the soft tissues of the neck
- Silicone- or water-based lubrication
- Endotracheal (ET) tube

Complications
- Bleeding
- Infection
- Failure to intubate
- Heat damage to mucosa

Procedure

1. Position the patient with slight extension of the head, allowing the epiglottis to lift away from the posterior pharyngeal wall.
2. Lubricate the distal end of the stylet with silicone spray or a water-based surgical lubricant.
3. Place the ET tube on the handle, and lock it in place with the clamp. The handle has a lever for adjusting to the size of the tube.
4. Place the wand and stylet through the ET tube and attach the wand to the reusable handle.
5. Align the numbers on the wand with the numbers on the ET tube.
6. Make a 90° to 120° angle 30 cm from the distal end of the wand, creating a "hockey stick."
7. Introduce the wand and ET tube setup into the oral pharynx from the side, and bring to midline behind the tongue using a pencil-like grip.
8. Pull the handle gently in a caudal direction until the soft tissue of the neck at the level of the hyoid is illuminated, indicating that the tip is in the vallecula. Small movements of the handle translate into large movements at the tip.
9. Once the anterior soft tissue of the neck is seen *(A)*, pull the handle again caudally and advance the wand and ET tube setup until the midline glow is seen in the anterior neck just below the thyroid prominence *(B)*.
10. Retract the stylet approximately 10 cm, and advance the wand and ET tube setup through the vocal cords.
11. Unlock the ET tube, and remove the wand.

Complications
- Bleeding
- Infection
- Failure to intubate
- Heat damage to mucosa

Discussion
- If a bright light is seen off midline, the tip of the light wand may lie in the piriform fossae. Rotation back toward the midline will correct this problem. When the esophagus is intubated, the transmitted glow from the wand is diffuse and not easily detected *(C)*.
- For nasotracheal intubations the same principle applies as for ET intubation, with these additions: the nasal passage requires preparation with vasoconstrictors, and the stylet should assume more of a J shape.
- A patient with possible cervical injury should remain in neutral position. For an obese patient or one with a short neck, a roll under the shoulders may improve exposure of the neck.
- The light is designed to emit a minimal amount of heat for short periods. After 30 seconds the light begins to blink.

Bibliography
Berns SD: Oral intubation using a lighted stylet vs. direct laryngoscopy in older children with cervical immobilization, *Acad Emerg Med* 3(1):34-40, 1996.

Cohn AI: Lighted stylet intubation: greasing your way to success, *Anesth Analg* 78(6):1205-1206, 1994.

Davis L: Lighted stylet tracheal intubation: a review, *Anesth Analg* 90:745-756, 2000.

Ellis DG: Success rates of blind orotracheal intubation using a transillumination technique with a lighted stylet, *Ann Emerg Med* 15(2):138-142, 1986.

Verdile VP: Nasotracheal intubation using a flexible lighted stylet, *Ann Emerg Med* 19(5):506-510, 1990.

A

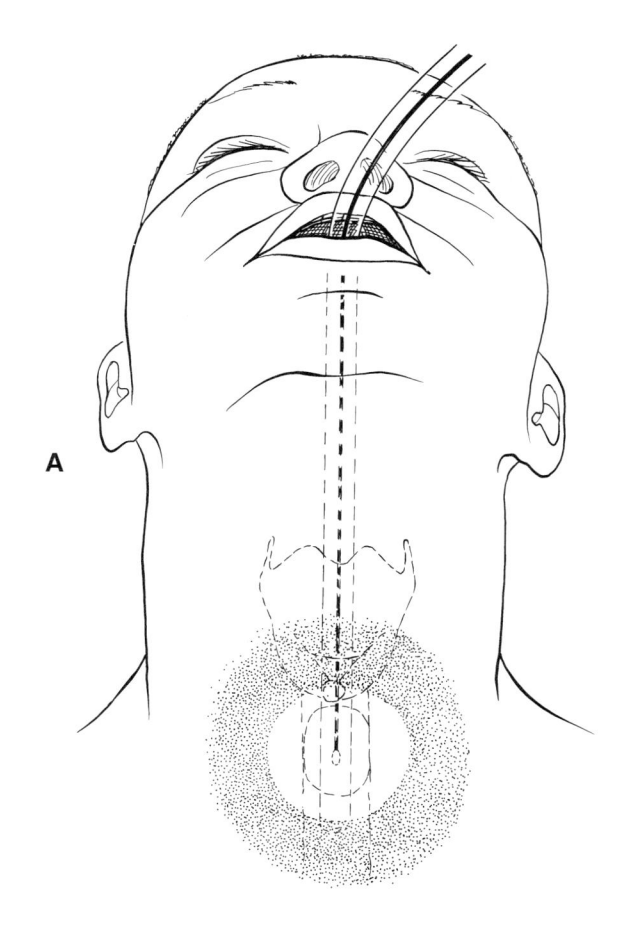

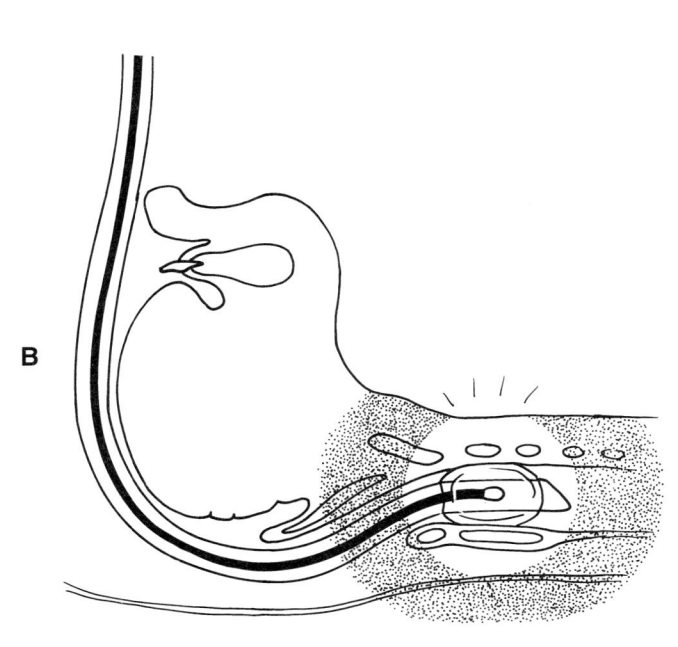

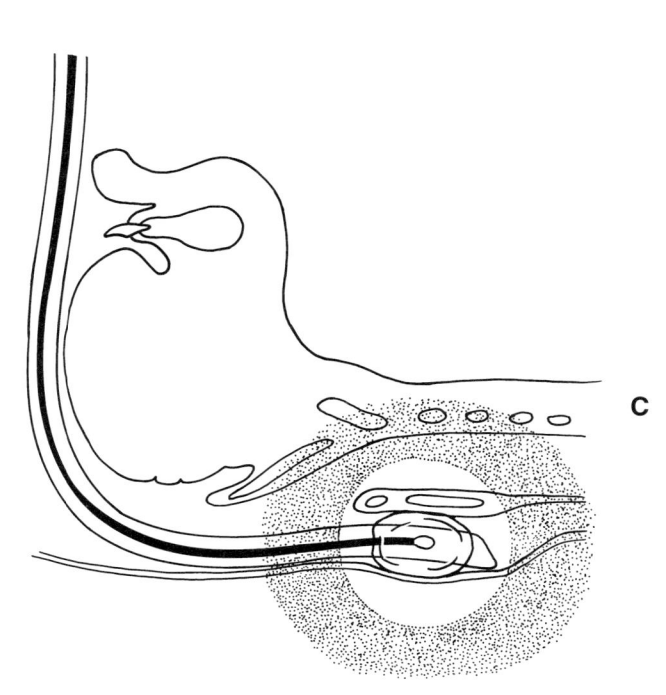

B
CORRECT PLACEMENT

C
INCORRECT PLACEMENT

Nasotracheal Intubation — Daniel F. Danzl

Indications
- Failure of direct laryngoscopy endotracheal intubation
- Contraindication to neuromuscular paralysis
- Respiratory distress
- Inability to perform orotracheal intubation (e.g., because of oral surgical procedures, trismus, mandibular dislocation)

Contraindications
- Apnea
- Maxillofacial deformities, fractures, or pathologic conditions (LeFort III fracture)
- Tracheobronchial injuries
- Mechanical obstruction by injury, neoplasm, infection, or foreign body
- Closed head injury
- Thrombolytic therapy
- Coagulopathy

Equipment
- Pulse oximetry and cardiac monitor
- Oxygen source
- Suction equipment
- Endotracheal (ET) tubes (0.5 mm smaller than tube used for orotracheal intubation):
  - Average adult man: 7.5 to 8 mm internal diameter
  - Average adult woman: 7 to 7.5 mm internal diameter
- 10-ml syringe
- Nasopharyngeal airways (variety of sizes)
- Topical vasoconstrictor spray (Neo-Synephrine 1%)
- Topical anesthetic and lubricant (lidocaine 2% jelly)
- Tube-securing material (e.g., twill tape, manufactured device)
- Confirmation equipment (e.g., end-tidal CO_2 device, esophageal detector device)
- Laryngoscope
- Magill forceps

Procedure

1. Initiate cardiac monitoring and pulse oximetry.
2. Spray both nares with topical vasoconstrictor.
3. Sequentially insert lubricated nasopharyngeal airways into the most patent naris in progressive fashion from smaller to larger airways. Initially insert the airway with the bevel facing the septum, then rotate so that the airway points down the nasopharynx while advancing.
4. Select an appropriate-size ET tube.
5. Check equipment, including ET tube cuff and suction.
6. Preoxygenate with 100% oxygen for 1 to 2 minutes.
7. Take a position alongside the patient.
8. Remove the last nasopharyngeal airway placed, and insert the ET tube at an angle 90° to the face (along the floor of nasal passage, not directed up along the septum) *(A)*.
9. Advance the tube into the retropharynx (using the curvature of the ET tube directed caudally) *(B)*.
10. While advancing the ET tube, listen for airflow from the patient's breathing through the tube.
11. During early inspiration, swiftly but gently advance the ET tube into the trachea.
12. If there is difficulty advancing or no airflow through the tube, slowly withdraw the tube until airflow is again audible. Then repeat step 11.
13. Once the tube is advanced into the trachea, air should flow through the tube as the patient breathes.
14. Inflate the cuff with 10 cc of air.
15. Confirm tube placement by checking bilateral breath sounds and using other available methods.
16. Secure the tube with available devices.

Complications

- Hypoxemia
- Hypercarbia
- Esophageal intubation
- Cardiac dysrhythmias
- Hypertension
- Elevated intracranial pressure
- Epistaxis
- Paranasal sinusitis
- Retropharyngeal abrasions or lacerations
- Laryngeal trauma
- Nasal septal or turbinate injury
- Piriform fossa injury

Discussion

- Patients often know which naris is more patent and can direct the operator to the appropriate side. If the airway is difficult to advance into the retropharyngeal space, the operator can attempt the intubation in the opposite naris.
- Estimate the depth of ET tube insertion by placing the tube along the side of the face and measuring from the thyroid cartilage to the tip of the nose.
- Directional tip ET tubes (Endotrol) that allow the operator to direct the tip of the tube anteriorly with a ring trigger can facilitate passage into the trachea, particularly in patients with an anteriorly placed airway.

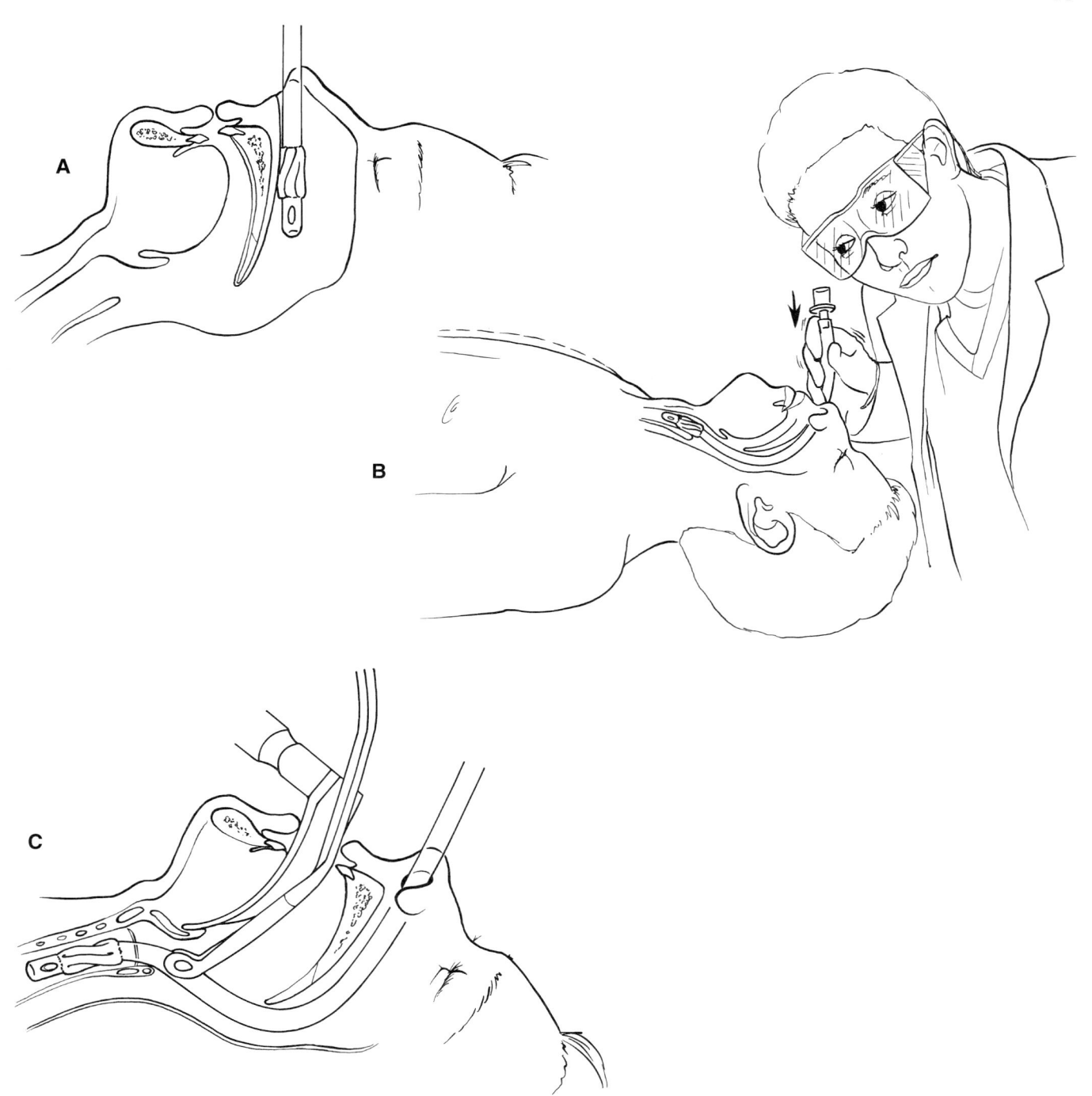

- The Magill forceps can be used to direct the ET tube into the larynx *(C)*.
- A number of devices, such as whistle caps and earpiece adapters, can be used to determine the presence of airflow in the ET tube during insertion.
- Most commonly patients are sitting up during nasotracheal intubation, but the procedure can be performed with the patient supine.
- Nasotracheal intubation can be performed in the field. Its use is dependent on agency protocol within a system.

Bibliography

Benumof JL: Management of the difficult adult airway, *Anesthesiology* 75:1087-1110, 1991.

Danzl DF, Thomas DM: Nasotracheal intubations in the emergency department, *Crit Care Med* 8:677-682, 1980.

Dorsey MJ, Jones BR: An inexpensive, disposable adapter for increasing the safety of blind nasotracheal intubations, *Anesth Analg* 69:135, 1989.

Holdgaard HO et al: Complications and late sequelae following nasotracheal intubation, *Acta Anaesthesiol Scand* 37:475-480, 1993.

Pediatric Endotracheal Intubation Ghazala Q. Sharieff

Indications
- Apnea
- Refractory bradycardia
- Shock
- Respiratory failure
- Cardiopulmonary arrest
- Inability to protect airway
- Altered level of consciousness
- Maintenance of patent airway

Contraindications
- Laryngotracheal injuries
- Maxillofacial trauma or deformities that prevent orotracheal intubation

Equipment
- Cardiac monitor and pulse oximeter
- Oxygen source
- Suction source and equipment
- Laryngoscope and blades:
  - Straight (Miller) blade:
    - Preterm neonates: size 0
    - Term neonates: size 1
    - Infants: size 2
    - Children: size 3
  - Curved (MacIntosh) blade:
    - Generally reserved for children 8 years or older
- Endotracheal (ET) tubes:
  - Less than 8 years of age: uncuffed tubes
  - Greater than 8 years of age: cuffed tubes
- Stylet
- 10-ml syringe
- Confirmation device (e.g., end-tidal CO_2 detector, esophageal intubation detector)
- Securing device (e.g., twill tape or manufactured device)

Procedure

1. Initiate cardiac monitoring and pulse oximetry.
2. Select appropriate-size ET tube, and insert stylet. Estimate appropriate ET tube size by the following:
   a. Formula of 4 + [Age in years/4]
   b. Approximation of ET tube diameter with little finger or naris of the patient
3. Check equipment, including ET tube cuff, laryngoscope light, and suction.
4. Evaluate the patient's airway anatomy: oral cavity size, neck mobility, teeth, and mentum-cricoid distance.
5. If cervical spine injury is not suspected, position the patient in the sniffing position and place a towel roll under the shoulders to align the oropharyngolaryngeal axes (A, B).
6. Preoxygenate with 100% oxygen for 1 to 2 minutes, and suction the oral cavity as necessary.
7. With operator at the head of the patient, adjust the height of the bed to a comfortable level for the operator.
8. Place the laryngoscope in the left hand and the ET tube in the right hand.
9. Insert the blade into the patient's oropharynx, and advance it to the base of the tongue.
10. Once the epiglottis is visualized, lift it upward and the vocal cords should come into view.
11. If a curved blade is used, the tip is placed in the vallecula and the epiglottis is lifted indirectly.
12. Insert the ET tube into the trachea past the vocal cords. The tube should not be passed unless the cords are visualized. The correct depth of insertion is approximately [10 + age in years] cm to the lips.
13. Carefully remove the stylet, and inflate the cuff with 10 cc of air.
14. Confirm tube placement by checking bilateral breath sounds and using other available methods.
15. Secure the tube with available devices.
16. Place a nasogastric tube for gastric decompression.

Complications
- Hypoxemia
- Hypercarbia
- Esophageal intubation
- Endobronchial intubation (most commonly right mainstem)
- Laryngospasm
- Dental trauma
- Direct mucosal injury

Discussion
- Medications, including sedative, induction, and paralytic agents, are commonly used to facilitate intubation. Operators should be familiar with the appropriate use, indications, contraindications, and complications of these medications.
- Selection of the type of laryngoscope blade is often personal preference. However, for children less than 8 years, the straight blade is preferred because the epiglottis is relatively large and floppy. For this age group, uncuffed tubes should be used because of the

A CORRECT POSITION

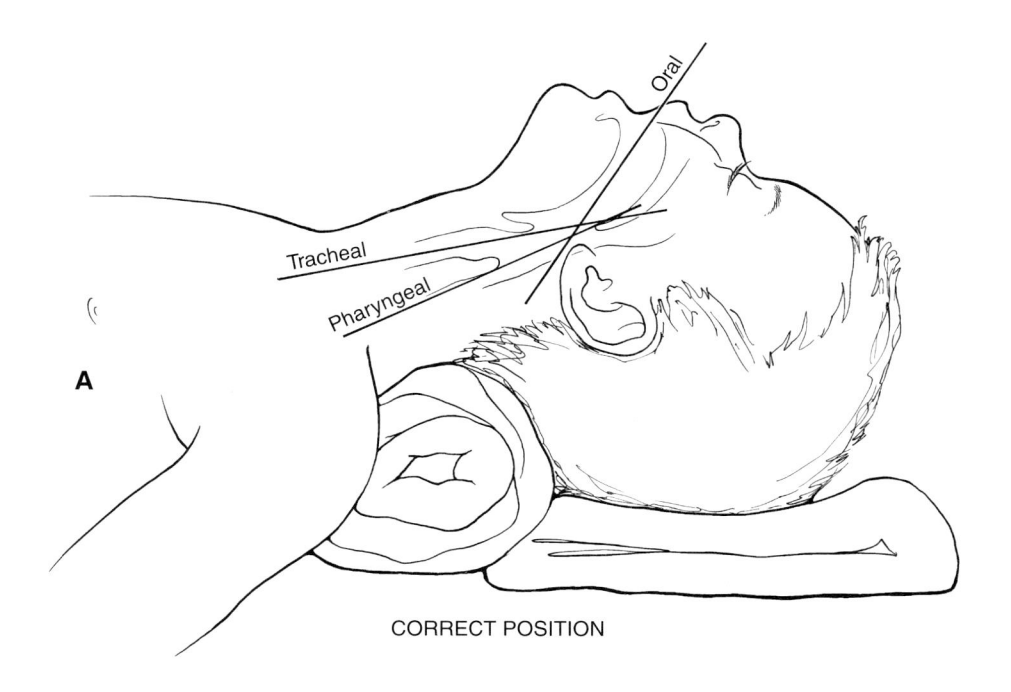

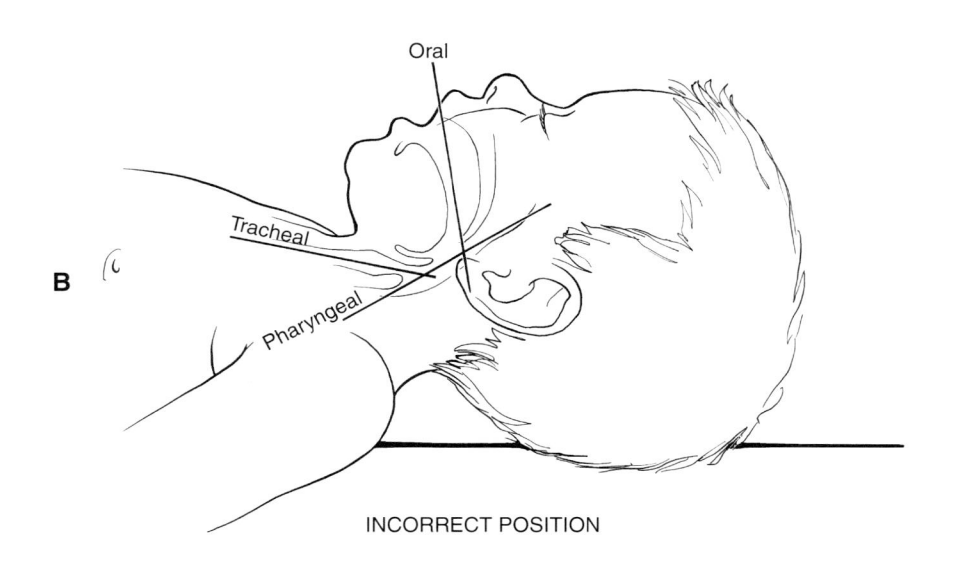

Tracheal, Pharyngeal, Oral

B INCORRECT POSITION

Oral, Tracheal, Pharyngeal

relatively narrow airway and the risk of subglottic stenosis.
- Some physicians prefer not to use stylets when intubating infants and young children because of the small ET tube size. For older children, stylets are recommended.
- Endotracheal intubation in pediatric patients is performed in the prehospital setting, although its utility is controversial. After intubation, children should be placed in full cervical spine immobilization to minimize the risk of tube dislodgment.

Bibliography

Baren JM, Seidel J: Emergency management of respiratory distress and failure. In Barkin RM, ed: *Pediatric emergency medicine*, ed 2, St Louis, 1997, Mosby.

Rivera B, Tibballs J: Complications of endotracheal intubation and mechanical ventilation in infants and children, *Crit Care Med* 20(2):193-199, 1992.

Walsh-Sukys M, Krug SE: *Orotracheal intubation and needle cricothyrotomy: procedures in infants and children*, Philadelphia, 1997, WB Saunders, pp 36-49.

Yamamoto LG: Rapid sequence anesthesia induction and advanced airway management in pediatric patients, *Emerg Clin North Am* 9:611-638, 1991.

Tracheal Suctioning ■ DANIEL F. DANZL

Indications
- Need to clear secretions, vomitus, or blood in an intubated patient
- Aspiration
- Endobronchial ball-valve obstruction

Contraindications
- None

Equipment
- Pulse oximeter and cardiac monitor
- Oxygen source
- Suction power source of at least 80 to 120 mm Hg
- Tubing
- Connectors
- Plastic rigid-tip Yankauer suction catheter
- Soft curved-tip and straight suction catheters

Procedure

1. Initiate cardiac monitoring and pulse oximetry.
2. Preoxygenate with 100% oxygen for 1 to 2 minutes.
3. Check the function of the suction power source and equipment.
4. Select an appropriate-size catheter, which should not be larger than half the endotracheal (ET) tube diameter.
   a. Average adult male: 14 Fr
   b. Average adult female: 12 to 14 Fr
   c. Newborn to 6 months (7 kg): 8 Fr
   d. Up to 2 years (12 kg): 10 Fr
   e. Older than 2 years: 12 Fr
5. Using sterile technique, insert and advance the catheter into the ET tube without covering the catheter sidehole port *(A)*.
   a. To enter the right mainstem bronchus, use a straight catheter.
   b. To enter the left mainstem bronchus, use a curved-tip catheter, turn the patient's head to the right, and rotate the catheter on entry.
6. Close the catheter side port with your thumb once the catheter is inserted.
7. Withdraw the catheter slowly with a rotating motion over 10 seconds *(B)*.
8. Reconfirm bilateral breath sounds after the suction catheter is removed.

Complications
- Hypoxemia
- Cardiac dysrhythmias
- Hypertension
- Elevated intracranial pressure
- Vagal stimulation with bradycardia and hypotension
- Pulmonic collapse
- Vomiting, coughing, or reflex bronchospasm
- Direct mucosal injury
- Simple or tension pneumothorax
- Infection

Discussion
- In patients with cough or reflex bronchospasm, consider using topical or IV lidocaine to blunt the response.
- If the catheter cannot be advanced, the ET tube may be kinked or partially occluded. Reposition the ET tube or deflate the cuff if you suspect cuff overinflation.
- Suctioning can be safely performed in the prehospital field.

Bibliography
American Heart Association: *Textbook of advanced cardiac life support,* Dallas, 1994, The Association.
Daya M et al: Basic life support. In Dailey RH et al, eds: *The airway: emergency management,* St Louis, 1992, Mosby.
Hoffman LA, Maszkiewicz RC: Airway management for the critically ill patient, *Am J Nursing* 87:39-43, 1987.
Marx GF et al: Endotracheal suction and death, *NY State J Med* 68:565-566, 1968.
Shim C et al: Cardiac arrhythmias resulting from tracheal suctioning, *Ann Intern Med* 71:1149-1153, 1969.

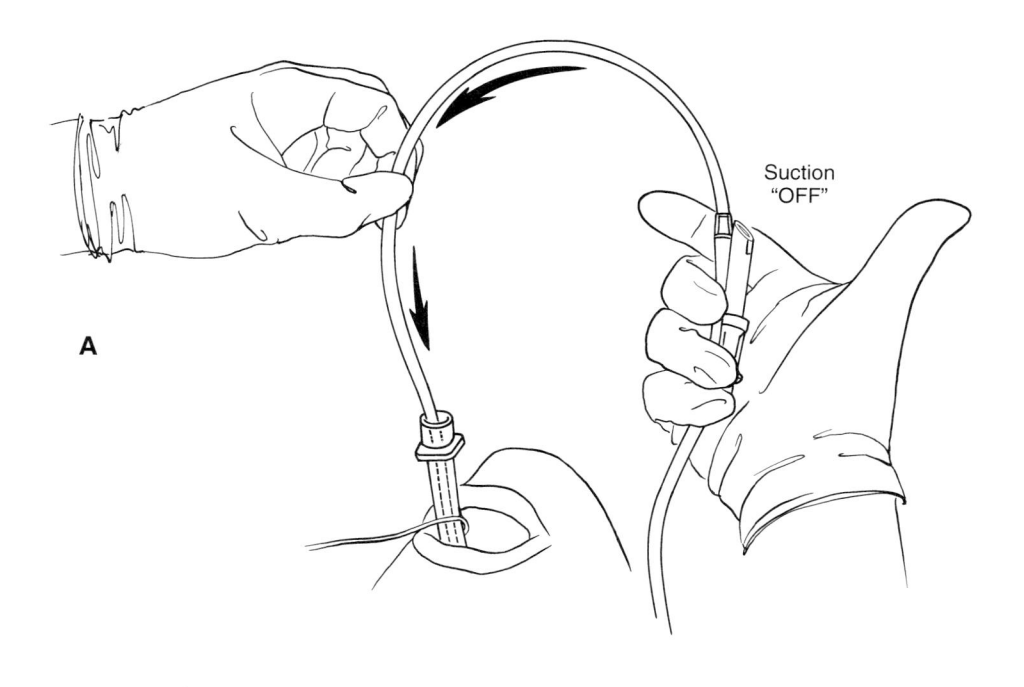

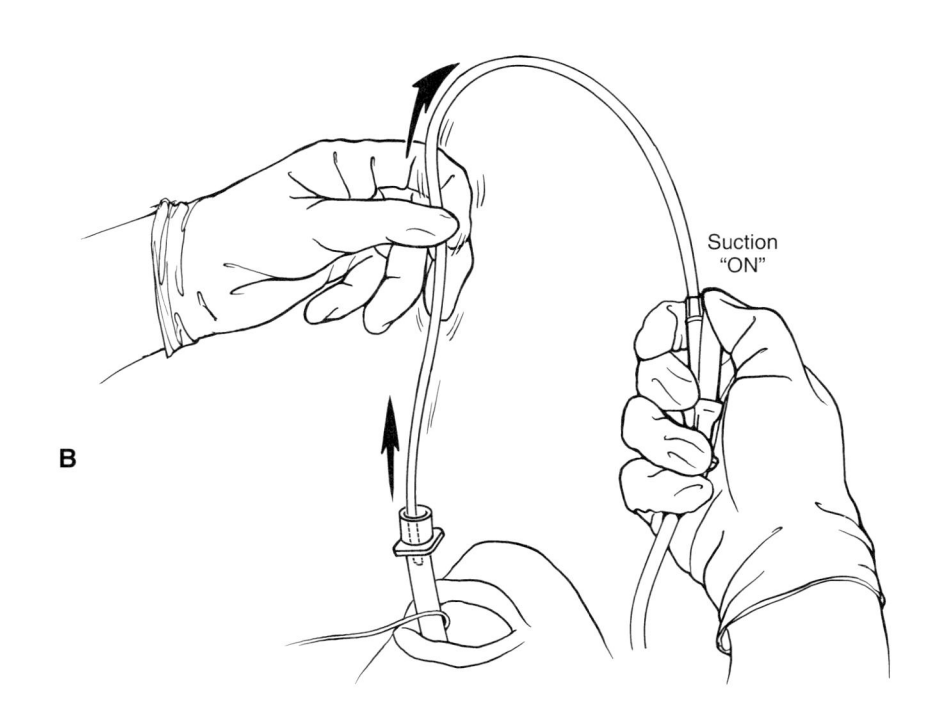

A

Suction "OFF"

B

Suction "ON"

Needle Cricothyrotomy ▪ KENNETH J. BRAMWELL

Indications
- Need for airway control
- Failure of or contraindication to orotracheal and nasotracheal intubation
- Patient age less than 8 years

Contraindications
- No absolute contraindications
- Relative contraindications:
  - Coagulopathy
  - Anterior neck hematoma
  - Overlying infection
  - Fractured larynx
  - Possible tracheal transection
  - Complete upper airway obstruction

Equipment
- Towel roll
- Betadine antiseptic solution
- 4 × 4 gauze pads
- 14- or 16-gauge angiocatheter
- 3- or 5-ml syringe
- Normal saline
- 2-0 silk suture material
- Hemostat
- 30-psi oxygen source and tubing

Procedure

1. If it is not contraindicated, place a towel roll under the patient's shoulders and lower neck to maximize exposure of the neck.
2. Identify the cricothyroid membrane. Begin palpation in the sternal notch and work cephalad in the midline. The cricothyroid membrane is the depression in the airway just cephalad to the cricoid cartilage. The thyroid cartilage is just cephalad to this membrane and is the only V-shaped cartilage in the neck.
3. Attach the angiocatheter to the syringe. Aspirate 1 to 2 ml of normal saline into the barrel of the syringe.
4. Prepare the anterior midline neck in sterile fashion. Locate the cricothyroid membrane again. Stabilize the thyroid cartilage with the thumb and middle fingers of the nondominant hand. Place the index finger of the nondominant hand on the cricothyroid membrane *(A)*.
5. Advance the angiocatheter through the skin and cricothryoid membrane into the larynx while maintaining negative pressure on the syringe. The appearance of bubbles in the barrel of the syringe should confirm proper location of the assembly.
6. Once into the larynx, advance the catheter over the needle in a caudad direction. Remove the needle and syringe, being careful to stabilize the catheter in place *(B)*.
7. Suture the catheter in place. Attach the catheter directly to the wall oxygen supply or jet ventilation source *(C)*.

Complications

- Improper placement
- Subcutaneous emphysema
- Inadequate ventilation
- Hemorrhage
- Aspiration
- Infection
- Barotrauma

Discussion

- The placement of normal saline into the barrel of the syringe is helpful for confirmation of proper location but is not essential to the procedure.
- In young patients the bony landmarks may be difficult to palpate because the thyroid cartilage does not become prominent until adolescence. For this reason the cricoid cartilage is the key landmark.
- Many commercially available kits for needle cricothyrotomy include essentially the same components as above with slight modifications.
- Needle cricothyrotomy is a temporizing measure. Preparations should be made for either fiberoptic intubation or formal tracheostomy.
- Needle cricothyrotomy is also a component of retrograde intubation. In addition, its equipment is incorporated into some of the adult cricothyrotomy kits rather than an open technique.
- The procedure can be done by prehospital personnel with advanced training and scope of practice.

Bibliography

American College of Surgeons: *Advanced trauma life support manual,* ed 6, Chicago, 1997, The College, pp 83-85.

American College of Emergency Physicians and American Academy of Pediatrics: *Advanced pediatric life support manual,* ed 3, Dallas, 1998, The College and The Academy, pp 263-264.

Greenfield RH: Percutaneous transtracheal ventilation. In Henretig FM, King C, eds: *Textbook of pediatric emergency procedures,* Baltimore, 1997, Williams & Wilkins, pp 239-249.

Peak DA, Roy S: Needle cricothyroidotomy revisited, *Pediatr Emerg Care* 15(3):224-226, 1999.

Cricoid space
Cricoid cartilage

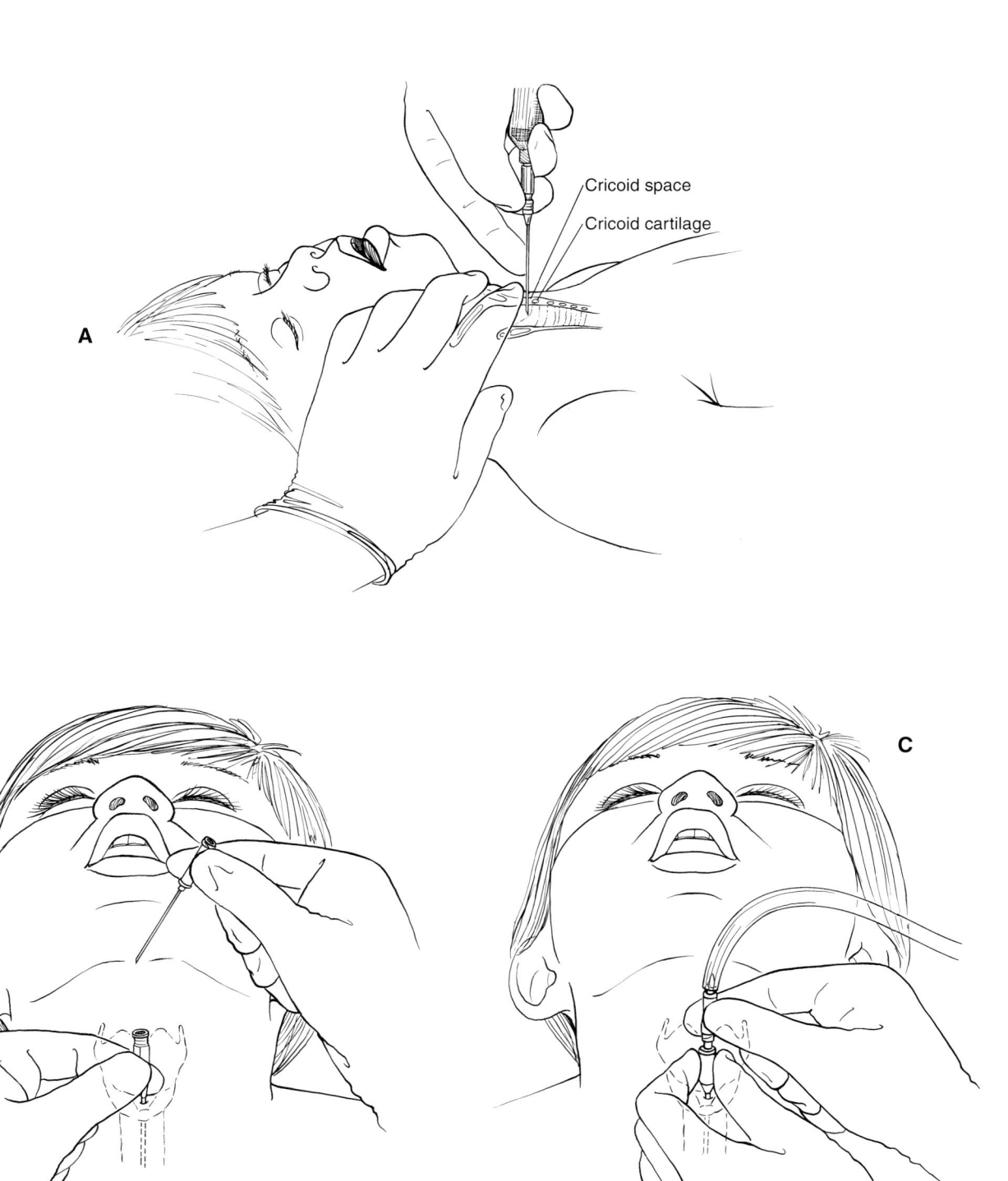

A

B

C

Cricothyrotomy ▪ RON M. WALLS

Indications
- Failure of orotracheal or nasotracheal intubation in a patient requiring definitive airway management
- Contraindication to orotracheal or nasotracheal intubation in a patient requiring definitive airway management
- Chemically paralyzed patient who cannot be given bag-valve-mask ventilation
- Destruction of the central face, mouth, or nose without means of maintaining the airway
- Severe supraglottic airway obstruction

Contraindications
- No absolute contraindications
- Relative contraindications:
  - Age less than 8 years
  - Anterior neck hematoma or infection
  - Previous cricothyrotomy
  - Coagulopathy
  - Tracheal tumor or mass

Equipment
- Scalpel with No. 11 blade
- Tracheal hook
- Trousseau dilator
- No. 4 Shiley cuffed tracheostomy tube with introducer and riser
- Betadine antiseptic solution
- 4 × 4 gauze pads
- 3-0 silk stay sutures or twill tape

Procedure

1. Identify the thyroid cartilage, the only V-shaped structure encountered when palpating up the neck. The cricothyroid space is the gap immediately caudad to the thyroid cartilage.
2. Prepare the neck in sterile fashion. With the nondominant hand holding the thyroid cartilage, make a vertical midline incision from the thyroid cartilage caudad about 3 to 4 cm *(A)*.
3. Place a tracheal hook through the cricothyroid space and hold cephalad traction with the nondominant hand *(B-D)*.

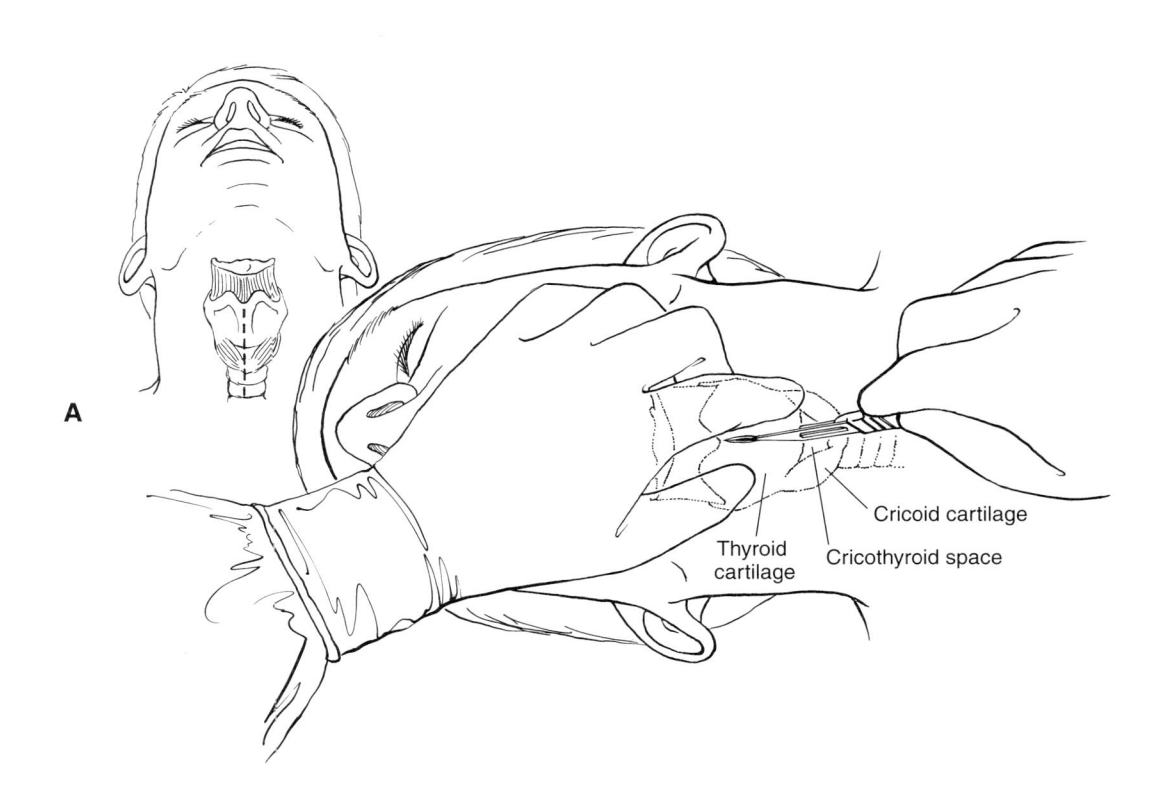

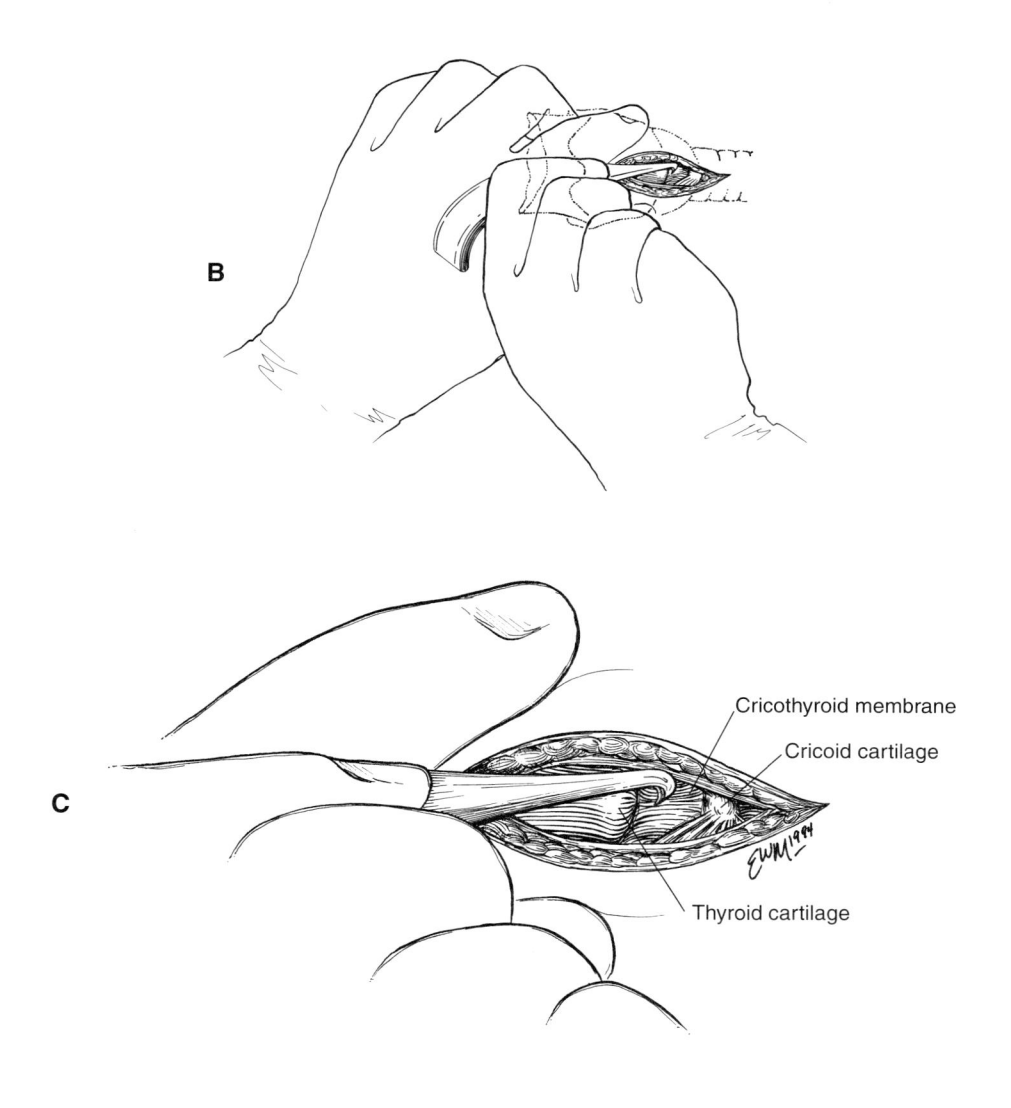

B

C
- Cricothyroid membrane
- Cricoid cartilage
- Thyroid cartilage

D
Left hand takes trachea hook from right hand

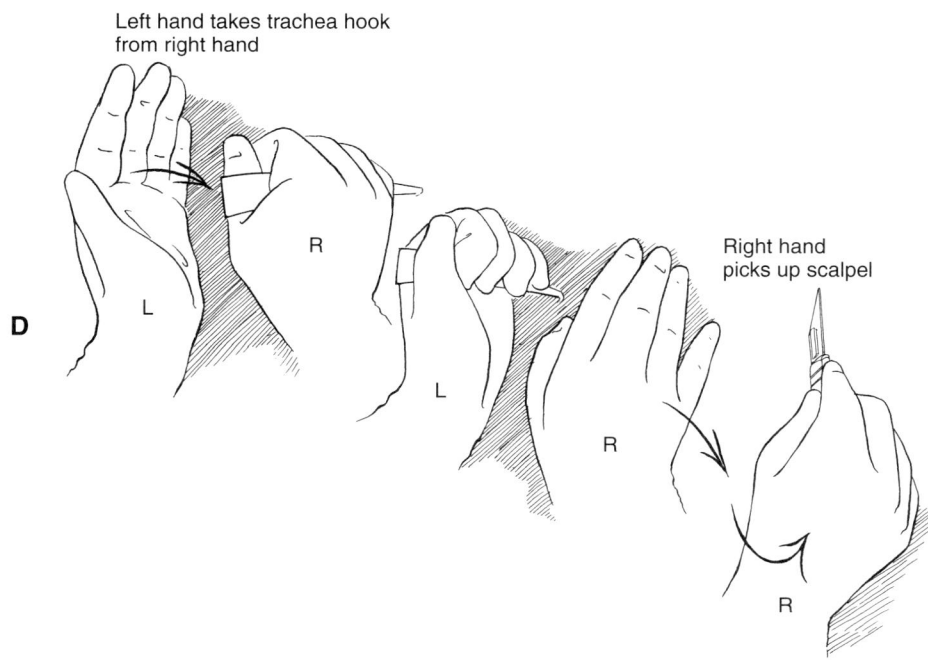

Right hand picks up scalpel

4. Make a transverse incision across the exposed cricothyroid membrane *(E, F)*. If time permits, insert stay sutures in the trachea *(G, H)*. Then dilate the space using the Trousseau dilator, while maintaining traction with the hook *(I-K)*.

5. Place a Shiley cuffed tracheostomy tube through the cricothyroid membrane, initially aiming posterior, then redirecting caudad once through the membrane *(L)*. Remove the hook before insertion to avoid damaging the tube.

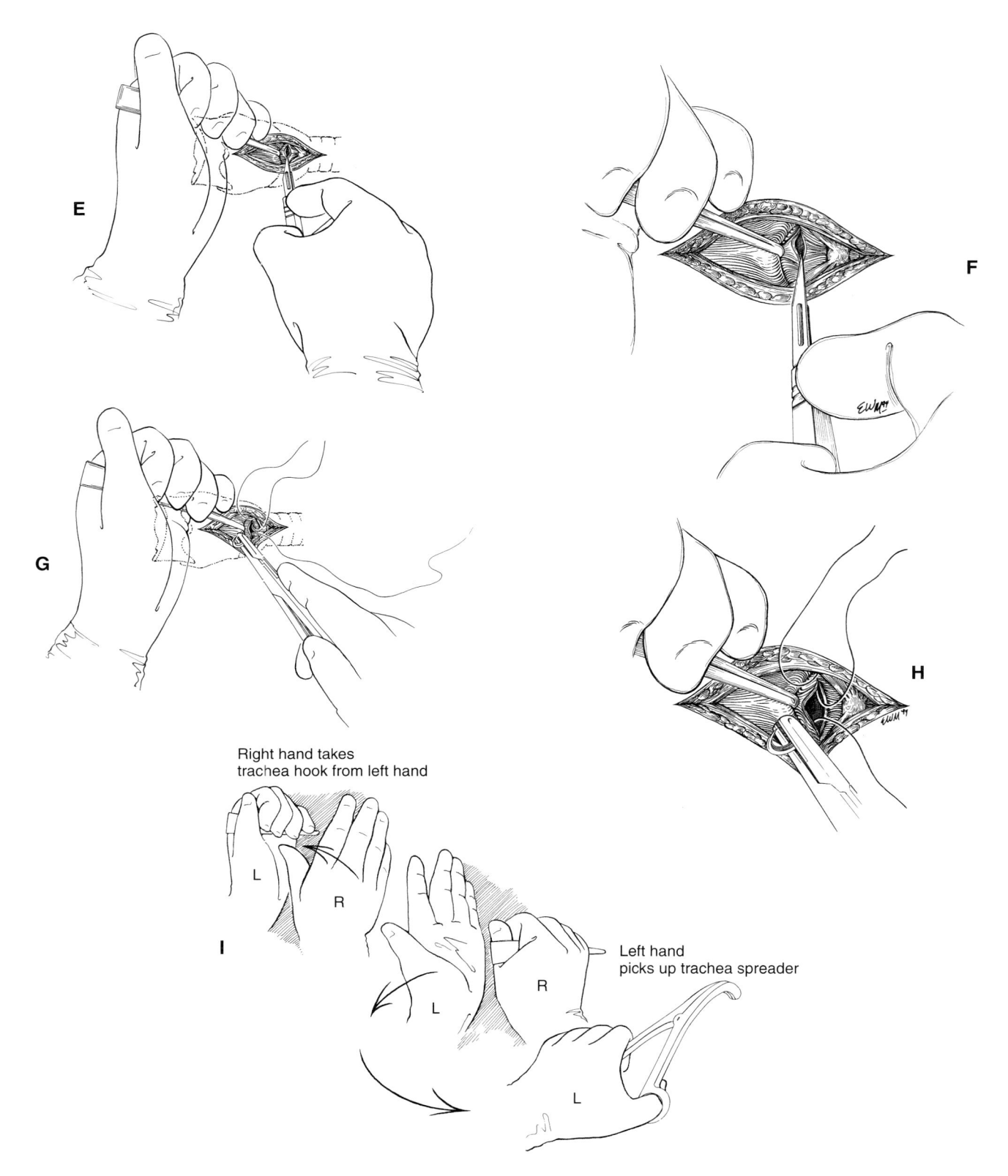

Right hand takes trachea hook from left hand

Left hand picks up trachea spreader

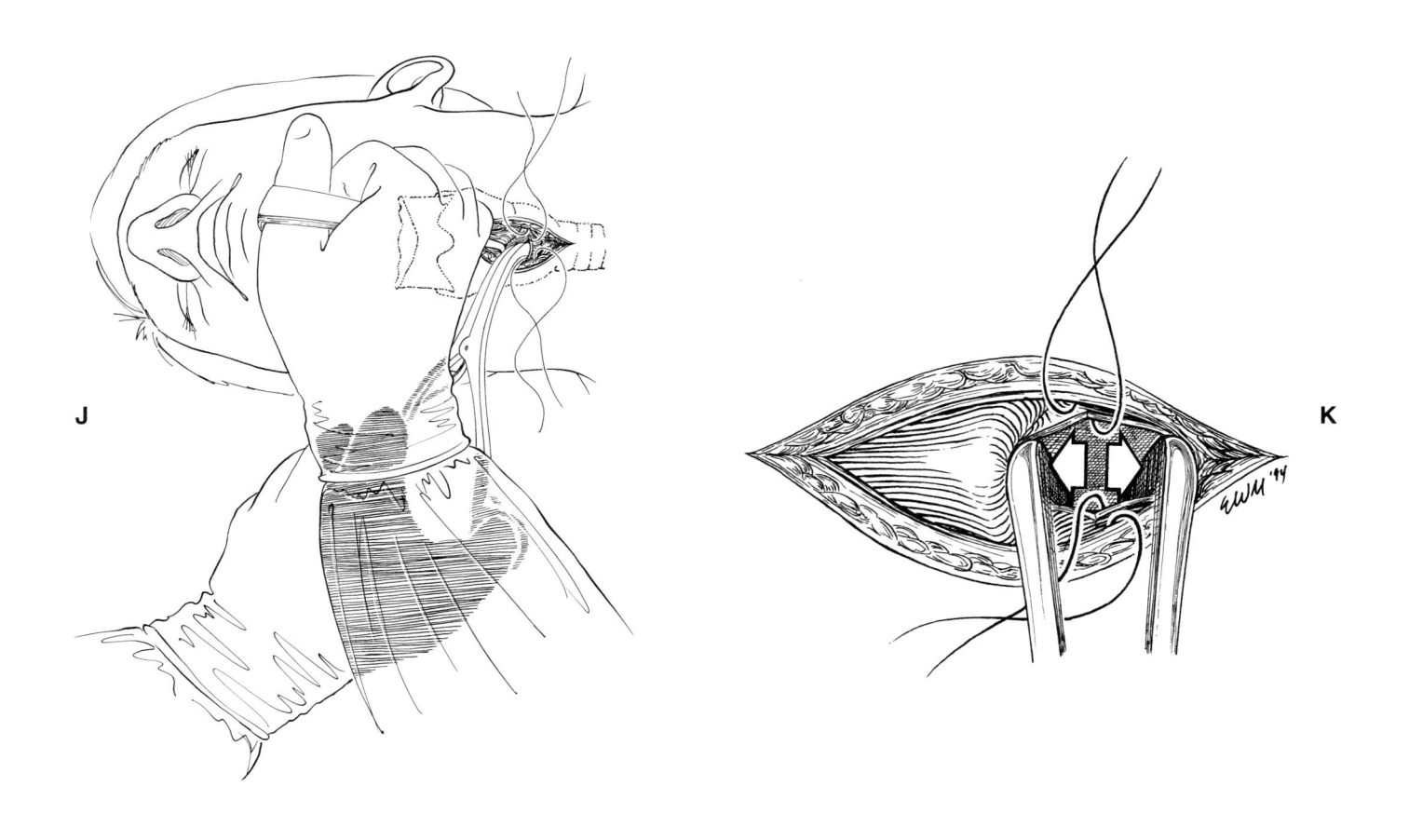

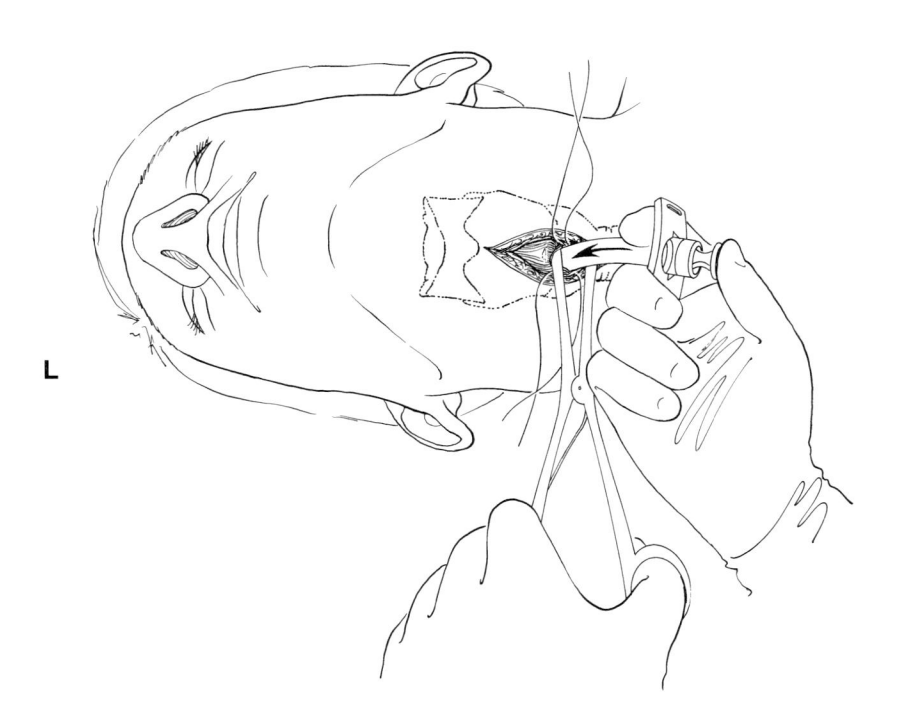

Airway

27

J

K

L

6. Inflate the balloon *(M)*, and remove the introducer *(N)*. Place the riser, attach an Ambu-bag, and secure the Shiley tube with sutures or twill tape *(O)*. The ventilator connector and weaning devices are shown in *P*.

Complications

- Thyroid gland damage
- Large vessel injury with hemorrhage
- Thyroid cartilage fracture
- Damage to adjacent anatomic structures
- Infection
- Aspiration

Discussion

- Some operators prefer a horizontal skin incision, but it increases the risk of tube misplacement and does not allow extension of the incision if greater exposure is needed. In addition, a horizontal incision increases the risk of lacerating the neck vessels, resulting in significant hemorrhage.
- The cricothyroid space can be dilated without the Trousseau dilator by inserting the scalpel handle into the cricothyroid space after incising the membrane and rotating 180°.
- Expect bleeding in the surgical field. Do not become fixated on obtaining hemostasis immediately. Bleeding will resolve slowly after placement of the tube.
- Some operators merely use the hook, dilate the opening, and then place the Shiley tube without removing the hook until the airway is secured.
- Cricothyrotomy can be safely performed in the prehospital field but is best left to personnel experienced in the procedure.

Bibliography

Bainton CR: Cricothyrotomy, *Int Anesthesiol Clin* 32(4):95-101, 1994.

Burkey B et al: The role of cricothyroidotomy in airway management, *Clin Chest Med* 12:561-571, 1991.

Salvino CK et al: Emergency cricothyroidotomy in trauma victims, *J Trauma* 34:503-505, 1993.

Walls RM: Cricothyrotomy, *Emerg Med Clin North Am* 6:725-736, 1988.

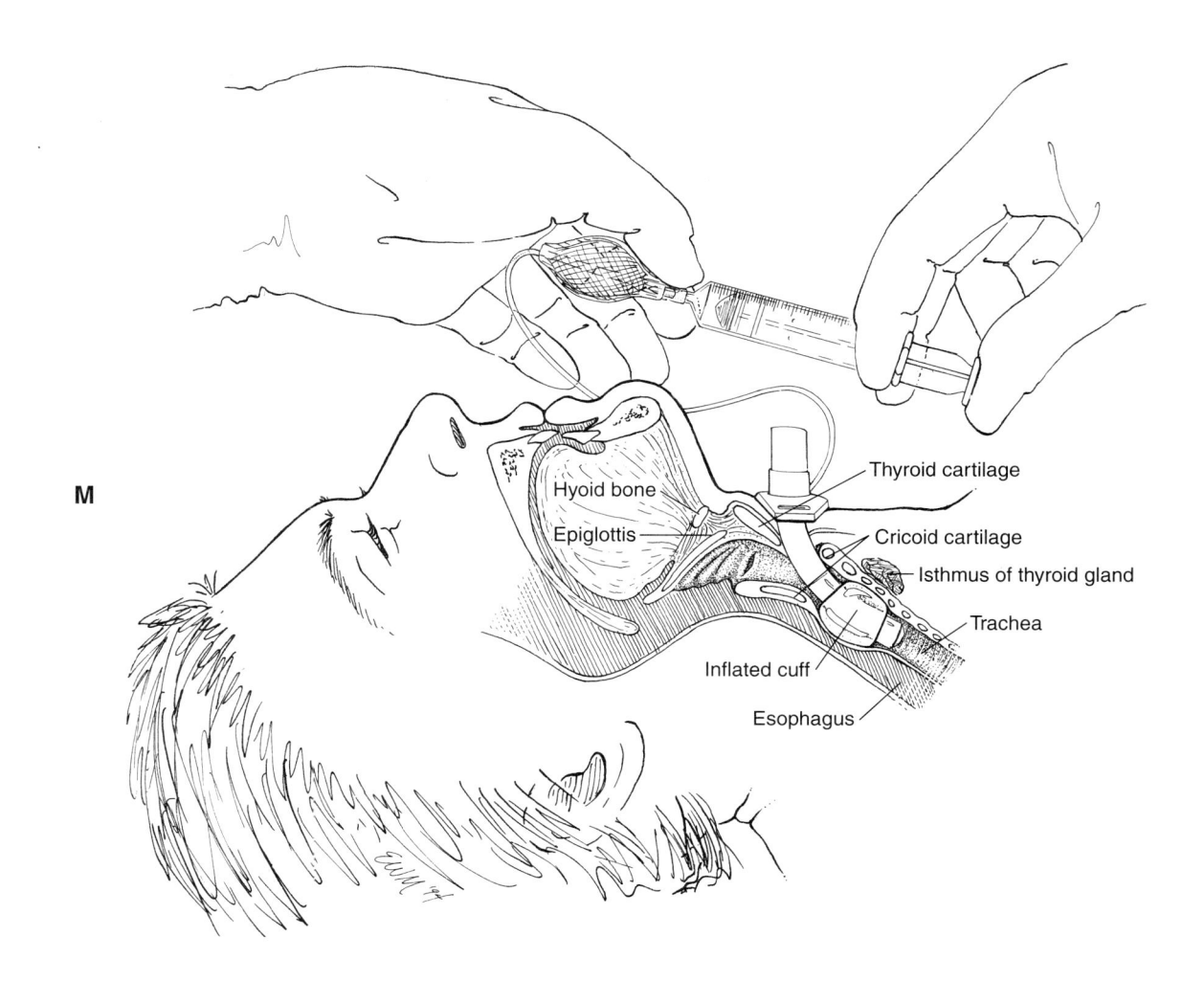

M

AIRWAY 29

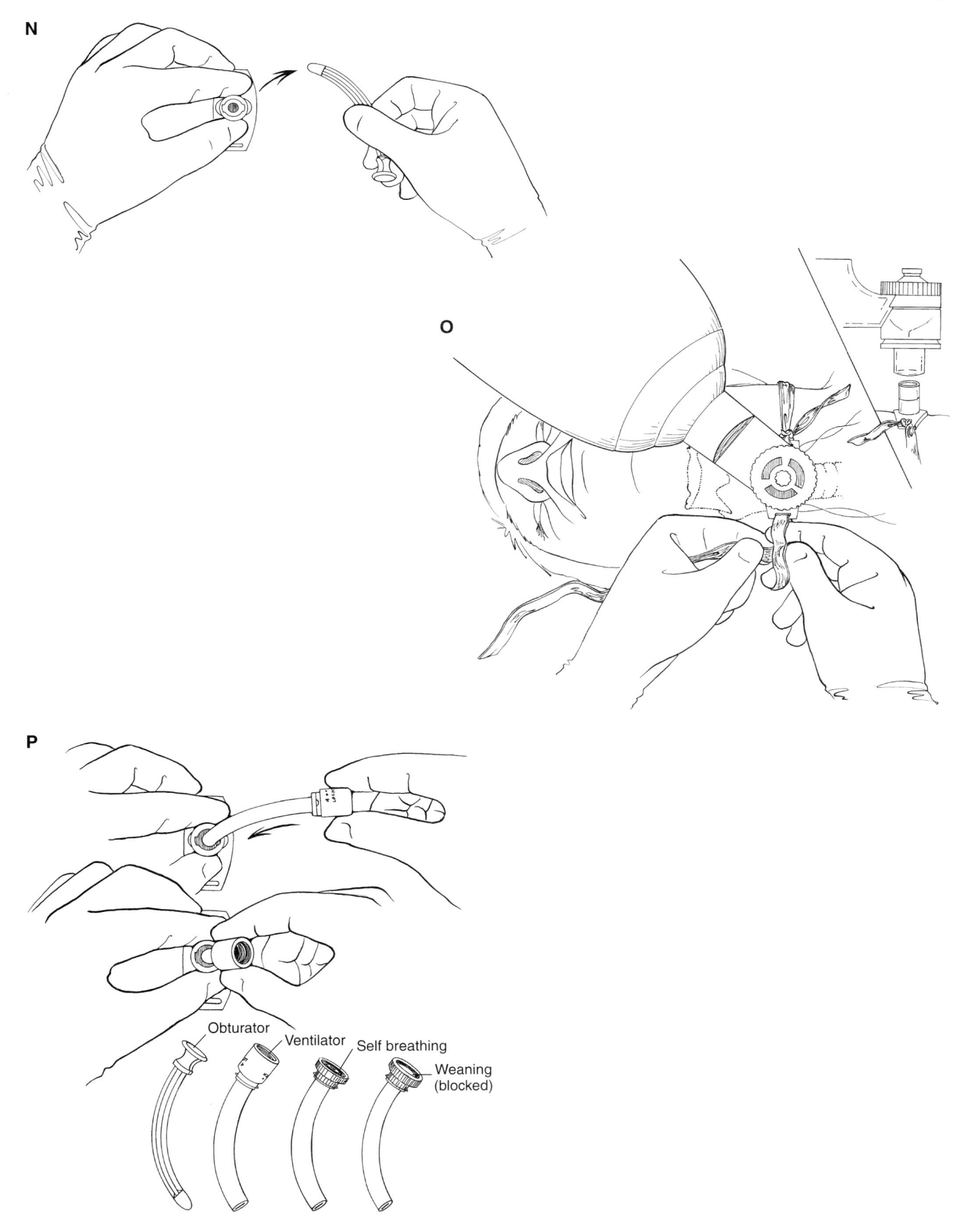

Obturator Ventilator Self breathing Weaning (blocked)

CHAPTER 2

THORAX

External Defibrillation ■ JAMES H. TRUONG AND MARK I. LANGDORF

Indications
- Ventricular fibrillation
- Pulseless ventricular tachycardia in an unresponsive patient

Contraindications
- Responsive patient
- Patient with a pulse
- Danger to operators from wet patient or surroundings
- Asystole or other signs of death (decomposition, decapitation, rigor mortis)

Equipment Needs
- Defibrillator with paddles or self-adhesive pads
- Conductive media (electrode gel or gel-pads)

Procedure

1. Place the patient in a supine position, expose the patient's chest, and remove any jewelry from the defibrillation field.
2. Check the equipment, and ensure a dry skin surface and surroundings.
3. Apply conductive gel or gel-pads to the chest.
   a. Anteroapical placement (for paddles): right sternal just below clavicle and left anterior or midaxillary lower left side of the chest *(A)*
   b. Anteroposterior placement (for self-adhesive pads): left lower sternal border and posterior below the left scapula; if unable to place the posterior pad, use anteroapical locations *(B)*
4. Check the rhythm on the defibrillator monitor, and confirm ventricular fibrillation or pulseless ventricular tachycardia.
5. Switch the defibrillator to unsynchronized mode, and charge it to 200 J *(C)*.
6. If using paddles, place paddles over gel or gel-pads and apply a minimum of 25 lb of pressure to each paddle *(D)*.
7. Call out, "All clear," and ensure that others are not in direct contact with the patient or gurney.
8. Discharge the defibrillation shock.
9. Reassess rhythm and treat as indicated, including increasing subsequent shocks to 300 and 360 J.

Complications
- Partial- or full-thickness skin burns
- Postdefibrillation dysrhythmias
- Inadvertent shock to others
- Defibrillation-induced myocardial damage

Discussion

- Presence of a pacemaker or automated internal cardiac defibrillator device is not a contraindication to external defibrillation. However, pads or paddles should be placed at least 12.5 cm (5 inches) away from the device to prevent its subsequent malfunction.
- If paddles are used, the conductive gel of each paddle should not be permitted to spread to within 5 cm of the gel for the other paddle. Self-adhesive pads should be placed in anteroapical positions if posterior placement would significantly delay defibrillation.
- Defibrillator batteries should be checked routinely. If the defibrillator is not discharging, the power supply should be checked and the monitor should be examined to see that it is in asynchronous mode and has been charged.
- Caution must be exercised in a wet environment such as rain or a case of near-drowning. The patient must first be brought into a dry area, and all wet clothing must be removed. Moisture must be wiped off the thorax before defibrillation is attempted.

Bibliography

Cobbe SM et al: "Heartstart Scotland"—initial experience of a national scheme for out of hospital defibrillation, *Br Med J* 302:1517-1520, 1991.

Dalzell GW, Adgey AJ: Determinants of successful transthoracic defibrillation and outcome in ventricular fibrillation, *Br Heart J* 65:311-316, 1991.

Kerber RE, Sarnat W: Factors influencing the success of ventricular defibrillation in man, *Circulation* 60(2):226-230, 1979.

Kerber RE et al: Transthoracic resistance in human defibrillation, *Circulation* 63(3):676-681, 1981.

Sedgwick ML et al: Performance of an established system of first responder out of hospital defibrillation, *Resuscitation* 26:75-88, 1993.

Thorax

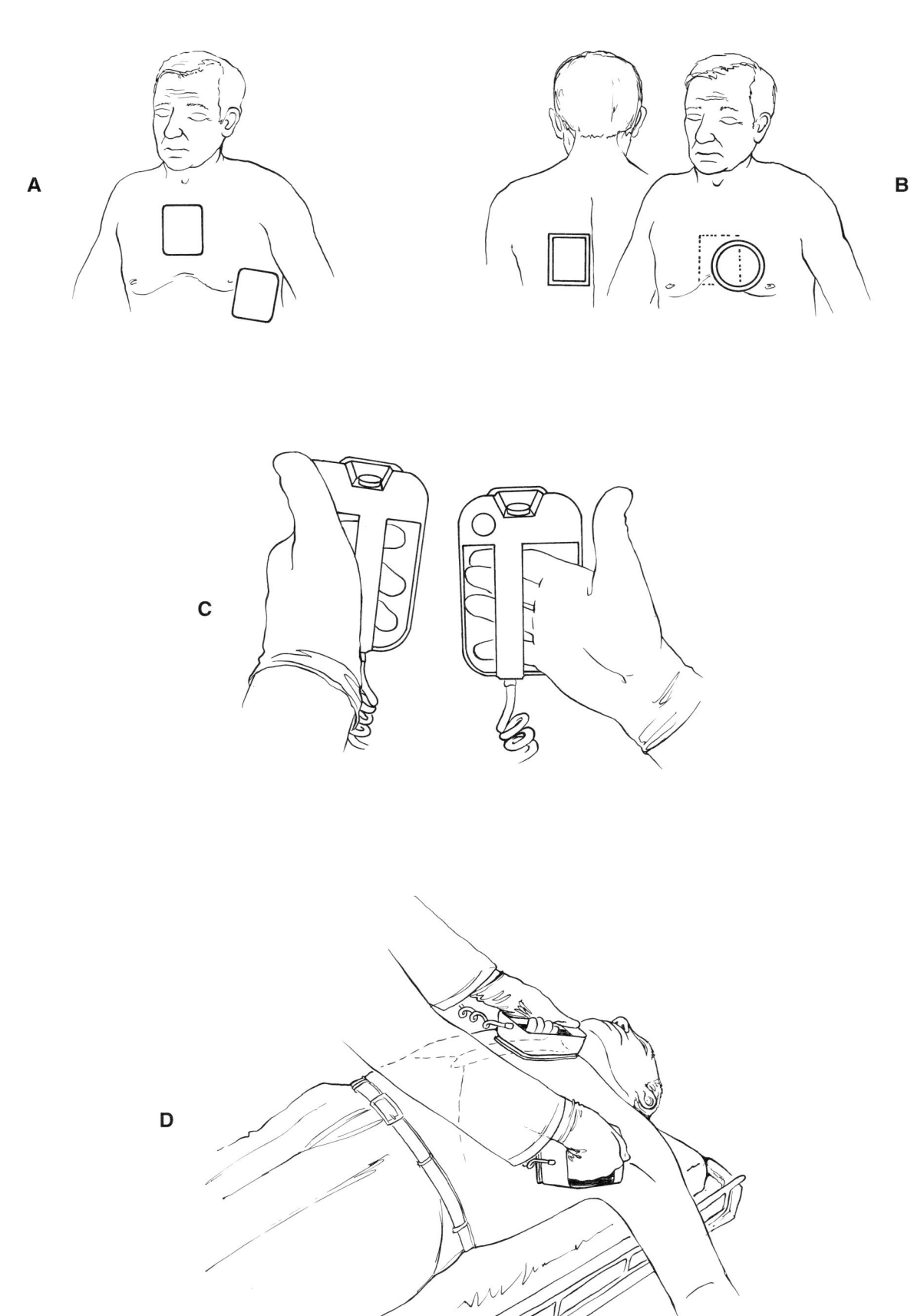

33

Intercostal Nerve Block ▪ ERIK D. BARTON

Indications
- Painful rib fractures

Contraindications
- Flail chest
- Overlying skin infection

Equipment
- Betadine antiseptic solution
- Sterile drapes and gloves
- 10-ml syringe
- 22- to 25-gauge 2-inch needles
- Anesthetic agents: bupivacaine with epinephrine or mixture of plain bupivacaine and lidocaine 1% with epinephrine

Procedure

1. Place the patient in sitting position, leaning forward on a Mayo stand *(A)*.
2. Locate the fractured rib, and follow the rib posteriorly to the costovertebral junction.
3. Prepare the area in a sterile fashion.
4. Draw 5 to 10 ml of the anesthetic agent into the syringe, and attach the smaller gauge needle.
5. Make a small skin wheal over the inferior aspect of the transverse process of the vertebra.
6. Insert the needle perpendicular to the skin and inferior to the transverse process of the vertebra *(B)*. Aspirate for blood or air.
7. Inject 2 to 5 ml of the anesthetic agent into the area *(C)*.
8. Remove the needle, obtain hemostasis, and observe the patient for complications for 30 minutes.
9. Block the ribs above and below the fractured rib in the manner described previously.

Complications
- Pneumothorax
- Lung puncture
- Hemothorax
- Iatrogenic infection
- Anesthesia toxicity
- Persistent bleeding
- Intrathecal or epidural injection of anesthetic

Discussion

- Patients with chronic obstructive pulmonary disease or other lung disease have an altered lung and pleural space architecture, resulting in a higher risk for pneumothorax. Greater caution is required.
- An alternative to the posterior approach is a lateral approach for anterior rib fractures. With this technique the needle is inserted over the lower third of the rib at a site proximal or posterior to the fracture (usually near the midaxillary line). However, this technique carries a higher risk of pneumothorax and hemothorax and does not provide as complete a block.

Bibliography
Hardy PA: Anatomical variation in the position of the proximal intercostal nerve, *Br J Anaesth* 61(3):338-339, 1998.
Johansson A et al: Multiple intercostals blocks by a single injection? A clinical and radiological investigation, *Acta Anaesthesiol Scand* 29(5):524-528, 1985.
Johnson MD et al: Bupivacaine with and without epinephrine for intercostal nerve block, *J Cardiothorac Anesth* 4(2):200-203, 1990.

Thorax

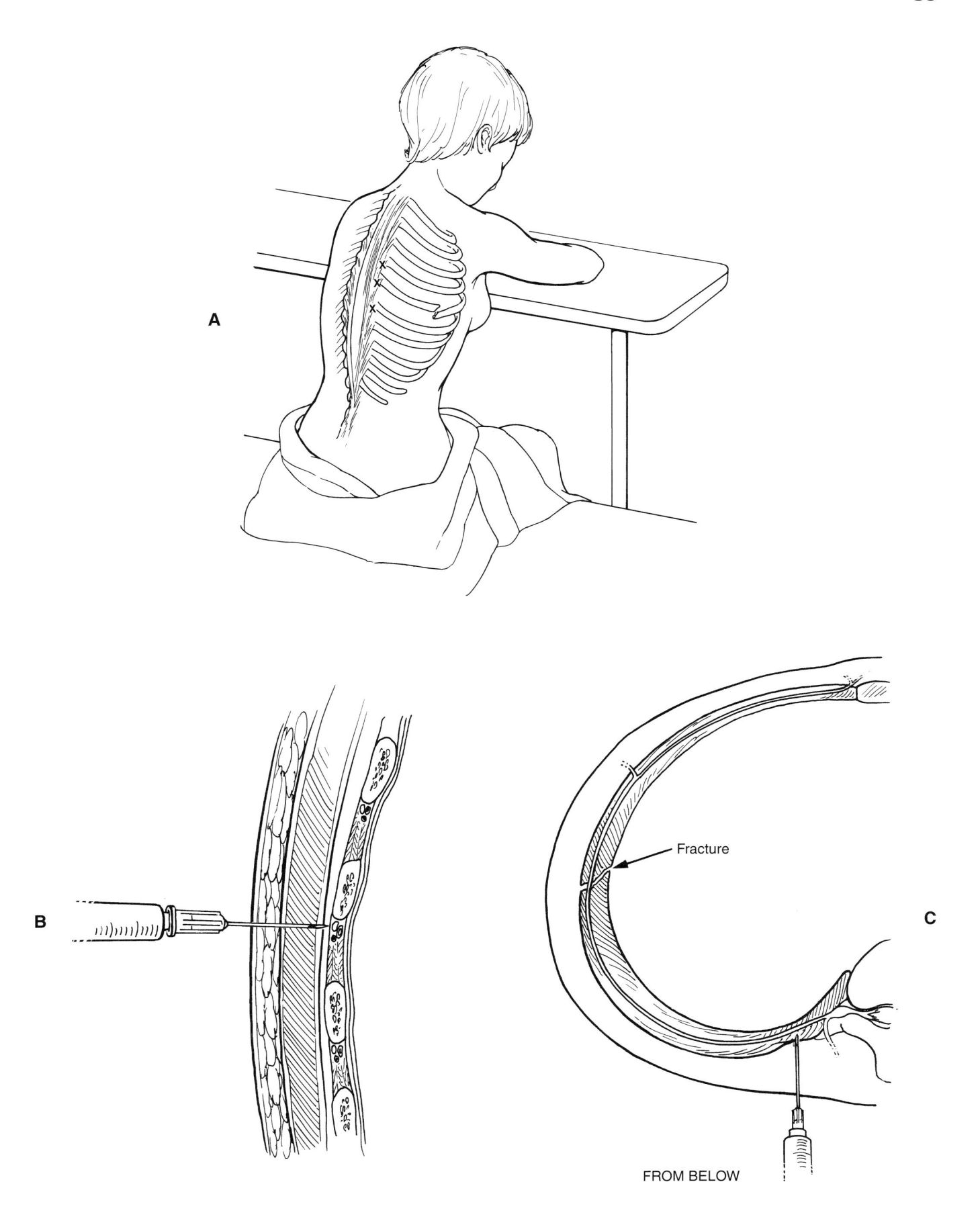

A

B

C Fracture

FROM BELOW

Thoracentesis • ERIK D. BARTON

Indications
- Diagnostic evaluation of pleural effusions
- Therapeutic drainage of a large pleural effusion or hydrothorax

Contraindications
- Bleeding disorder or anticoagulation therapy
- Hemothorax
- Empyema
- Ruptured diaphragm
- Overlying skin infection
- Loculated effusions

Equipment
- Commercially available thoracentesis aspiration set, or the following:
  - 16- to 20-gauge angiocatheters
  - 60-ml syringe
  - Local anesthetic agent (1% lidocaine with epinephrine) with syringe and needles
  - Betadine antiseptic solution
  - Sterile drapes and gloves
  - Sterile tubing with three-way stopcock
  - Fluid collection bottles

Procedure

1. Place the patient in sitting position, leaning forward on a Mayo stand *(A)*.
2. Stand behind the patient.
3. Percuss the back to locate the effusion, and perform sterile preparation of the area two intercostal spaces below at the posterior axillary or midscapular line.
4. Palpate the superior edge of the rib nearest the site, which should be no lower than the 9th rib.
5. Infiltrate this area with local anesthetic (3 to 5 ml).
6. Attach an angiocatheter with a needle to a syringe.
7. Slowly insert the angiocatheter directly over the upper third of the rib until it strikes the bone.
8. Gently apply upward tension on the skin, and guide the angiocatheter with your finger over the upper rib border.
9. With the angiocatheter directed slightly inferiorly, advance it into the pleural space and aspirate for fluid *(B)*.
10. For diagnostic purposes, remove the appropriate amount of fluid required and then remove the angiocatheter.
11. For therapeutic purposes, remove the needle, leaving the angiocatheter in place. Directing the patient not to inspire, place a thumb over the angiocatheter hub after needle removal to maintain a closed system. Attach a stopcock and proximal tubing to the angiocatheter, and attach distal tubing to the collection bottle, at which time the patient can resume respiration.
12. Withdraw the desired amount of fluid while maintaining a closed system at all times, and then remove the catheter *(C)*.
13. Observe the patient for 30 to 60 minutes after the procedure, and obtain a postprocedure chest radiograph.

Complications

- Pneumothorax
- Coughing
- Lung puncture or laceration
- Hemothorax
- Diaphragmatic injury
- Reexpansion pulmonary edema
- Retained catheter fragment
- Iatrogenic infection

Discussion

- Real-time ultrasonography can be used to locate pleural effusions and direct the needle insertion to a location that minimizes the risk of complications.
- Patients with chronic obstructive pulmonary disease or other lung disease have an altered lung and pleural space architecture, resulting in higher risk for pneumothorax. Greater caution is required, and smaller volumes should be removed.
- When the angiocatheter is used, the needle should never be reinserted into the catheter because of the risk of shearing the catheter tip in the pleural space.
- For diagnostic thoracentesis a standard hollow-bore needle can be used in lieu of the angiocatheter.
- For therapeutic thoracentesis many kits have a needle-over-catheter configuration that allows the operator to maintain a closed system at all times. These kits use a breakaway needle that can be removed after catheter placement is secure. Many collection systems include vacuum bottles that facilitate fluid collection for large effusions.

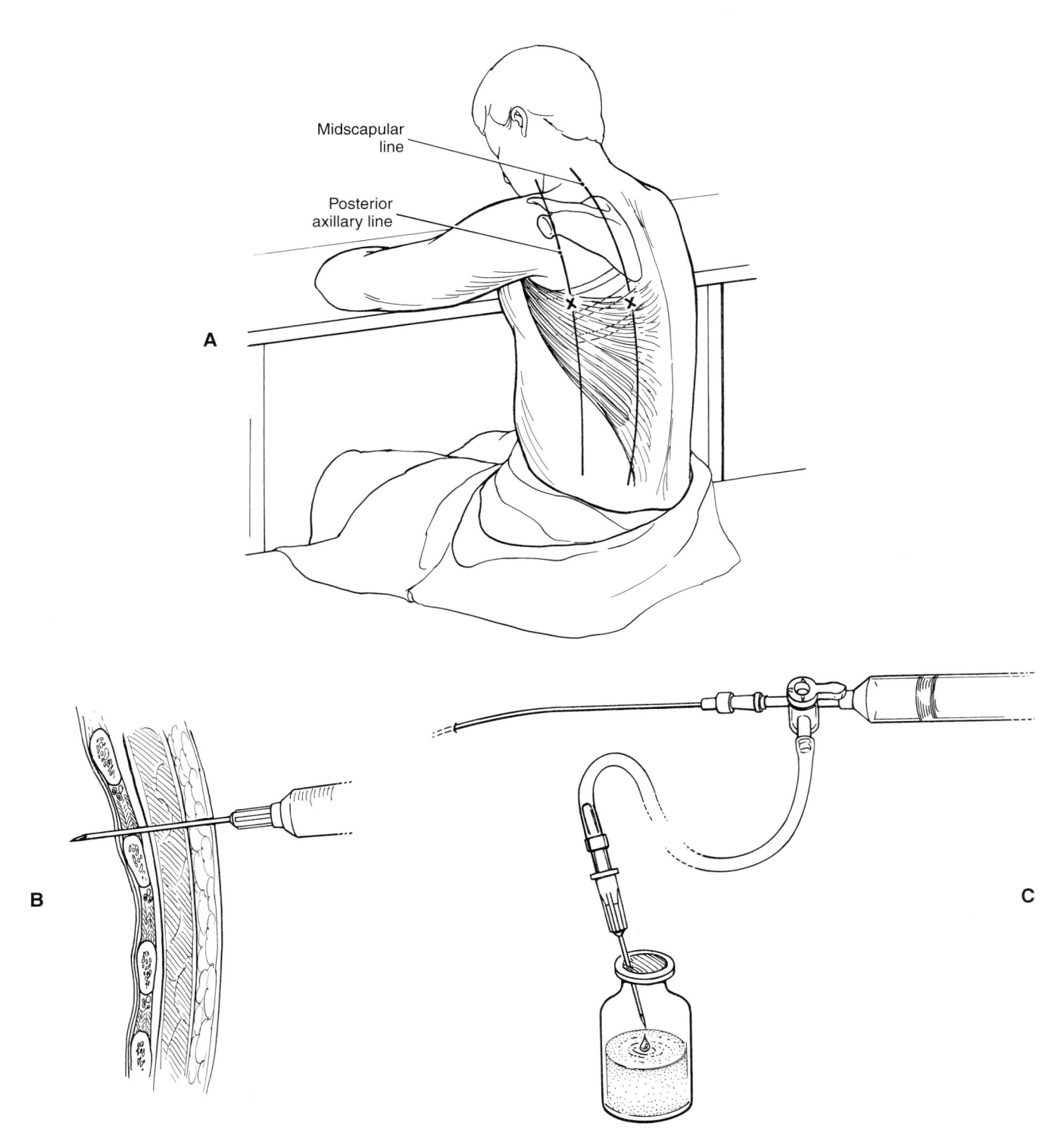

Bibliography

Collins TR, Sahn SA: Thoracentesis: clinical value, complications, technical problems, and patient experience, *Chest* 91:817-822, 1987.

Doyle JJ et al: Necessity of routine chest roentgenography after thoracentesis [see comments], *Ann Intern Med* 124(9):816-820, 1996.

McCartney JP et al: Safety of thoracentesis in mechanically ventilated patients, *Chest* 103(6):1920-1921, 1993.

Qureshi N et al: Thoracentesis in clinical practice, *Heart Lung* 23(5): 376-383, 1994.

Raptopoulos V et al: Factors affecting the development of pneumothorax associated with thoracentesis [see comments], *Am J Roentgenol* 156(5):917-920, 1991.

Needle Thoracostomy • MICHAEL B. WOLFE AND REBECCA SMITH-COGGINS

Indications
- Clinical evidence of tension pneumothorax

Contraindications
- None

Equipment
- 3- to 6-cm-long 14-gauge angiocatheter
- Betadine antiseptic solution

Procedure

1. Identify the 5th intercostal space at the midaxillary line on the affected side *(A)*.
2. Prepare the area in sterile fashion.
3. Insert the catheter through the chest wall at the 5th intercostal space, just over the 6th rib, until the parietal pleura has been entered. This is usually signaled by a "pop" and a rush of air *(B)*.
4. Remove the needle, leaving the angiocatheter in place.

Complications

- Pneumothorax
- Lung puncture or laceration
- Hematoma
- Retained catheter fragment
- Iatrogenic infection
- Failure to decompress

Discussion

- If the patient is still awake and not deteriorating, a local anesthetic (e.g., lidocaine) can be administered before placement of the angiocatheter.
- When an angiocatheter is used, the needle should never be reinserted into the catheter because of the risk of shearing the catheter tip in the pleural space.
- Needle thoracostomy is only temporizing, and definitive treatment with a chest tube thoracostomy is needed urgently. The catheter tip will quickly become occluded by blood if a hemothorax is present.
- A midaxillary insertion site is used to avoid penetration of the internal mammary artery, as well as to avoid the large muscle groups of the chest that are encountered with the midclavicular approach.
- This procedure is often performed in the prehospital setting by ground paramedics and flight personnel.

Bibliography

Barton ED: Prehospital needle aspiration and tube thoracostomy in trauma victims: a six-year experience with aeromedical crews, *J Emerg Med* 13(2):155-163, 1995.

Britten S, Palmer SH: Needle thoracentesis in tension pneumothorax: insufficient cannula length and potential failure, *Injury* 27(5):321-322, 1996.

Coats TJ et al: Prehospital management of patients with severe thoracic injury, *Injury* 26(9):581-585, 1995.

Thorax

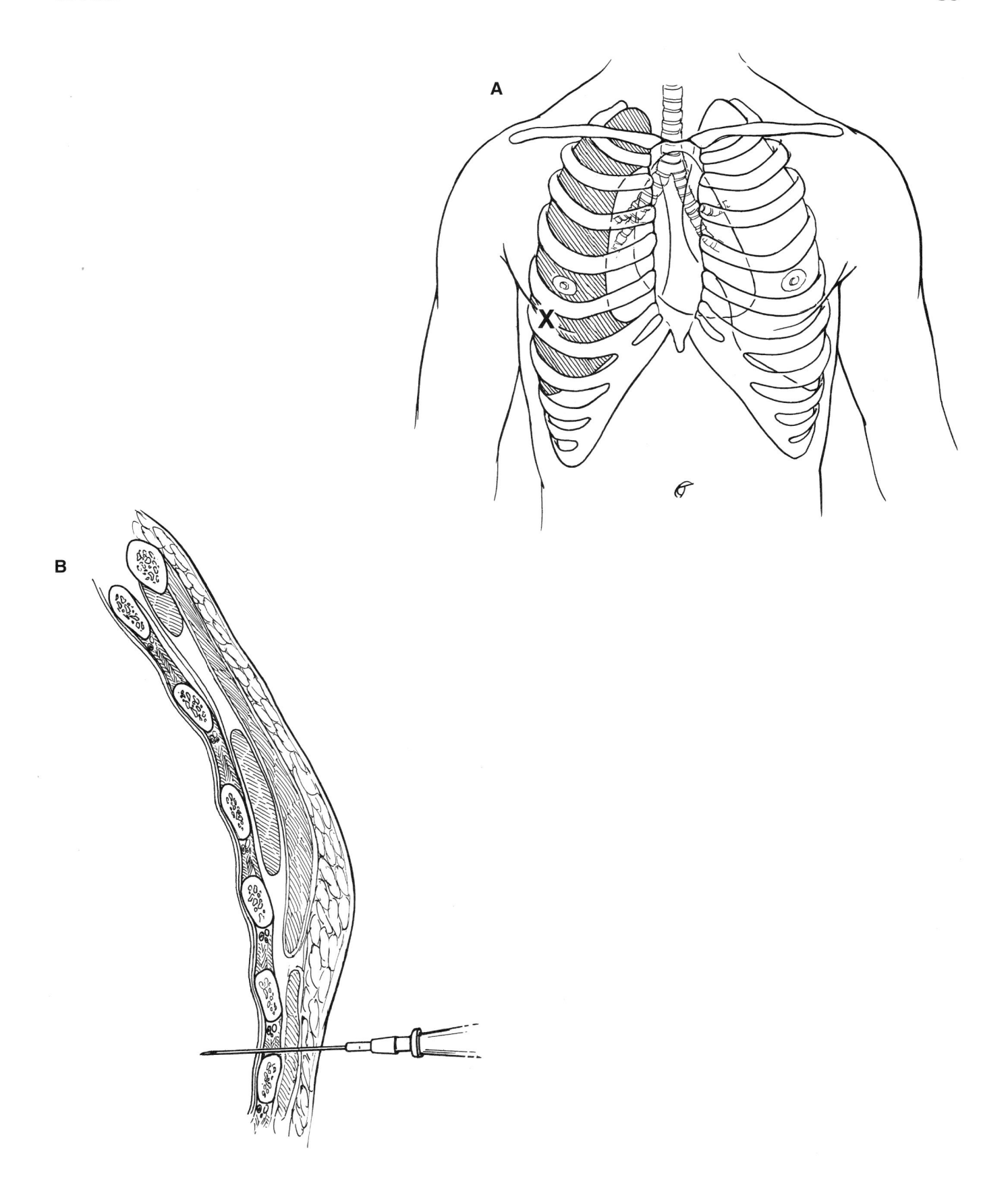

Tube Thoracostomy ▪ KIM M. FELDHAUS

Indications
- Tension pneumothorax
- Simple pneumothorax
- Hemothorax
- Pleural effusions
- Empyema
- Chylothorax

Contraindications
- Multiple pulmonary adhesions
- Large pulmonary bullae or blebs
- Need for open thoracostomy
- Massive hemothorax before fluid resuscitation
- Coagulopathy

Equipment
- Local anesthetic agent (1% lidocaine with epinephrine) with syringe and needles
- Betadine antiseptic solution
- Sterile drapes and gloves
- Scalpel with No. 10 blade
- Large curved Mayo scissors
- Large Kelly clamps
- Medium Kelly clamps
- Chest tube:
  - 16 to 24 Fr in children
  - 28 to 40 Fr in adults
- Water-seal apparatus (Pleur-evac) with clear tubing, serrated connector, and suction
- Needle driver
- Large cutting needle with 0 or 1-0 silk
- Vaseline-impregnated gauze
- 4 × 4 gauze pads
- Wide cloth adhesive tape

Procedure
1. Place the patient in a semierect position (or supine if the patient's condition is unstable).
2. Elevate the arm above the head on the ipsilateral side for the procedure.
3. Mark the site for insertion at the 4th intercostal space at the anterior axillary line *(A)*.
4. Prepare and drape the skin in sterile fashion.
5. Raise a wheal with anesthetic over the insertion site.
6. Infiltrate deeper with the lidocaine, using the 25-gauge needle to anesthetize the subcutaneous tissue, intercostal muscles, and parietal pleura *(B)*.
7. An awake patient will require 10 to 20 ml of lidocaine.
8. Make a 2- to 3-cm incision over the 5th rib, running parallel to the rib.
9. Bluntly dissect the subcutaneous tissues, using the Kelly clamp or Mayo scissors.
10. Dissection should be caudad, over the top of the 4th or 5th rib *(C)*.
11. Using a closed clamp or scissors, bluntly penetrate the parietal pleura with steady pressure *(D)*.

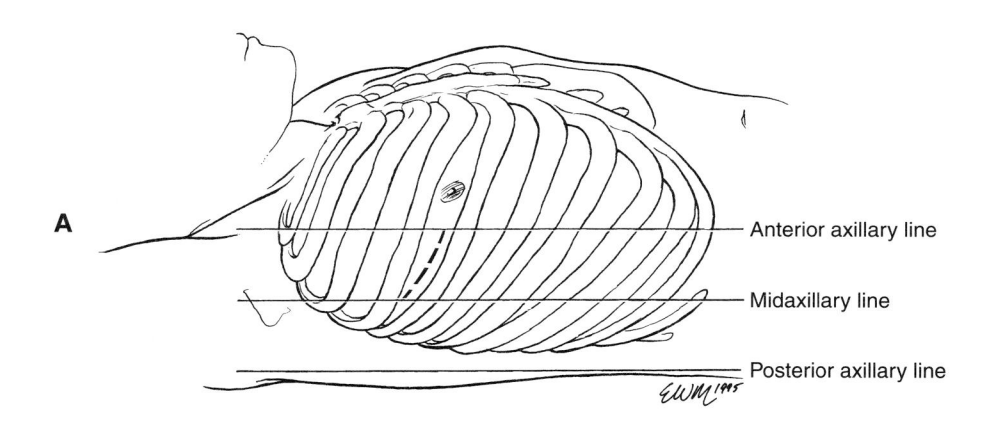

Thorax

B

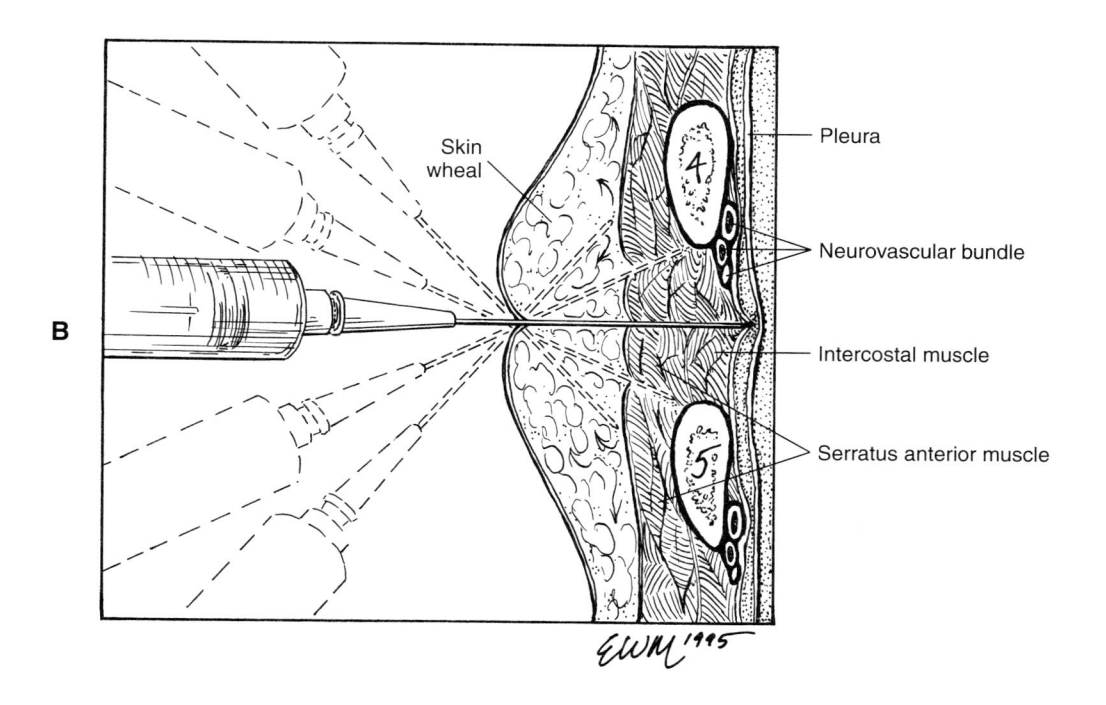

- Skin wheal
- Pleura
- Neurovascular bundle
- Intercostal muscle
- Serratus anterior muscle

C

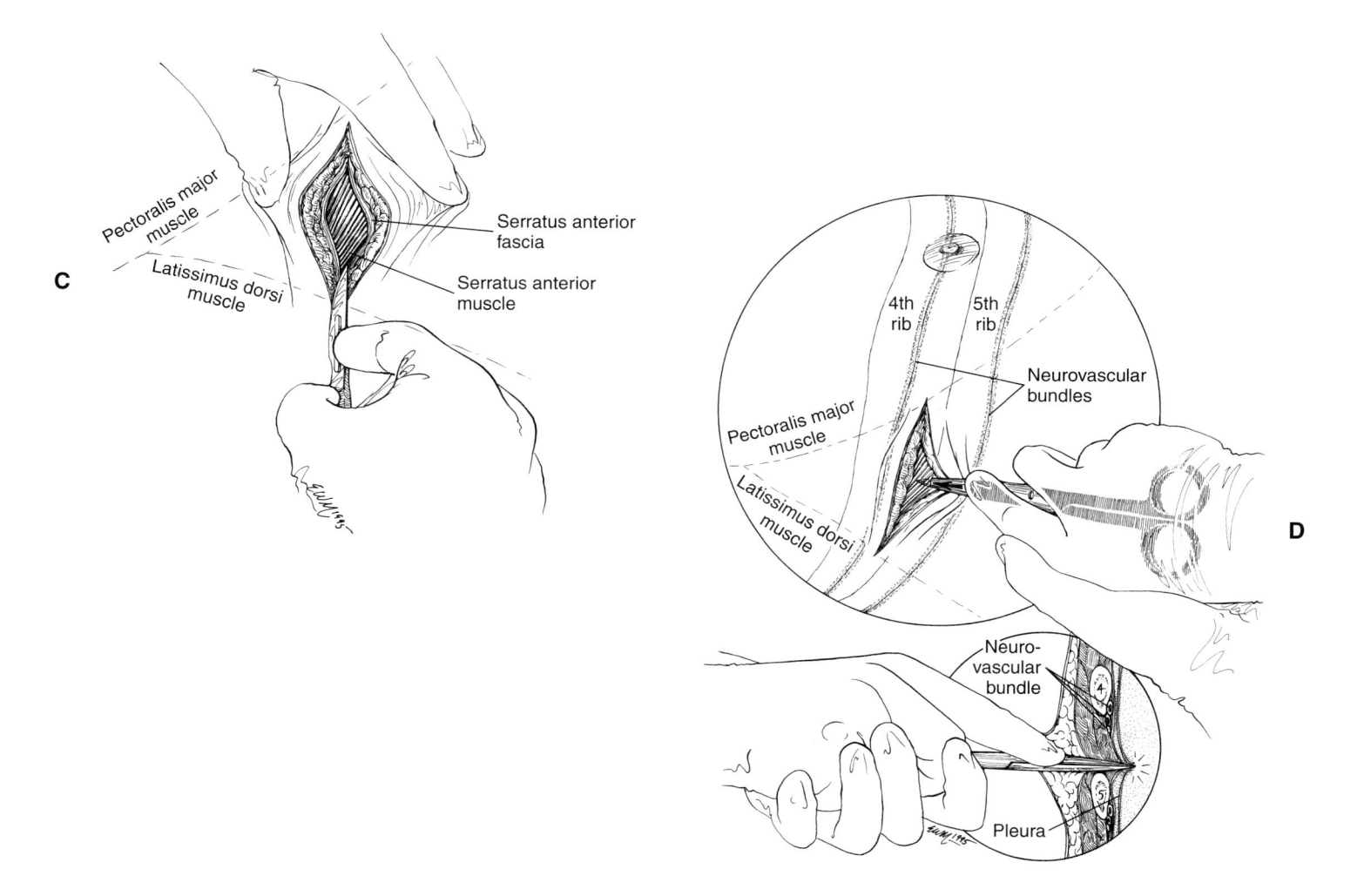

- Pectoralis major muscle
- Latissimus dorsi muscle
- Serratus anterior fascia
- Serratus anterior muscle

D

- 4th rib
- 5th rib
- Pectoralis major muscle
- Latissimus dorsi muscle
- Neurovascular bundles
- Neurovascular bundle
- Pleura

12. Open the instrument wide after penetrating the pleura *(E)*, and remove with the instrument still open to widen the size of the opening.
13. Insert a gloved finger through the pleural opening to verify position and absence of adhesions or abdominal organs *(F)*.
14. Guide an appropriate-size chest tube into place, using fingers and a Pean clamp on the end *(G)*.
15. Direct the tube posteriorly and cephalad until all holes are within the thoracic cavity *(H)*.

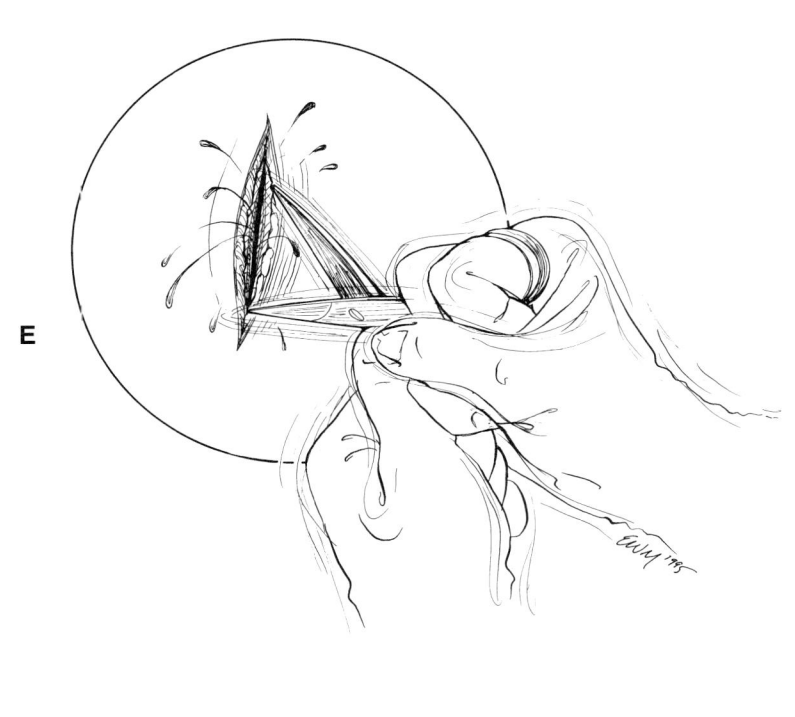

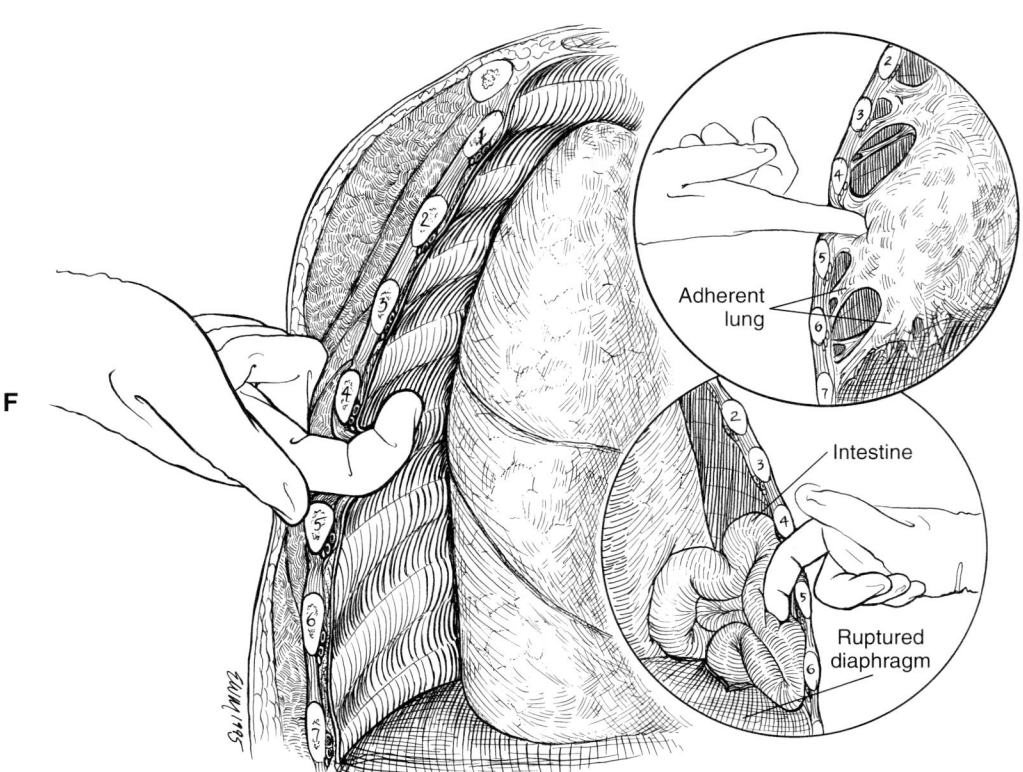

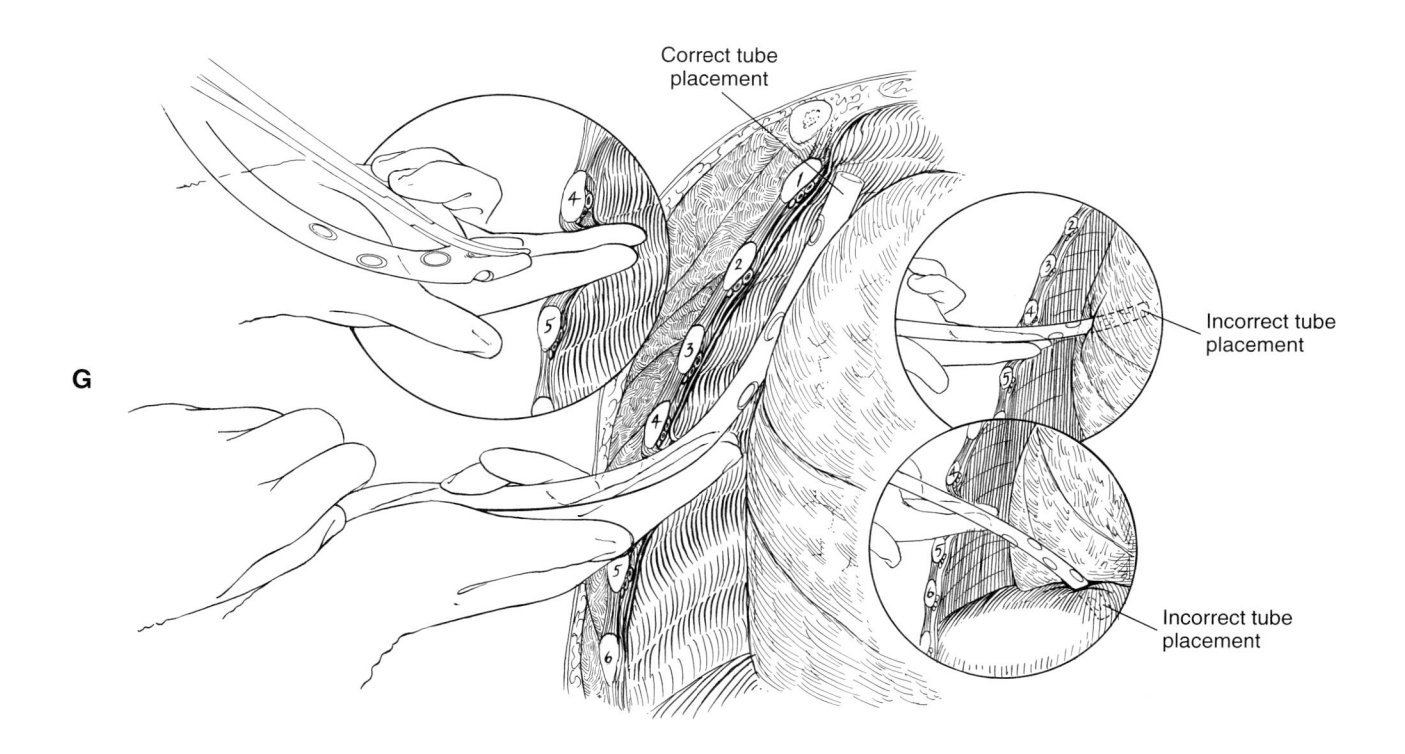

Thorax

Correct tube placement

Incorrect tube placement

Incorrect tube placement

G

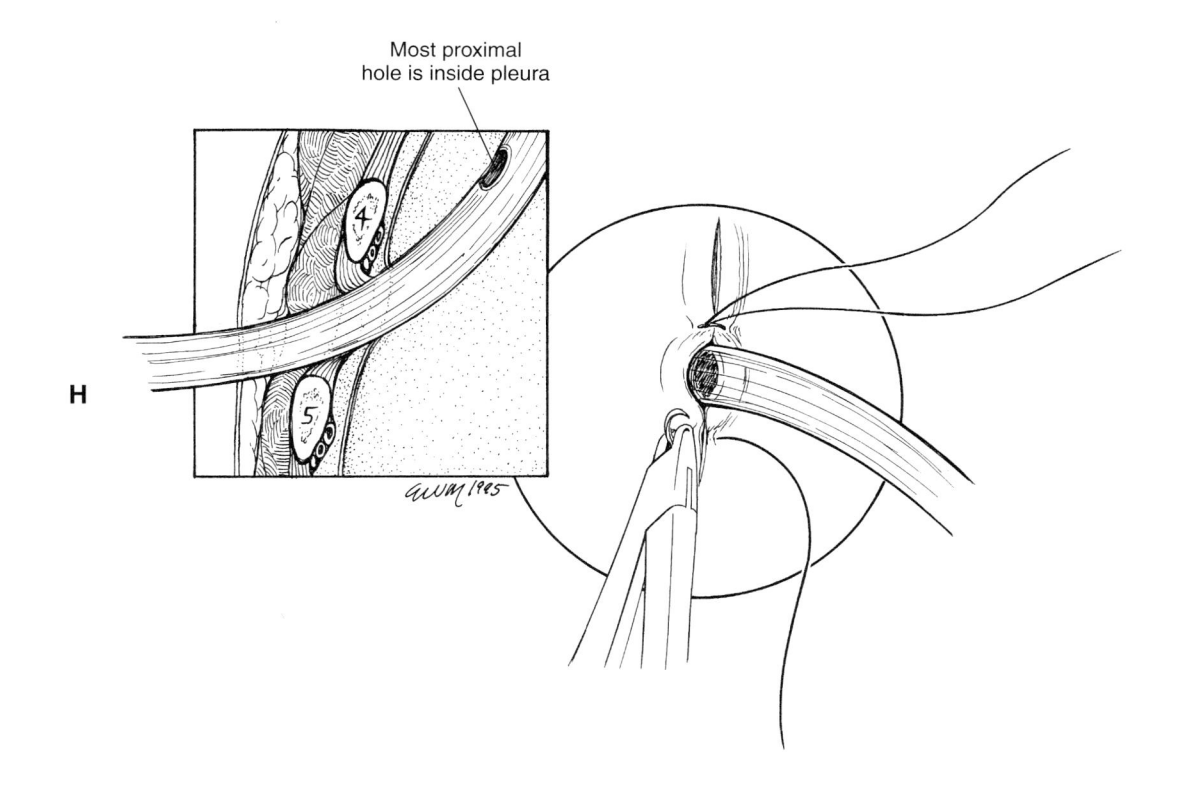

Most proximal hole is inside pleura

H

16. Connect the tube to a water-seal apparatus. If the system is patent, bubbles should appear when the patient coughs.
17. Secure the tube with suture in purse-string fashion and cover with Vaseline-impregnated dressing, 4 × 4 gauze pads, and adhesive tape *(I-K)*.

Complications

- Incorrect placement
- Infection
- Laceration of lung, liver, or other abdominal organs
- Injury to intercostal bundle
- Injury to long thoracic nerve

Discussion

- Smaller tubes (20 to 32 Fr) may be used for a pneumothorax. Larger tubes (36 to 40 Fr) are used if fluid drainage is needed. Pediatric sizes vary based on age and size. For an awake patient, parenteral sedation and analgesia should be considered.
- Some authors recommend placement of a tube thoracostomy in the 2nd intercostal space in the midclavicular line for air and in the posterior axillary line for fluid. We prefer the approach between the pectoral and latissimus dorsi muscles in the midaxillary line. Placement is easier in this location because there is less muscle mass requiring incision and more accurate because the operator can more easily palpate the tube going between the ribs.
- If the patient has a significant coagulopathy and the procedure is not an emergency, correct the coagulation status before placing the tube.
- Tube thoracostomies can be safely placed in the prehospital setting by appropriately trained personnel.

Bibliography

Barton ED: Prehospital needle aspiration and tube thoracostomy in trauma victims: a six-year experience with aeromedical crews, *J Emerg Med* 13(2):155-163, 1995.

THORAX

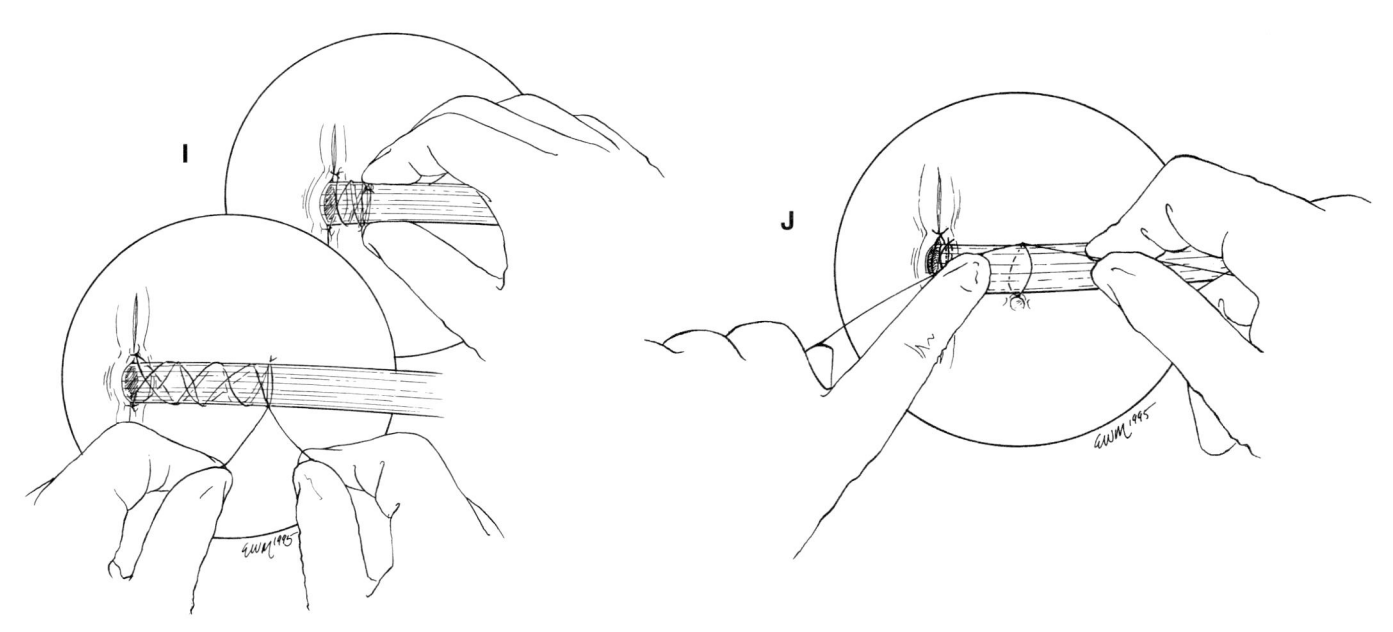

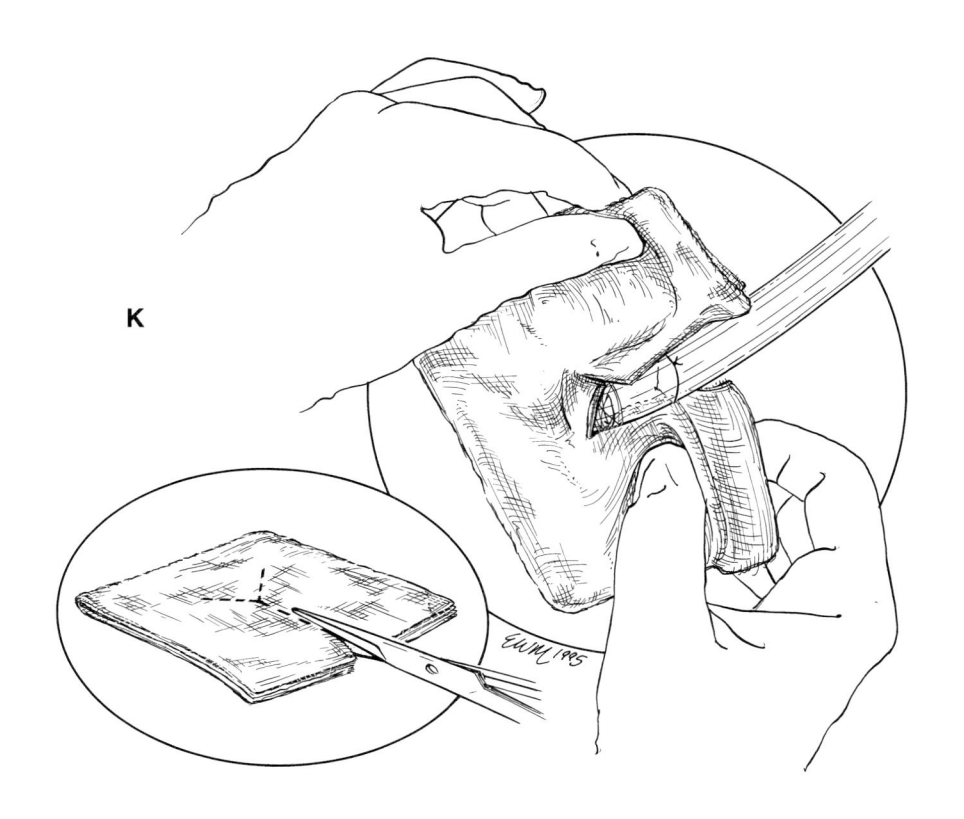

45

I

J

K

Thoracotomy ■ KENNETH C. JACKIMCZYK AND GARY J. ORDOG

Indications
- Penetrating trauma with loss of vital signs during transport or in the emergency department
- Penetrating trauma resulting in profound shock or rapid clinical deterioration that does not respond to aggressive fluid resuscitation
- Blunt trauma with loss of vital signs in the emergency department or hospital

Contraindications
- Clinically stable patient
- Obvious signs of death (e.g., rigor mortis, decapitation)
- Blunt trauma resulting in cardiopulmonary arrest in the field

Equipment
- Prep items
  - Sterile towels
  - Betadine solution
- Essential items
  - No. 10 scalpel
  - Rib spreader
  - Mayo scissors, curved, 6.25 inch
- Additional items
  - Metzenbaum scissors, curved, 9 to 10 inch
  - Mayo-Harrington scissors
  - Tissue forceps, 5½ and 10 inch
  - Pean and Crile hemostats
  - Satinsky vascular clamps
  - Lebsche knife with mallet
  - Hegar needle holders
  - Lap sponges
  - Raytec sponges
  - Jumbo applicators
  - 3-0 cardiovascular suture

Procedure

1. Place the patient in a supine position, and prepare the entire chest in sterile fashion.
2. Locate the left 5th intercostal space (just below the nipple in men, inframammary line in women) *(A)*.
3. Make an incision laterally, starting just left of the sternum and proceeding along the intercostal space to the midaxillary line. The incision should be made along the upper portion of the left 6th rib (parallel to the rib) to avoid the neurovascular bundle. The initial incision should be carried down through the pectoralis muscles and serratus fibers *(B, C)*.
4. Once the pleura is exposed, make a small incision in it with the scalpel *(D)*.

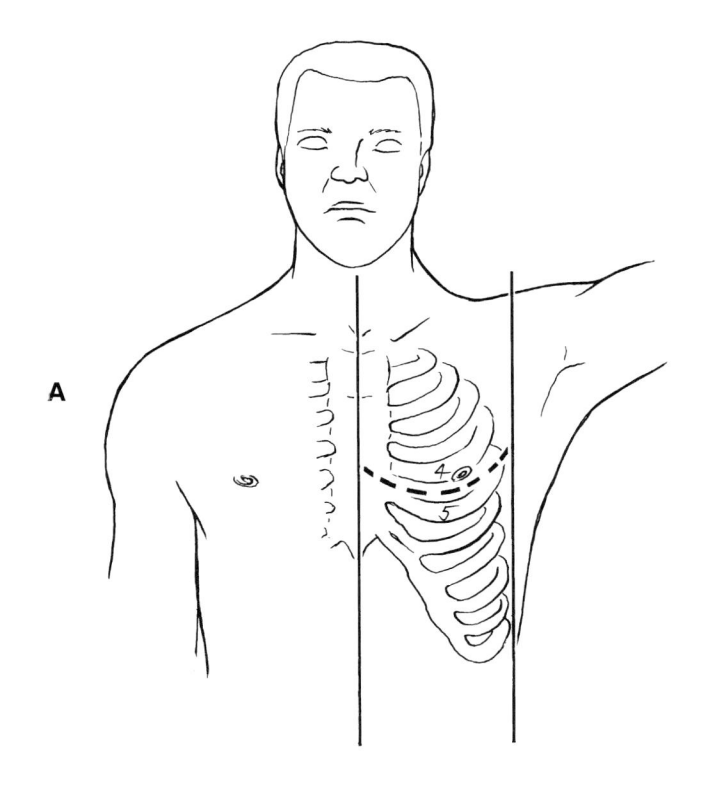

B

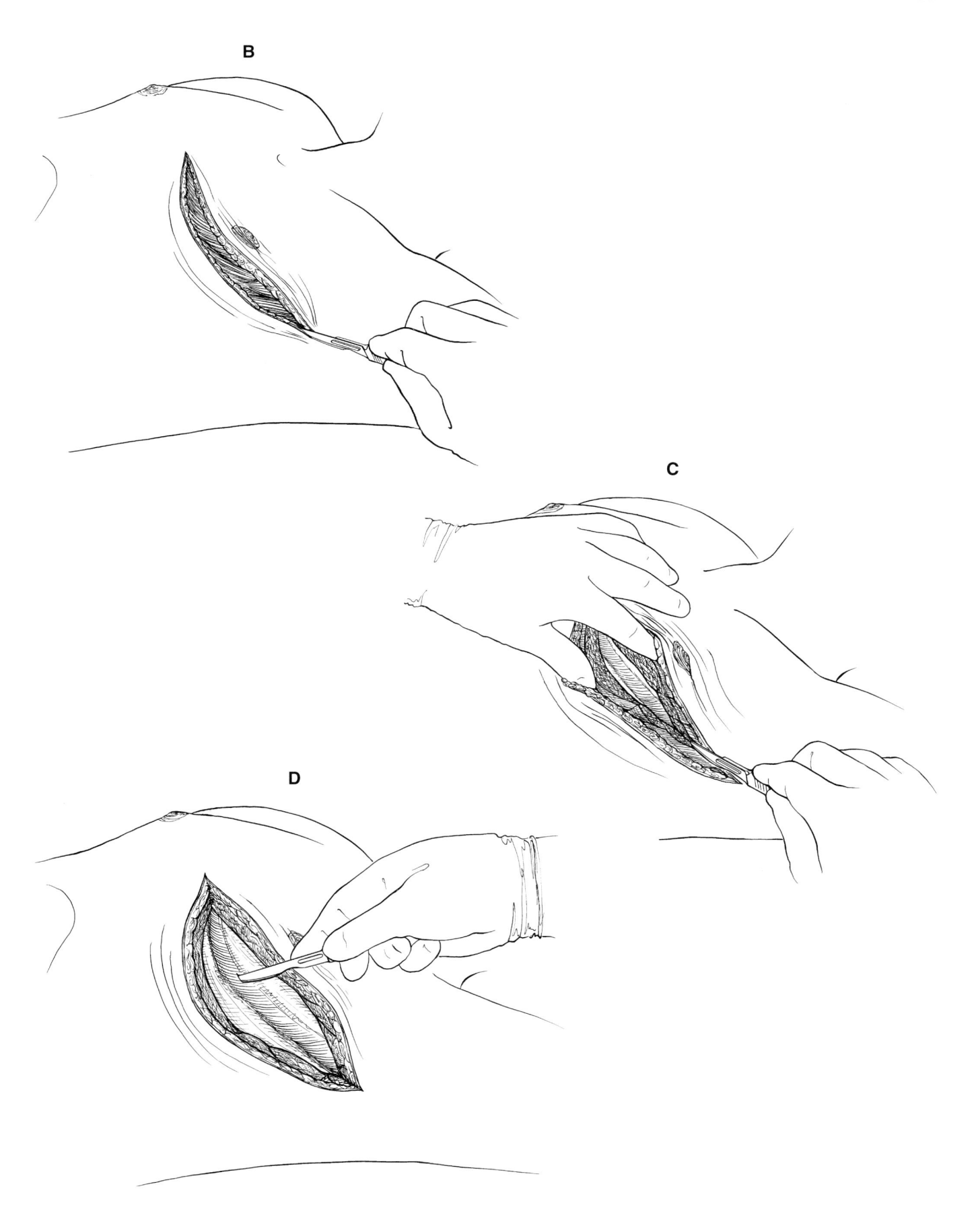

C

D

5. Open the remainder of the pleura in each direction from the initial incision with scissors *(E)*. Care should be taken to avoid injuring underlying structures.
6. Place a rib spreader in the chest incision with the handle of the spreader directed posteriorly *(F)*. The blades of the spreader should initially be closed when placed against the two sides of the chest incision.
7. Turn the handle of the rib spreader so that the two blades separate, widening the chest incision and spreading the 5th and 6th ribs apart. This will expose and afford access to the underlying structures *(G, H)*.
8. Additional sponges, clamps, hemostats, and other items can be used to isolate various underlying structures as described in the sections on aortic cross-clamping and cardiorrhaphy.

Complications

- Laceration of thoracic structures (heart, coronary arteries, lung, phrenic nerve)
- Infection
- Dysrhythmias
- Pericarditis
- Postpericardectomy syndrome

Discussion

- If exposure of the right side of chest is needed, the chest incision may be extended across the sternum, with use of a Lebsche knife or Gigli saw to cut through the sternum. If this is done, the internal mammary arteries must be identified and ligated. After the sternum is transected, a similar intercostal incision is made on the right side of the chest with a scalpel and scissors.
- Once the chest is opened, the operator can perform open cardiac massage, internal defibrillation, cardiorrhaphy, wound repair, or aortic cross-clamping (see appropriate sections).

Bibliography

Bodai BIO et al: Emergency thoracotomy in the management of trauma: a review, *JAMA* 249:1891-1896, 1983.

Boyd M et al: Emergency room resuscitative thoracotomy: when is it indicated? *J Trauma* 33(5):714-720, 1992.

Brown SE et al: Penetrating chest trauma: should indications for emergency room thoracotomy be limited? *Am Surg* 62(7):530-534, 1996.

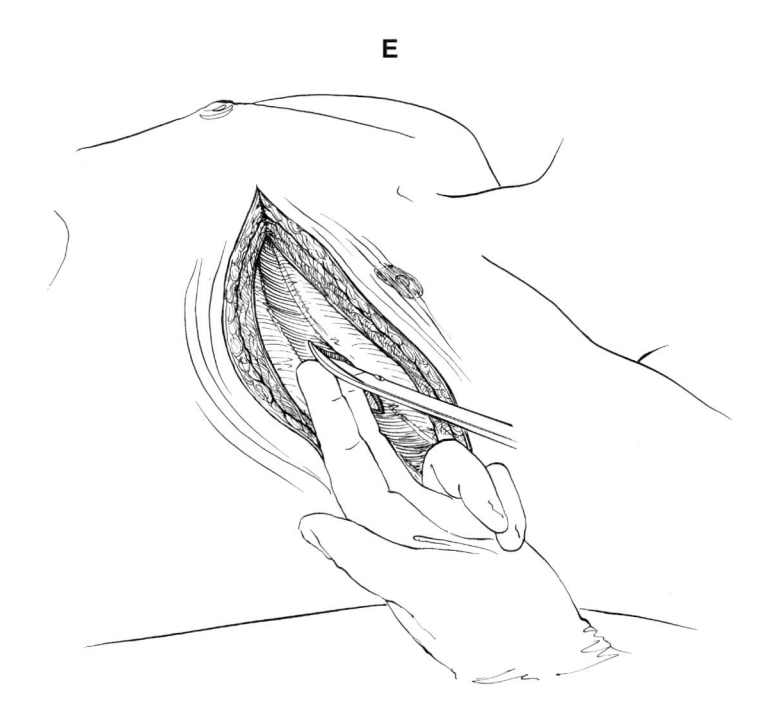

E

THORAX 49

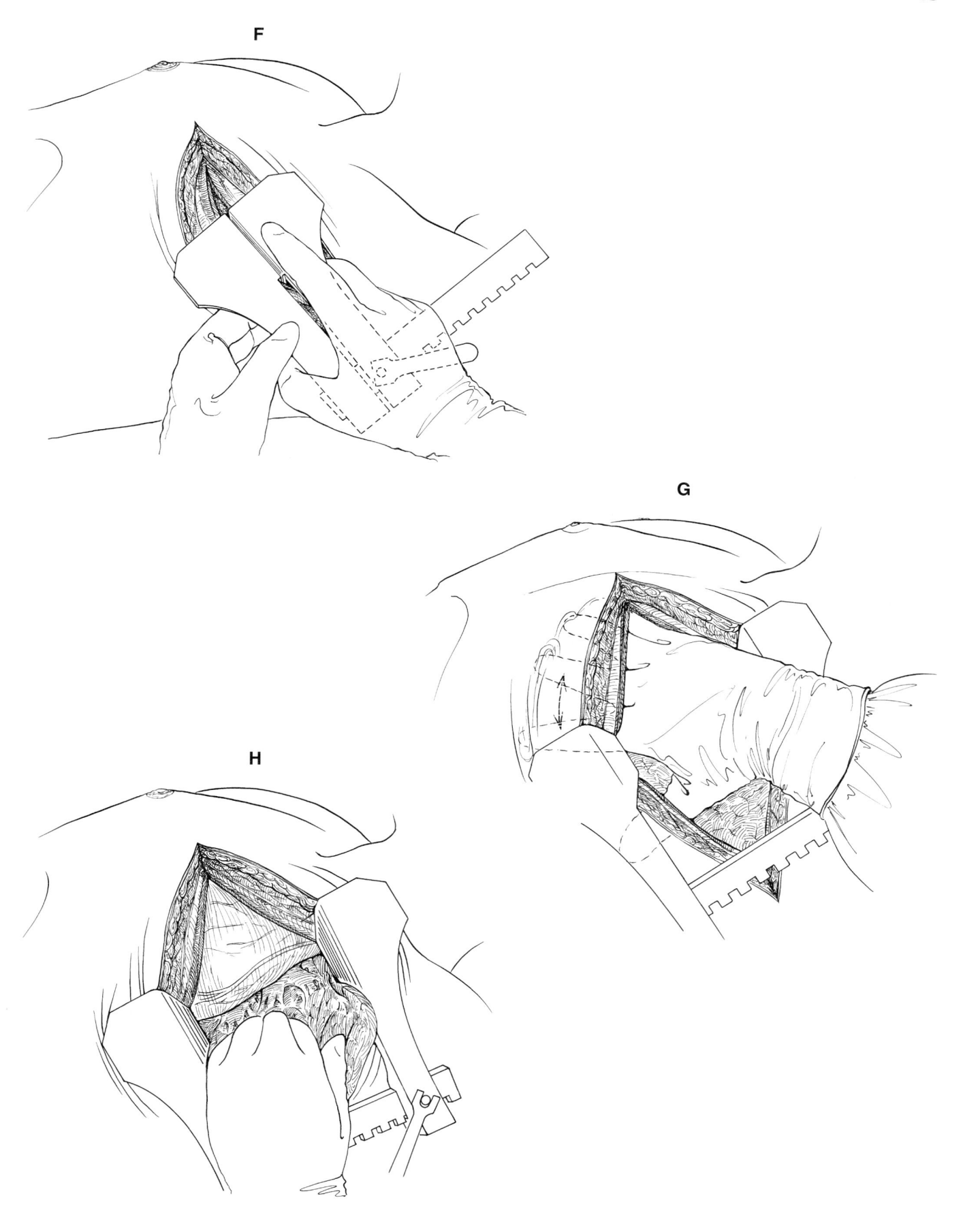

F

G

H

Cardiac Massage ▪ KENNETH C. JACKIMCZYK

Indications
- Absent or inadequated cardiac activity noted during open thoracotomy

Contraindications
- Patient with a pulse

Equipment
- See thoracotomy equipment
- Sterile gloves

Procedure

1. Complete open thoracotomy as described in an earlier section.
2. Gloved, cupped hands, with thumbs kept close to fingers, should be placed anterior and posterior to the heart (A-C).

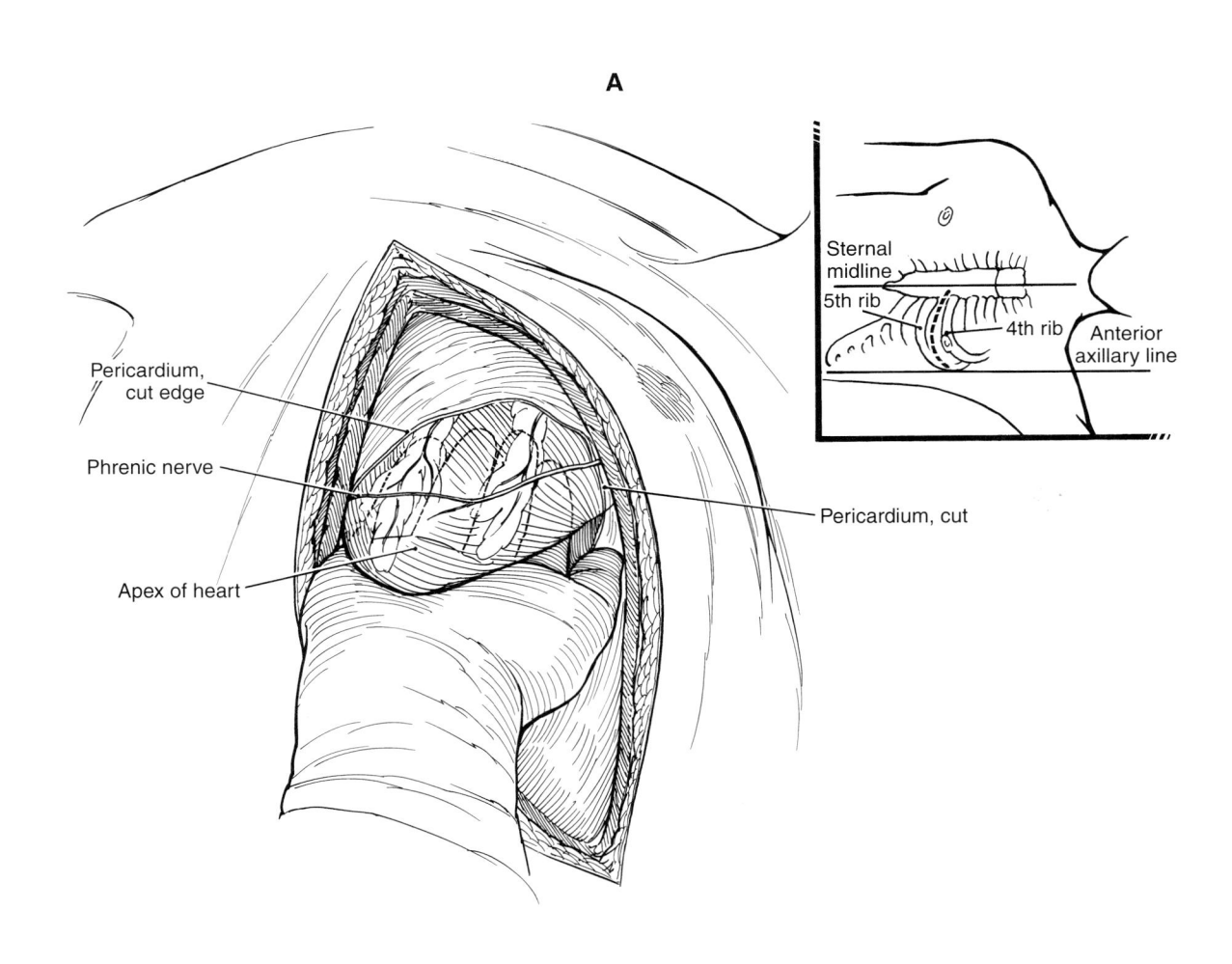

B

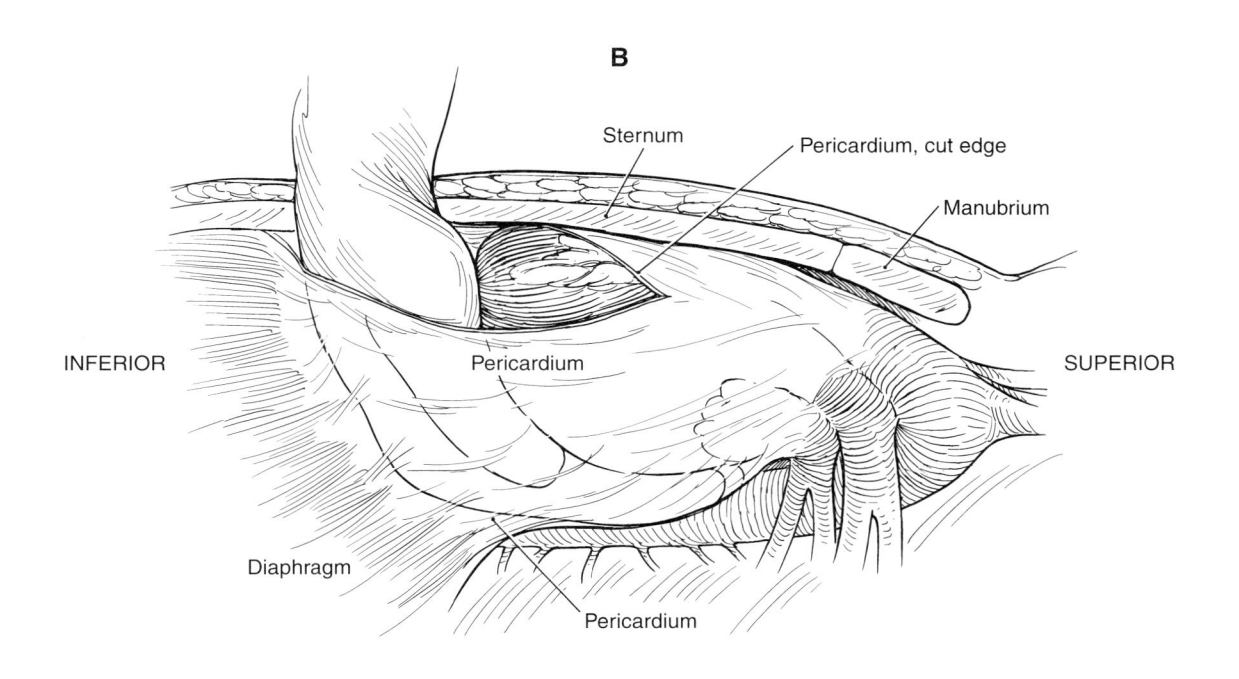

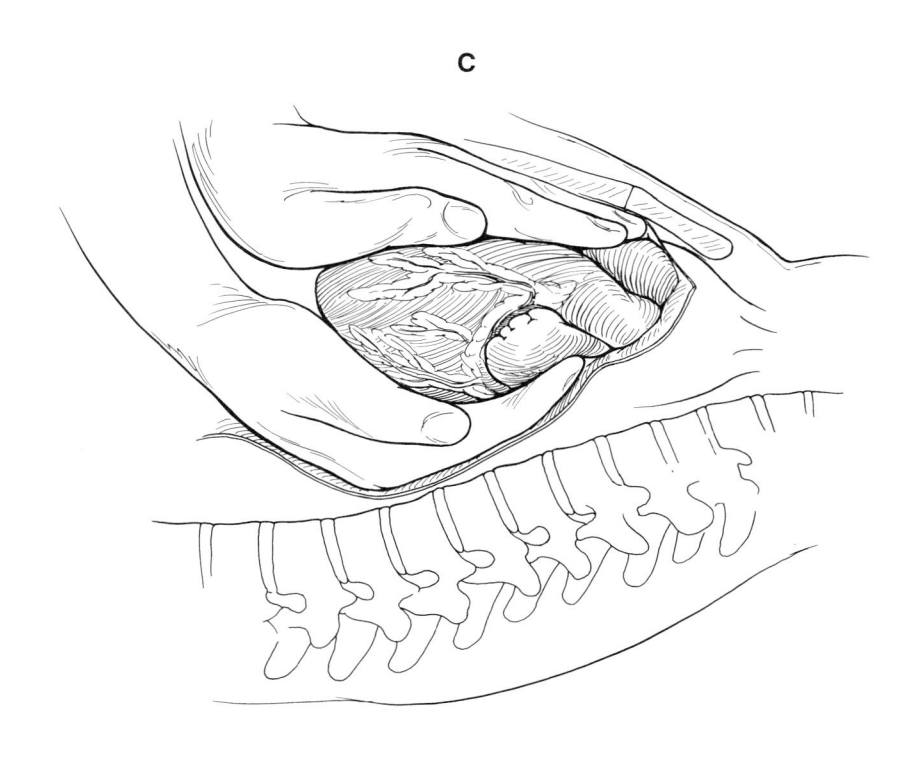

Sternum
Pericardium, cut edge
Manubrium
INFERIOR
Pericardium
SUPERIOR
Diaphragm
Pericardium

C

3. The hands are squeezed firmly together, mimicking the normal cardiac contractions *(C, D)*.

Complications

- Cardiac perforation
- Infection

Discussion

- Care must be taken to keep thumbs close to fingers and not squeeze the heart in between, which can cause cardiac perforation.
- Before massage, clots should be evacuated from within the pericardium and cardiac wounds should be repaired.
- A one-handed variation can be performed in which the right hand, located posteriorly, compresses the anterior aspect of the heart against the posterior aspect of the sternum *(E)*.
- The heart should not be compressed by fingers alone, since this increases the risk for perforation *(F, G)*.

Bibliography

Geehr EC, Auerbach PS: Open-chest cardiac massage for victims of medical arrest, *Ann Emerg Med* 14:498, 1985.

Sanders AB et al: Improved resuscitation from cardiac arrest with open-chest massage, *Ann Emerg Med* 13:672-675, 1984.

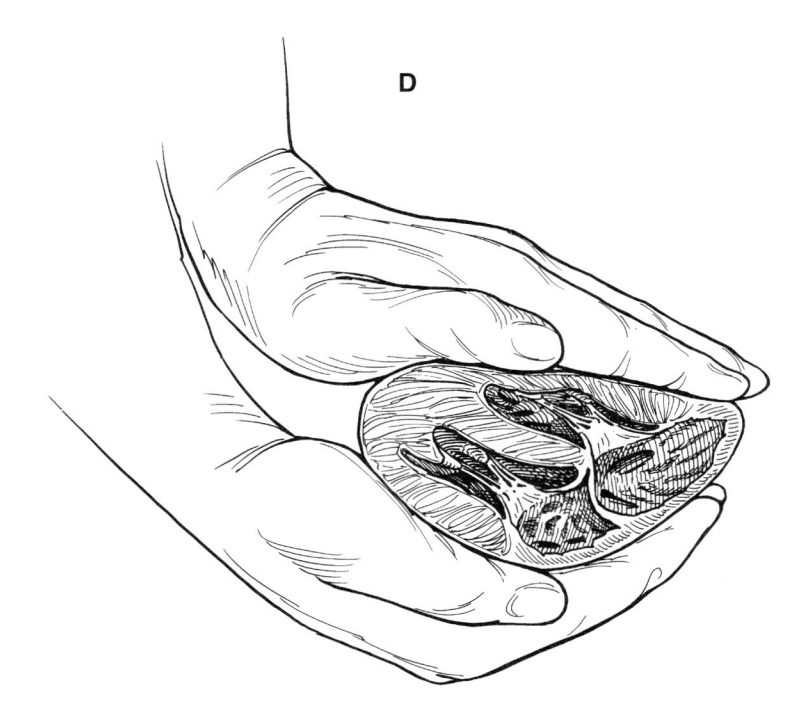

D

E

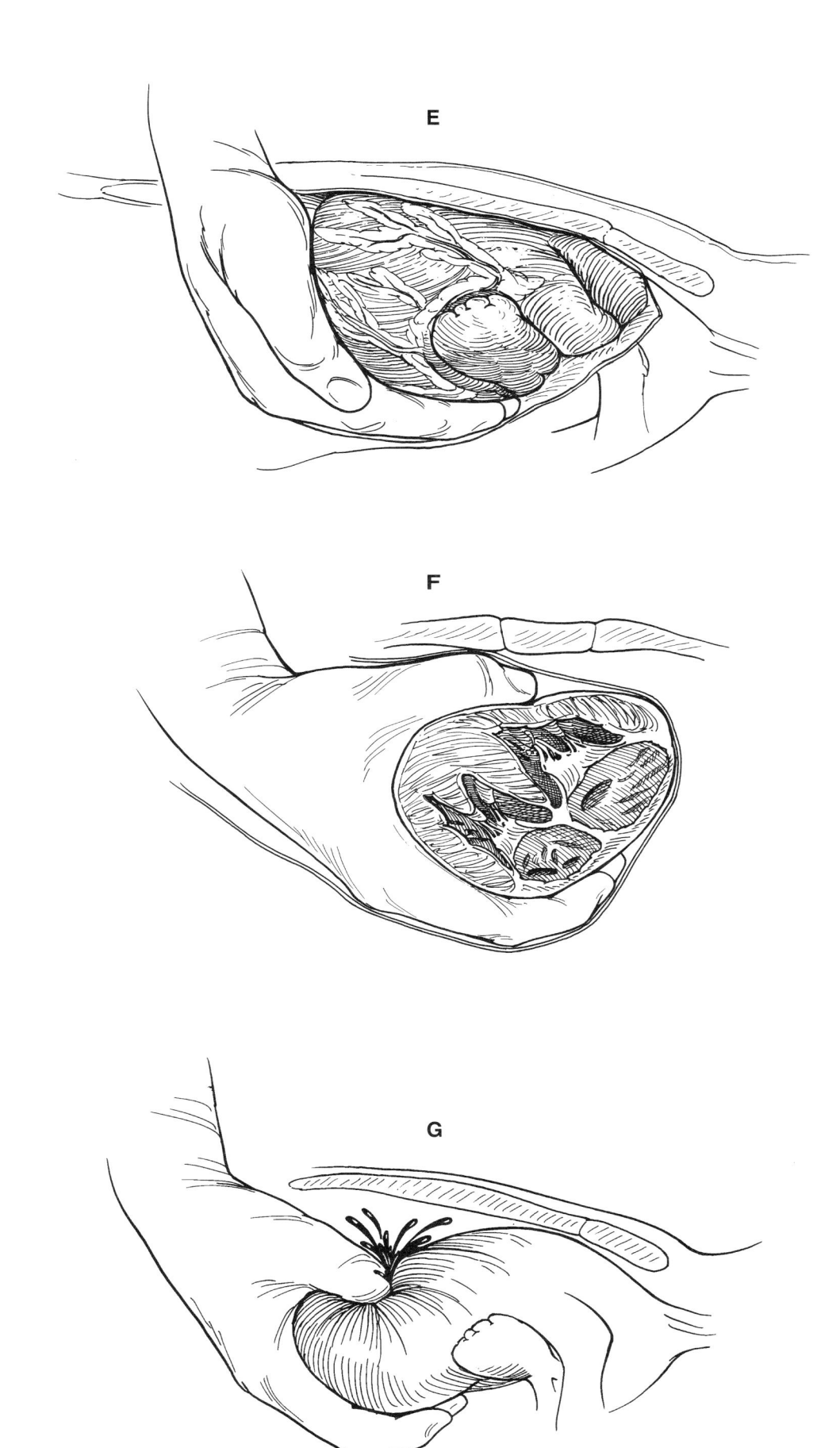

F

G

Cardiorrhaphy • GARY J. ORDOG

Indications
- Penetrating injury to the heart, necessitating emergency repair

Contraindications
- Obvious signs of death (e.g., rigor mortis, decapitation)

Equipment
- Thoracotomy equipment
- Satinsky vascular clamp
- Vascular clamps
- Sponges (lap and Raytec)
- Tissue forceps
- Mayo scissors
- Metzenbaum scissors, curved
- Teflon pledgets
- 3-0 Ethibond cardiovascular suture
- 3-0 Ethibond pledgetted cardiovascular suture
- Needle holders

Procedure

1. Complete open thoracotomy as described in an earlier section.
2. Locate the pericardium once underlying structures are exposed.
3. Identify the phrenic nerve lying along the pericardium and running in an superior-inferior direction.
4. Open the pericardium by grasping the tissue with a toothed forceps and nicking the pericardium with a scalpel, being careful to avoid the phrenic nerve.
5. Extend the incision in an cephalocaudad direction using blunt-tipped scissors.
6. Remove any clot and blood from the pericardium.
7. Explore the myocardium for any penetrating injuries.
8. Once the open wound is found, a finger may be inserted into the opening as a temporizing measure *(A)*.
9. Cardiovascular suture may be used to attempt wound closure while awaiting definitive treatment. Teflon pledgets should be used to avoid causing further laceration of the friable myocardium *(B-E)*. Care must be taken not to place sutures through the coronary arteries, which are easily identified.

Complications

- Infection
- Damage to adjacent structures
- Injury to coronary arteries, resulting in myocardial ischemia
- Myocardial rupture
- Irreversible hemorrhage or shock
- Dysrhythmias

Discussion

- A Foley catheter balloon may be inserted into a penetrating myocardial wound as a temporizing measure. First insert the uninflated catheter into the wound. Then inflate the balloon with normal saline and retract gently against the wound to tamponade bleeding and close the opening. Blood, IV fluids, and medications can be effectively infused directly into the cardiac chamber via the catheter.
- Lacerations of the auricular appendages can be effectively treated by clamping the appendage until more definitive closure can be obtained.

Bibliography

Adkins RB Jr et al: Penetrating chest wall and thoracic injuries, *Am Surg* 51:140-148, 1985.
Mattox KL et al: Cardiorrhaphy in the emergency center, *J Thorac Cardiovasc Surg* 69:886-895, 1974.
Moore EE: Prognostic factors in the emergency department thoracotomy for trauma, *Curr Concepts Trauma Care,* Fall 1982, pp 5-9.
Rohman M et al: Emergency room thoracotomy for penetrating cardiac injuries, *J Trauma* 23:570-576, 1983.

THORAX

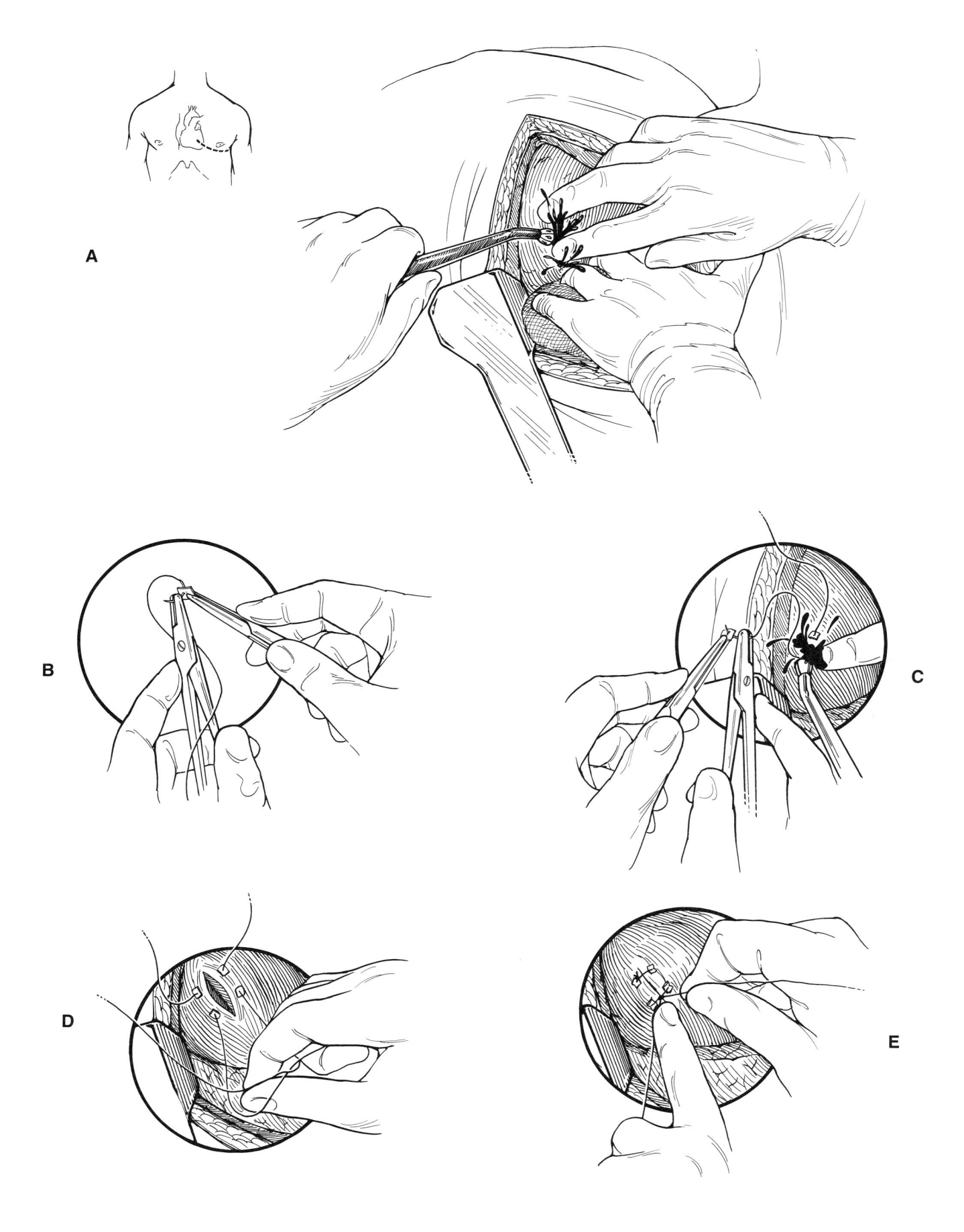

A

B

C

D

E

Internal Defibrillation ▪ KENNETH C. JACKIMCZYK

Indications
- Ventricular fibrillation in a patient with an open thoracotomy
- Pulseless ventricular tachycardia in a patient with an open thoracotomy

Contraindications
- Patient with a pulse

Equipment
- Internal defibrillator paddles
- Saline

Procedure

1. The patient should already be in a supine position with the heart exposed by an open thoracotomy.
2. Check equipment.
3. Paddles should be moistened with saline if they are gauze covered.
4. Place one paddle posteriorly over the left ventricle and the other anteriorly over the right ventricle (A).
5. Squeeze the paddles against the myocardium to allow firm tissue contact.
6. Defibrillate with 10 to 40 J until a normal rhythm is restored.

Complications

- Postdefibrillation dysrhythmias

Discussion

- Presence of a pacemaker or automated internal cardiac defibrillator device is not a contraindication to internal defibrillation.
- Defibrillation batteries and power supply should be checked routinely.

A

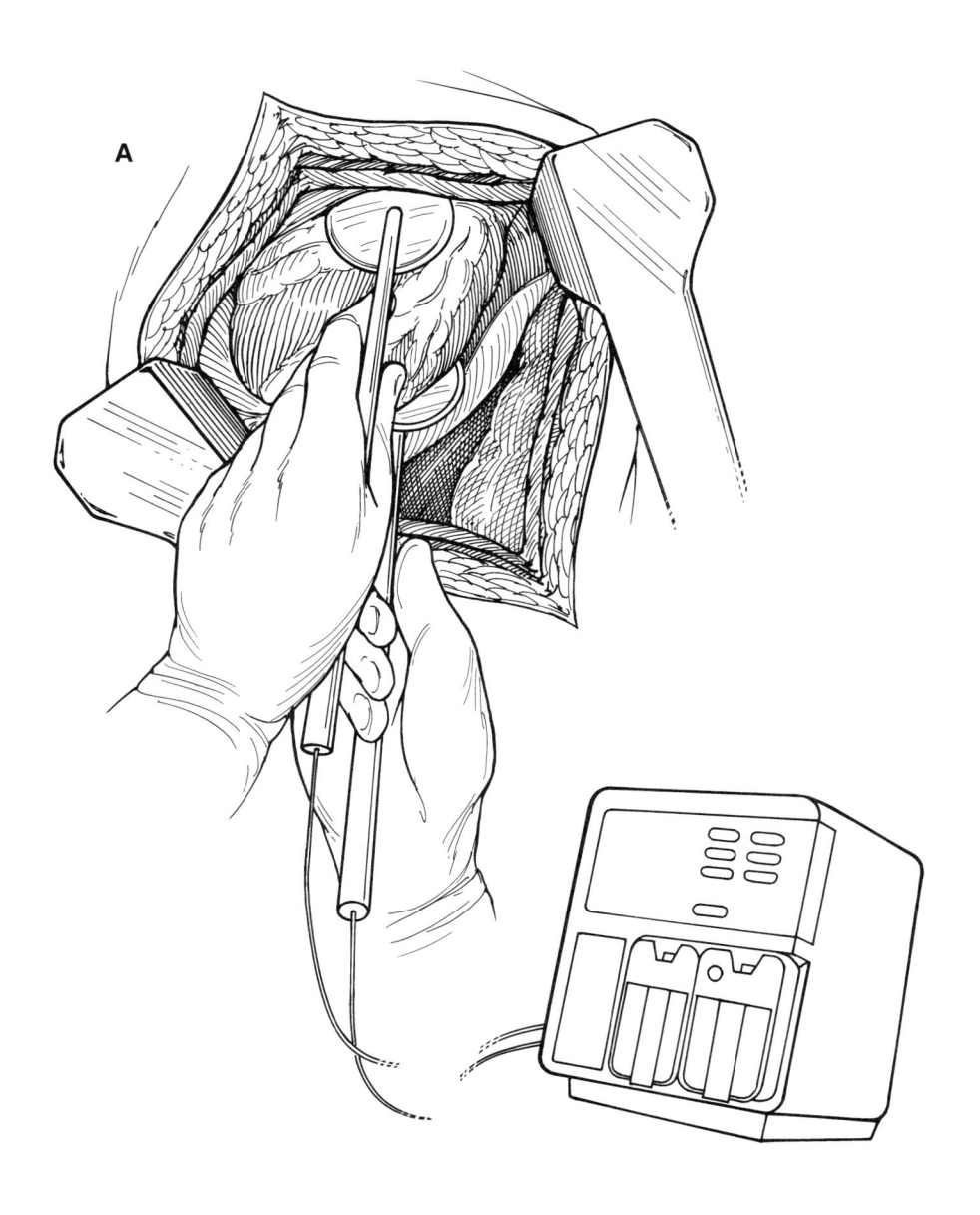

Aortic Cross-Clamping ▪ GARY J. ORDOG

Indications

- Aortic cross-clamping diverts all blood flow below the diaphragm to preserve blood flow to the brain and heart. Indications are similar to those for emergency thoracotomy:
  - Penetrating trauma with loss of vital signs during transport or in the emergency department
  - Penetrating trauma, resulting in profound shock or rapid clinical deterioration that does not respond to aggressive fluid resuscitation
  - Blunt trauma with loss of vital signs in the emergency department or hospital

Contraindications

- Obvious signs of death (e.g., rigor mortis, decapitation)

Equipment

- See thoracotomy equipment
- Satinsky vascular clamp

Procedure

1. Complete open thoracotomy as described in an earlier section *(A)*.
2. Retract the left lung by inserting the left hand posterior to the lung base and gently lifting anteriorly *(B)*.
3. Insert the right hand along the posterior thoracic cage toward the vertebral column inferior to the hilum.
4. Feel for the structures overlying the vertebral column, and use the fingers to bluntly dissect the tissue planes between the aorta and esophagus. The aorta is the pulsatile, muscular structure directly anterior to the esophagus.
5. Hook the index finger around the aorta (the aorta may be manually clamped at this point).
6. After the aorta has been isolated, obtain the Satinsky clamp. The clamp can be guided along the operator's arm to the aorta. The fingers can then ensure proper placement of the clamp tips on the aorta *(C, D)*.

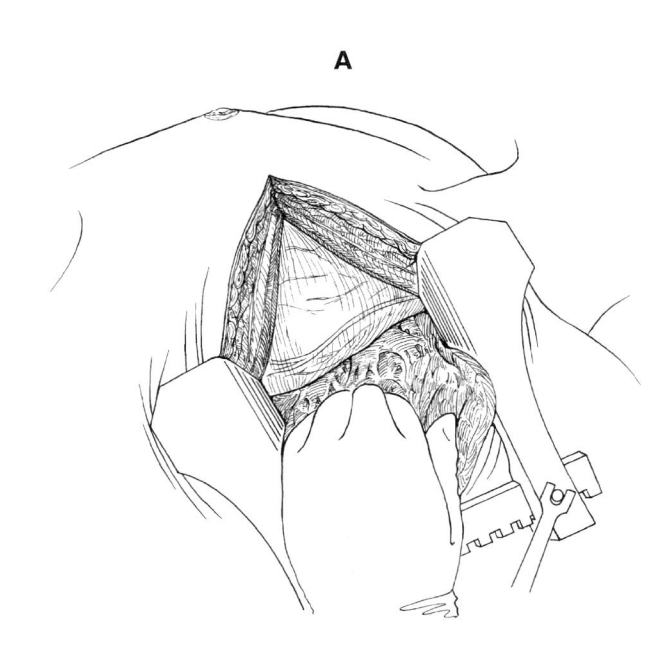

A

B

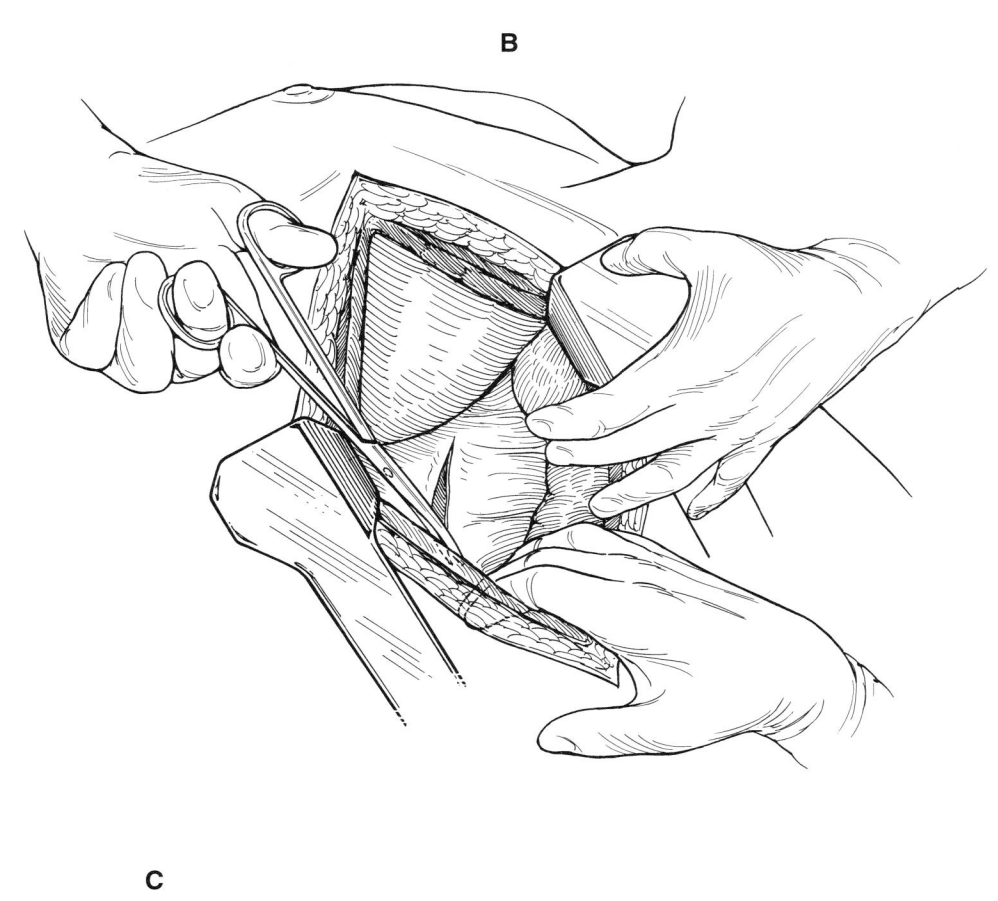

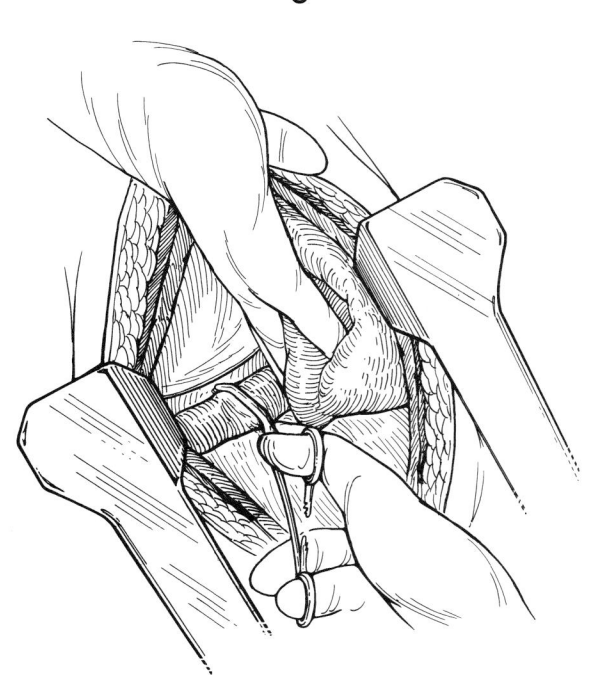

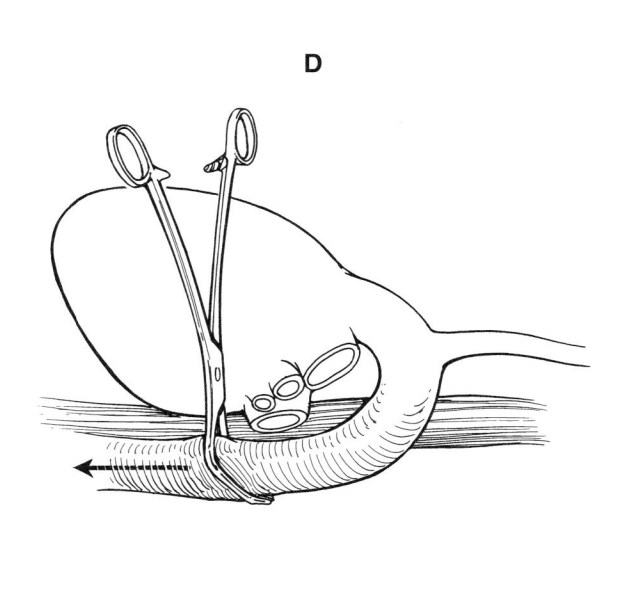

C

D

Complications

- Infection
- Damage to adjacent structures
- Paraplegia
- Renal failure
- Irreversible postclamping shock

Discussion

- Care must be taken to clamp only the aorta because other structures, including the vena cava and esophagus, are in the same vicinity.

Bibliography

Dunn EL et al: Hemodynamic effects of aortic occlusion during hemorrhagic shock, *Ann Emerg Med* 11:238-241, 1982.

Millikin JS, Moore EE: Outcome of resuscitative thoracotomy and descending aortic occlusion performed in the operating room, *J Trauma* 24:387-392, 1984.

Moore EE: Emergency thoracotomy and aortic cross-clamping. In Moore EE et al: *Critical decisions in trauma*, St Louis, 1984, Mosby, pp 524-529.

CHAPTER 3

CARDIOVASCULAR SYSTEM

Radial Artery Cannulation ▪ JOHN L. KENDALL

Indications
- Frequent arterial blood sampling
- Continuous arterial blood pressure monitoring

Contraindications
- Decrease in or absence of collateral blood flow (positive Allen test)
- Skin infection at site
- Previous surgery in the area
- Severe injury to the extremity
- Anticoagulation
- Coagulopathy
- Atherosclerosis

Equipment
- Betadine antiseptic solution
- Local anesthetic (1% lidocaine without epinephrine), syringe, and needles
- Arm board
- Sterile gloves and drapes
- 20-gauge, 2-inch catheter-over-the-needle (arterial guidewire kit)
- Pressure tubing
- Three-way stopcock
- Pressure transducer
- Silk or 4-0 nylon suture on a curved needle
- Needle driver
- Adhesive tape
- Connecting wire
- Heparinized saline solution
- Pressure blood infuser, set up with a continuous flush device

Procedure

1. Perform the Allen test on the selected wrist to assess for radial and ulnar artery patency *(A)*.
   a. Palpate and compress both arteries on the volar aspect of the wrist while the patient repeatedly makes a tight fist.
   b. Have the patient open the hand, and observe for blanching of the palm.
   c. Release compression of the ulnar artery (maintain compression of the radial artery) and assess for perfusion, noting the time duration for the blanching to resolve.
   d. The hand should refill with blood briskly, and the blanching should resolve within 5 to 10 seconds. If perfusion is delayed (positive Allen test), radial artery cannulation should not be performed at this site.
   e. If both radial and ulnar arteries demonstrate patency, the wrist may be used for arterial puncture and cannulation.
2. Position the patient's wrist on a short arm board, palm side up, in 60° extension. Proper support, such as a folded towel, should be placed under the wrist. The fingers can be taped to the board in extension to facilitate positioning *(B)*.
3. Prepare and drape the site in sterile fashion.
4. Palpate the radial artery near the radial styloid *(C)*.
5. Anesthetize the skin overlying the radial artery, injecting a small amount of 1% lidocaine without epinephrine *(D)*.
6. Remove the protective shield from the catheter-over-the needle unit. Test the advance and retraction of the spring-wire guide through the needle to ensure proper feeding. Retract the wire proximally as far as possible so that blood flashback is not inhibited.

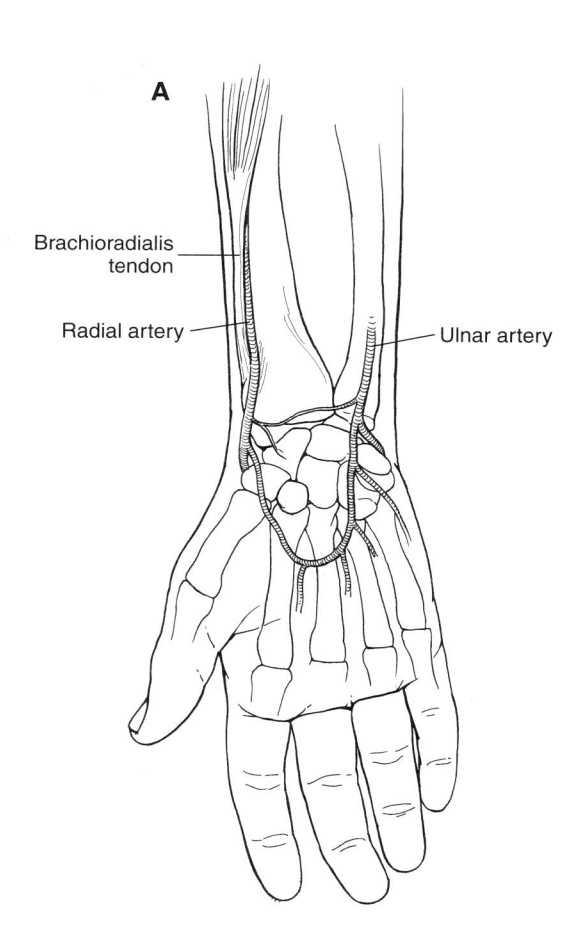

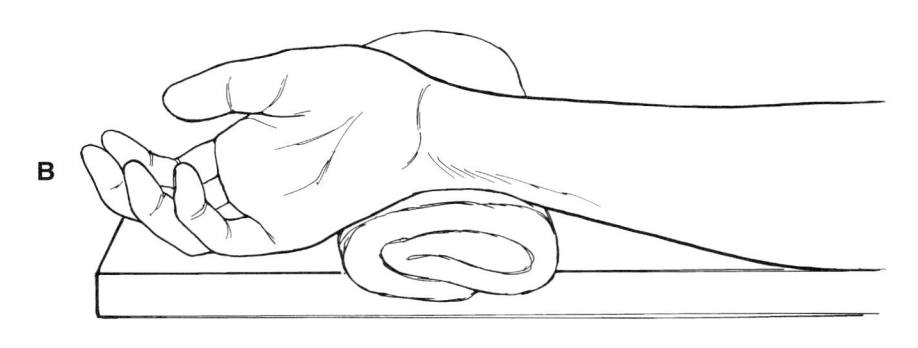

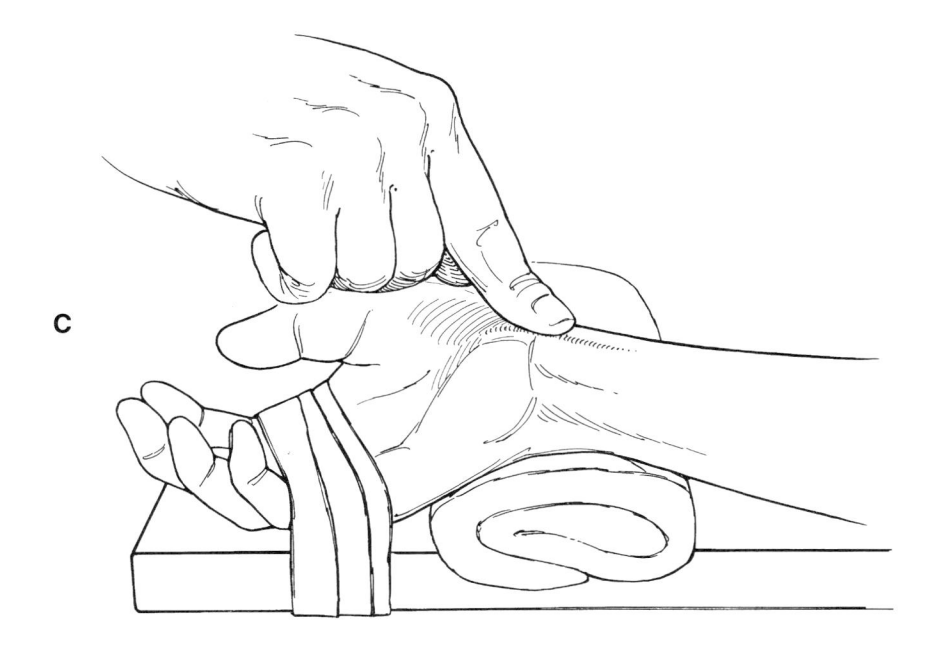

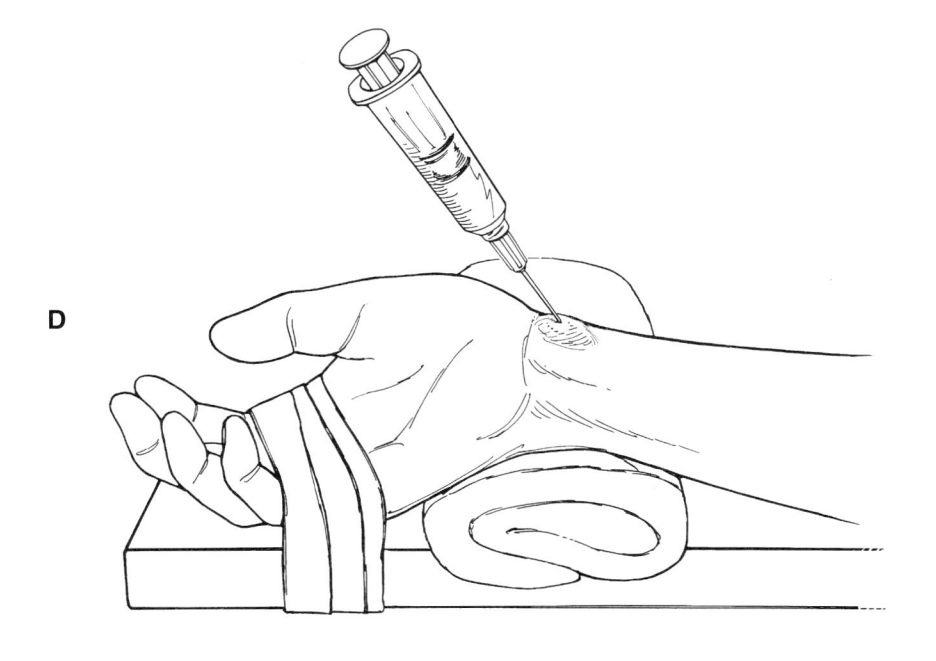

Cardiovascular System

B

C

D

7. Hold the catheter-over-the-needle unit at a 45° angle pointing cephalad, and puncture the radial artery at a point medial to the radial styloid *(E)*.
8. Slowly advance the needle until an arterial blood flashback is seen in the clear hub of the introducer needle.
9. After a flash of blood is visualized, decrease the angle of the catheter-over-the-needle unit to 20° and slowly advance the guidewire into the artery *(F, G)*.
10. Once the guidewire has been inserted into the artery, firmly hold the clear transducer needle hub in position and advance the catheter forward over the wire *(H)*. If difficulty is encountered during catheter placement, a slight rotating motion of the catheter hub may be helpful.
11. Hold the catheter in place, and remove the introducer needle, spring-wire guide, and clear tube assembly. Pulsatile flow of blood indicates successful placement into the vessel.
12. Attach a stopcock and injection tubing to the catheter hub. Flush with heparinized saline solution, and attach the blood pressure infuser.
13. Secure the catheter at two sites, using suture on a curved cutting needle, and place a sterile dressing over the site.

Complications

- Hematoma formation at puncture site
- Infection
- Thrombosis of vessel
- Catheter occlusion
- Catheter embolization
- Skin necrosis

Discussion

- Entering the skin at a site proximal to the radial styloid is not recommended because the artery is more mobile and lies deeper beneath the skin surface.
- Avoid hyperextension of the wrist because this may limit the ability to palpate a radial pulse by placing too much traction on the skin and radial artery.
- The cutdown technique provides an alternative approach, permitting direct visualization of the artery before cannulation. After the selected area is prepped, draped, and anesthetized, the skin over the artery is incised and subcutaneous tissue dissected. The artery is exposed, and two silk sutures are slid underneath the vessel to control it. The skin is punctured by the catheter-over-the-needle unit just distal to the incision and advanced into the surgical site. While the two silk sutures control the artery, the needle tip punctures the vessel wall and the catheter is threaded into the vessel lumen, after which the skin incision can be closed.

Bibliography

Frezza EE, Mezghebe H: Indications and complications of arterial catheter use in surgical or medical units: analysis of 4932 patients, *Am Surg* 64(2):127-131, 1998.

Gronbeck C 3d, Miller EL: Nonphysician placement of arterial catheters: experience with 500 insertions, *Chest* 104(6):1716-1717, 1993.

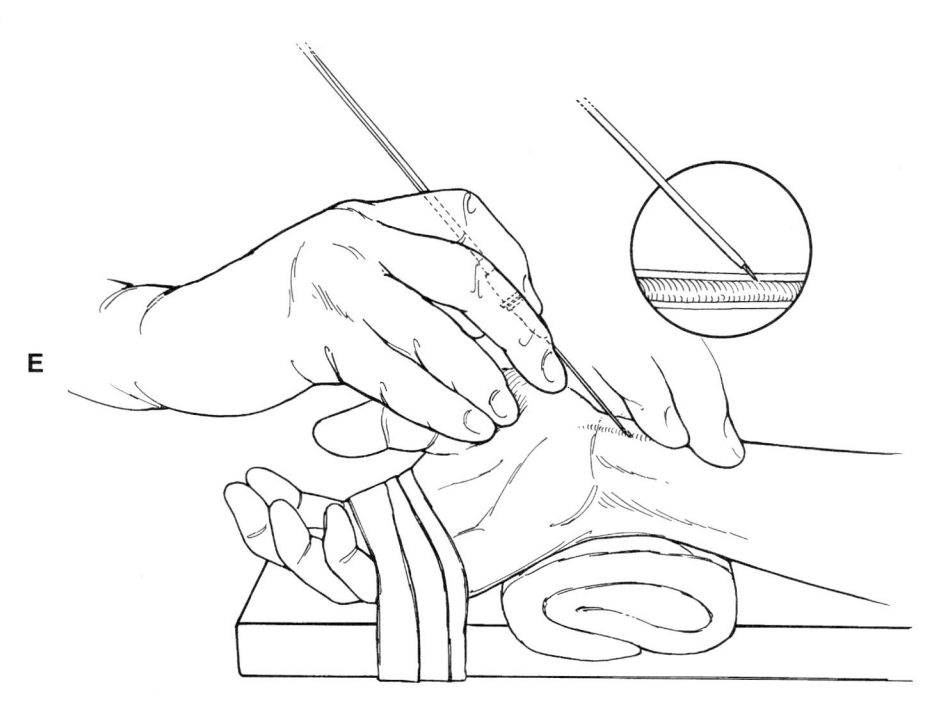

E

CARDIOVASCULAR SYSTEM 65

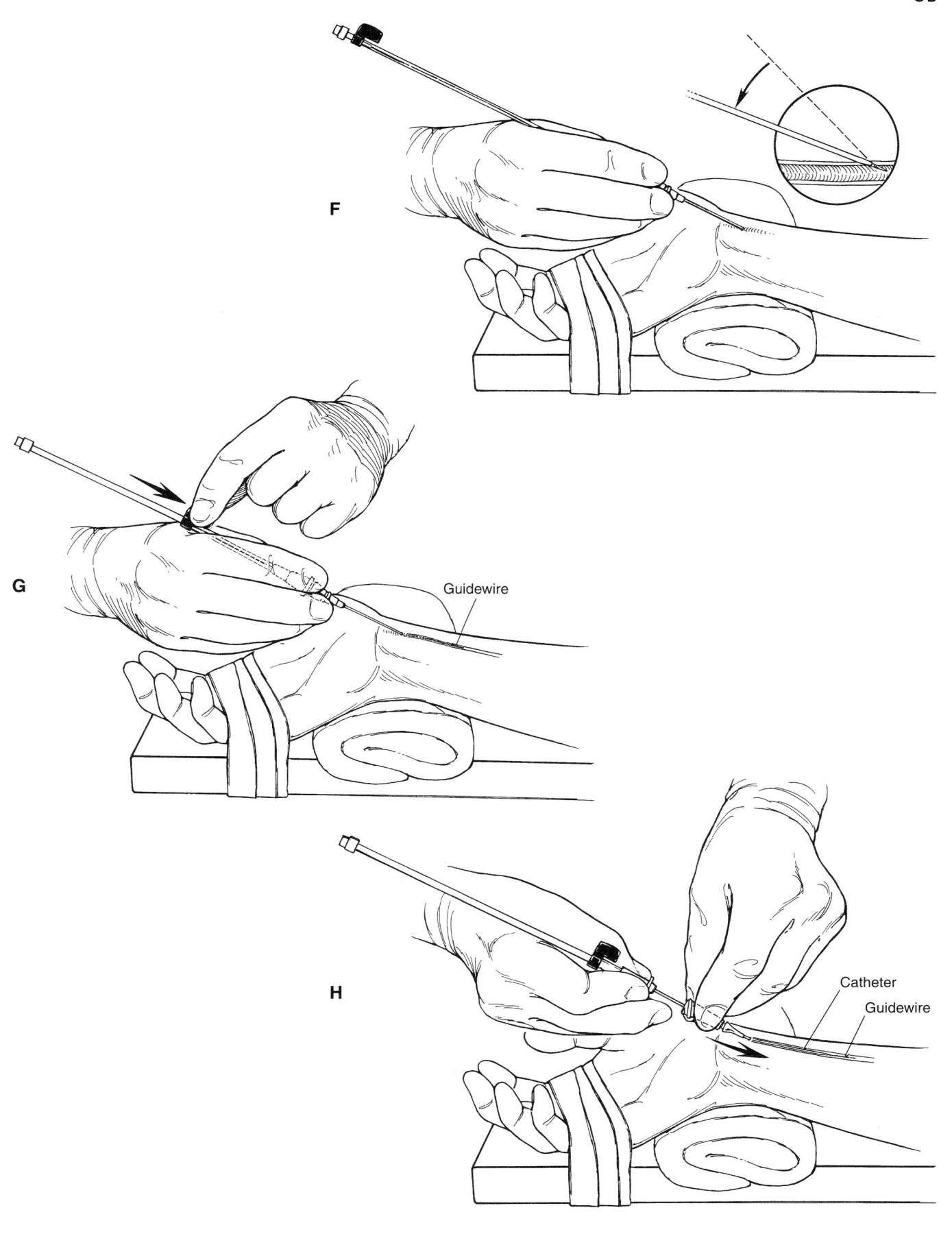

F

G Guidewire

H Catheter
Guidewire

Pericardiocentesis ▪ VINCENT J. MARKOVCHICK

Indications
- Pericardial tamponade with decompensation
- Cardiac arrest with pulseless electrical activity

Contraindications
- Patient in whom bedside ultrasound has not demonstrated pericardial effusion
- Coagulopathy (relative)

Equipment
- Sterile gloves
- Pericardiocentesis tray:
  - 50-ml syringe
  - Three-way stopcock
  - 18-gauge spinal needle
  - Betadine antiseptic solution
  - Wire with alligator clips on each end

Procedure

1. Prepare the skin in the subxiphoid area and epigastrium in sterile fashion.
2. Attach the three-way stopcock between the hub of the syringe and the spinal needle.
3. Attach one end of the alligator clip to the hub of the spinal needle and the other end to lead V of an electrocardiogram (ECG) or the MCL_1 lead.
4. While observing the ECG, advance the needle under the xiphoid process, directing it toward the tip of the right scapula.
5. On penetration of the skin the needle becomes a lead V electrode and cardiac complexes should become visible.
6. If premature ventricular contractions or an acute current of injury manifested as ST segment elevation is noted as the needle is being advanced, withdraw the needle slowly until these changes disappear and then aspirate.
7. Aspirate as much fluid as possible, using the three-way stopcock in patients with large effusions.
8. Remove the needle after the procedure.

Complications

- Development of pericardial effusion and tamponade

Discussion

- If the procedure is being performed in the prehospital setting without an ECG, gently aspirate as the needle is being advanced toward the right scapula. Aspirate as much blood as possible, at least 10 to 20 ml. If the patient's clinical condition improves, this is most likely due to release of pericardial pressure. If the patient's condition does not change, the blood is most likely from the ventricle.
- Bedside ultrasound can be used to assist guidance of the needle.
- If a significant delay will occur in getting the patient to the operating room, an angiocatheter may be advanced into the pericardial space by use of the same technique as above. The needle is removed and the catheter left for repeated aspirations if fluid reaccumulates.

Bibliography
Markovchick VJ, Wolfe RW: *Thoracic trauma in emergency medicine, concepts and clinical practice*, ed 4, St Louis, 1997, Mosby.

Cardiovascular System

A

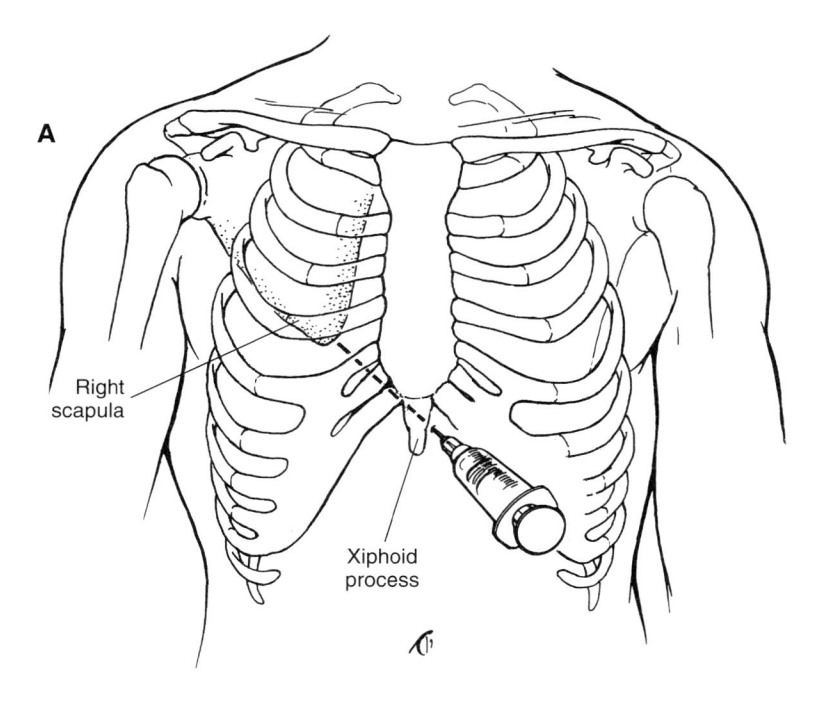

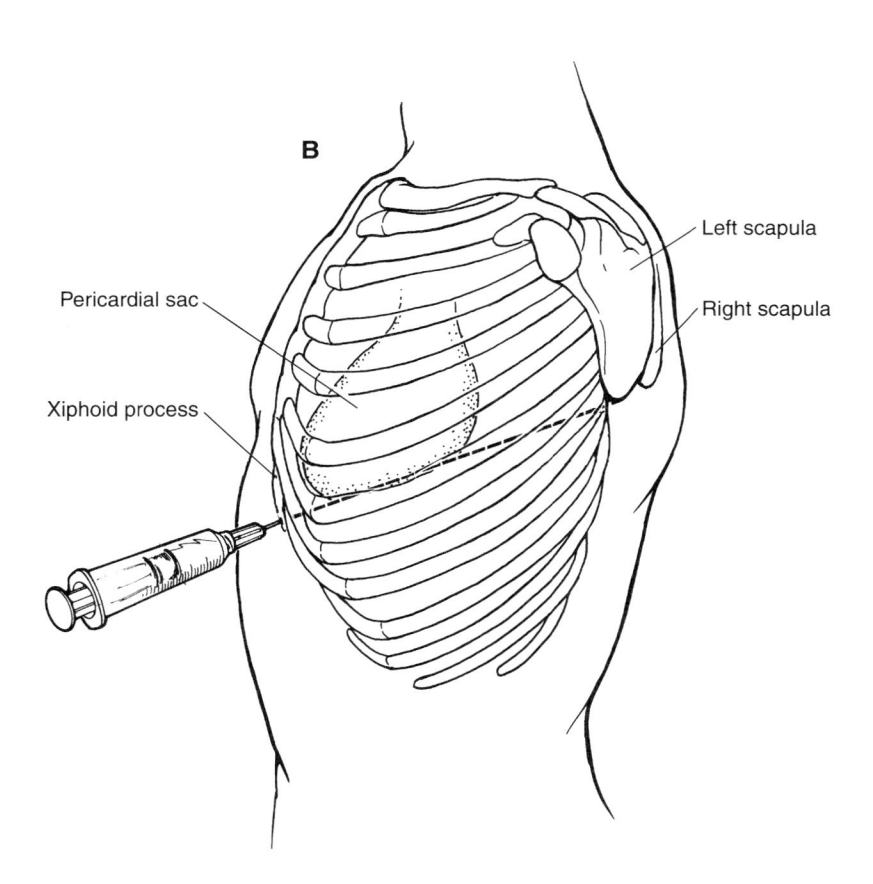

Right scapula

Xiphoid process

B

Left scapula

Pericardial sac

Right scapula

Xiphoid process

Peripheral Venous Access

PERIPHERAL VENIPUNCTURE CHRISTOPHER F. RICHARDS

Indications
- Vascular access for fluid or drug therapy

Contraindications
- If other sites are available, the access site should not be in the region of burns, cellulitis, phlebitis, thrombosis, arteriovenous fistulas, or lymphatic insufficiency.

Equipment
- Gloves
- Betadine antiseptic solution
- Tourniquet
- Angiocatheter
- IV tubing set
- IV fluid
- Sterile dressing
- Tape

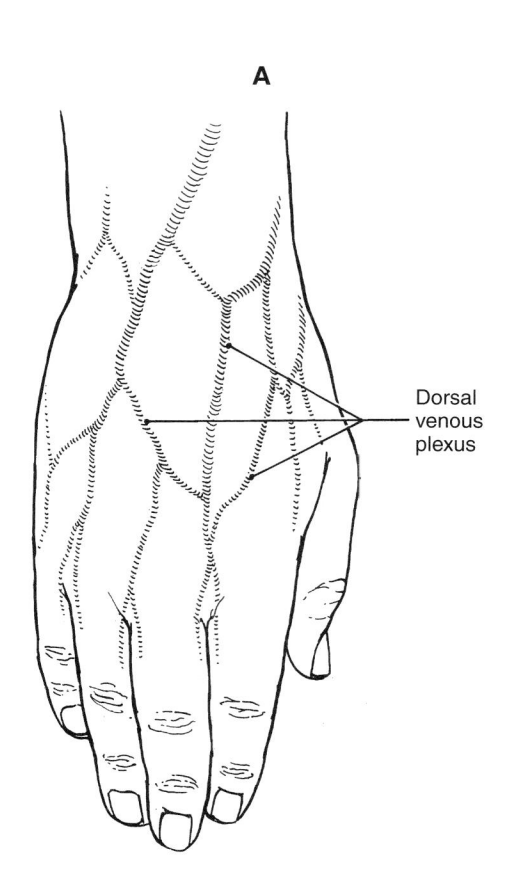

Procedure

Hand and Arm Venipuncture

- Hand venipuncture is shown in *A, C, E,* and *F.* Arm venipuncture is shown in *B, D,* and *G.*
1. Prepare the IV fluid bag with IV tubing set, and have the line flushed and ready to use.
2. Place a tourniquet on the upper arm, and search for an appropriate site on the lower arm, usually the basilic, cephalic, or dorsal hand vein *(A)*.
3. Prepare the site in sterile fashion *(B)*.
4. Use your nondominant hand to pull the skin taut and stabilize the vein.
5. Using sterile technique, puncture the skin with the angiocatheter, keeping the bevel up and entering at a 30° angle from the surface *(C, D)*. The skin should be punctured a few millimeters distal to the intended vein site, aiming proximally.
6. Once the vein is entered, blood will appear in the "flash chamber" of the angiocatheter.
7. Hold the needle steady, and advance the angiocatheter over the needle into the vein.
8. Remove the needle while holding proximal pressure over the vein at the distal end of the catheter *(E)*.

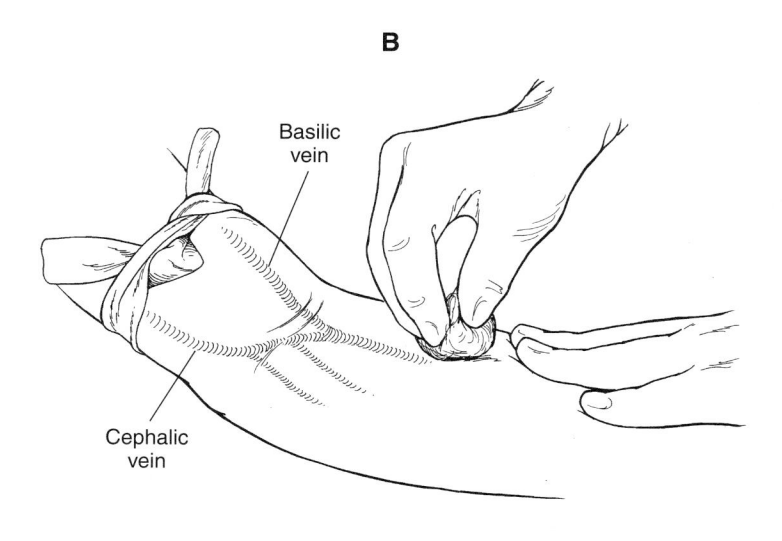

A

Dorsal venous plexus

B

Basilic vein

Cephalic vein

Cardiovascular System

C

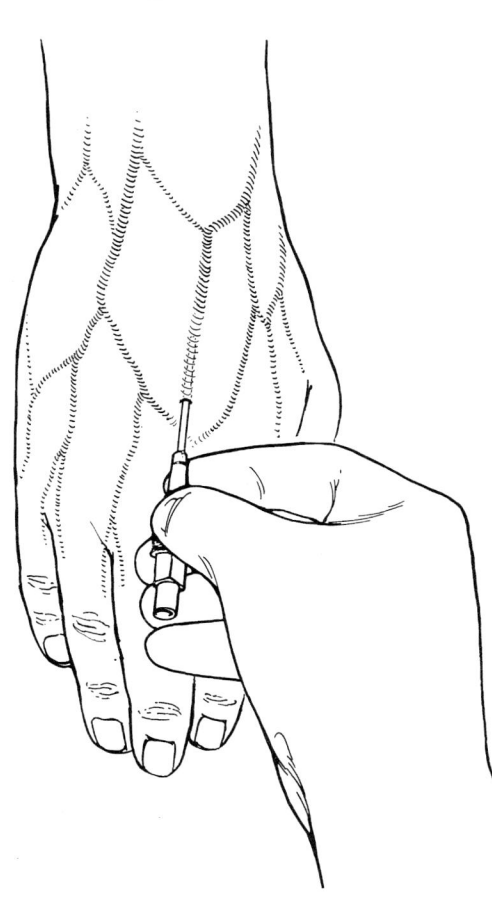

D

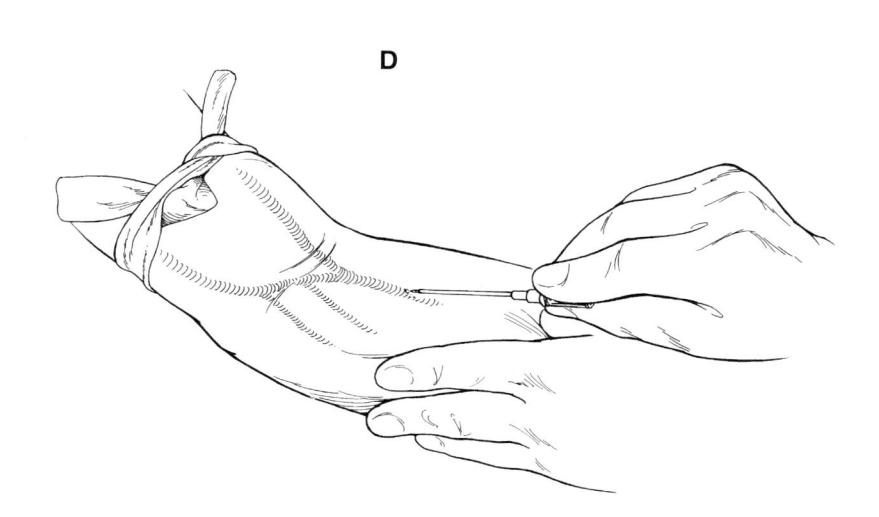

E

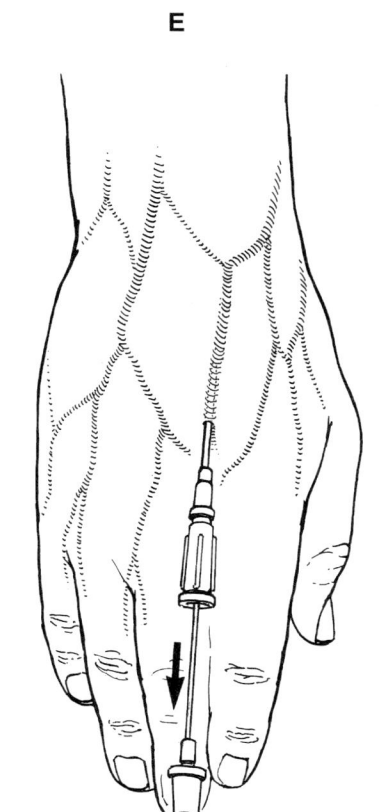

9. Attach the IV line and remove the tourniquet. Fluids should flow freely *(F, G)*.
10. Apply a sterile dressing and tape it into place.

External Jugular Vein
1. Prepare the IV fluid bag with the IV tubing set, and have the line flushed and ready to use.
2. Place the patient in the Trendelenburg position, and apply light pressure to the supraclavicular fossa while the patient performs a Valsalva maneuver.
3. Prepare the site in sterile fashion.
4. Use your nondominant hand to pull the skin taut and stabilize the vein.
5. Using sterile technique, puncture the skin with the angiocatheter, keeping the bevel up and entering at a 30° angle from the surface. The skin should be punctured a few millimeters distal to the intended vein site, aiming proximally *(H, I)*.
6. Once the vein is entered, blood will appear in the "flash chamber" of the angiocatheter.
7. Hold the needle steady, and advance the angiocatheter over the needle into the vein.
8. Remove the needle while holding proximal pressure over the vein at the distal end of the catheter.
9. Attach the IV line. Fluids should flow freely *(J)*.
10. Apply a sterile dressing, and tape it into place.

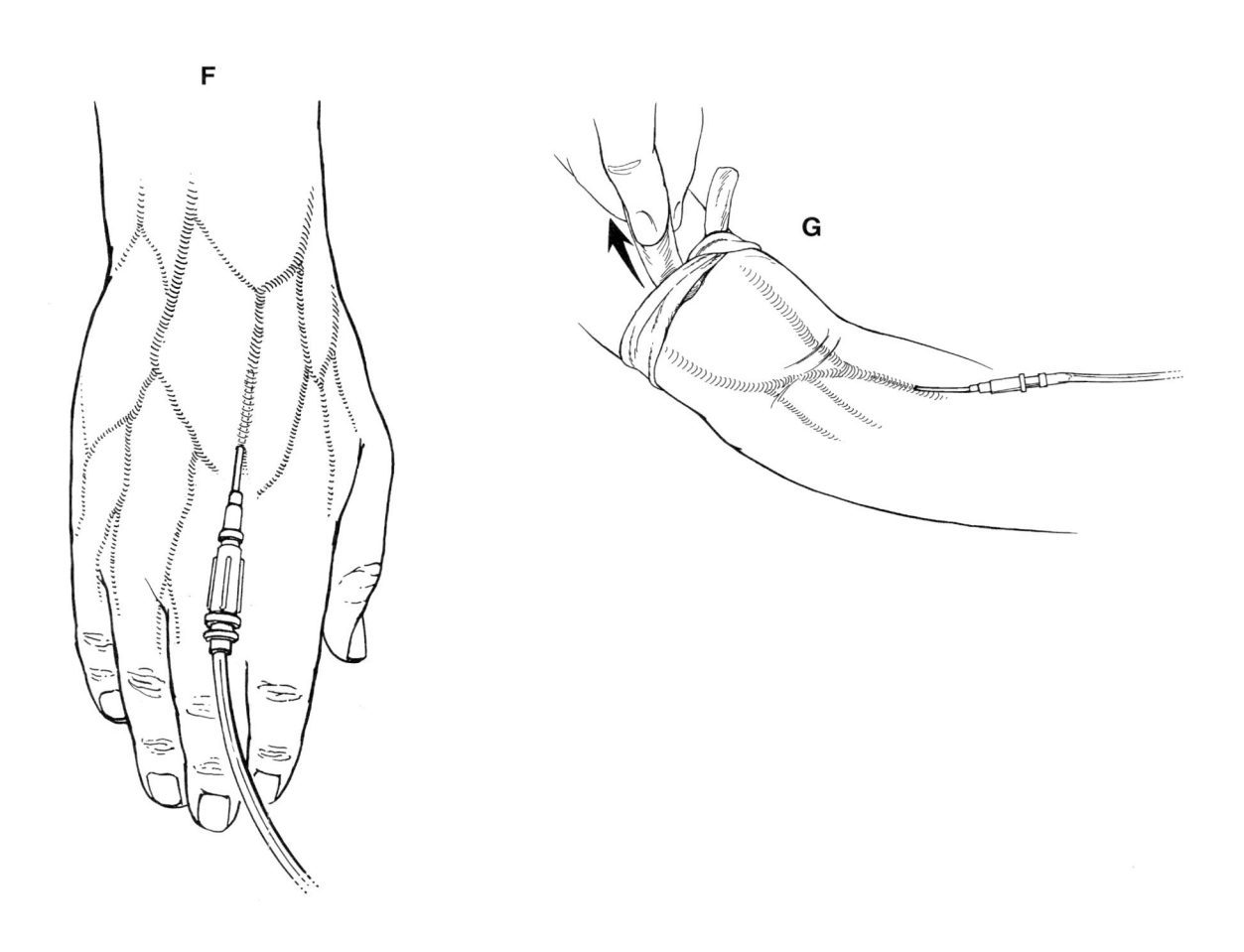

H

External jugular vein

Sternocleidomastoid muscle

I

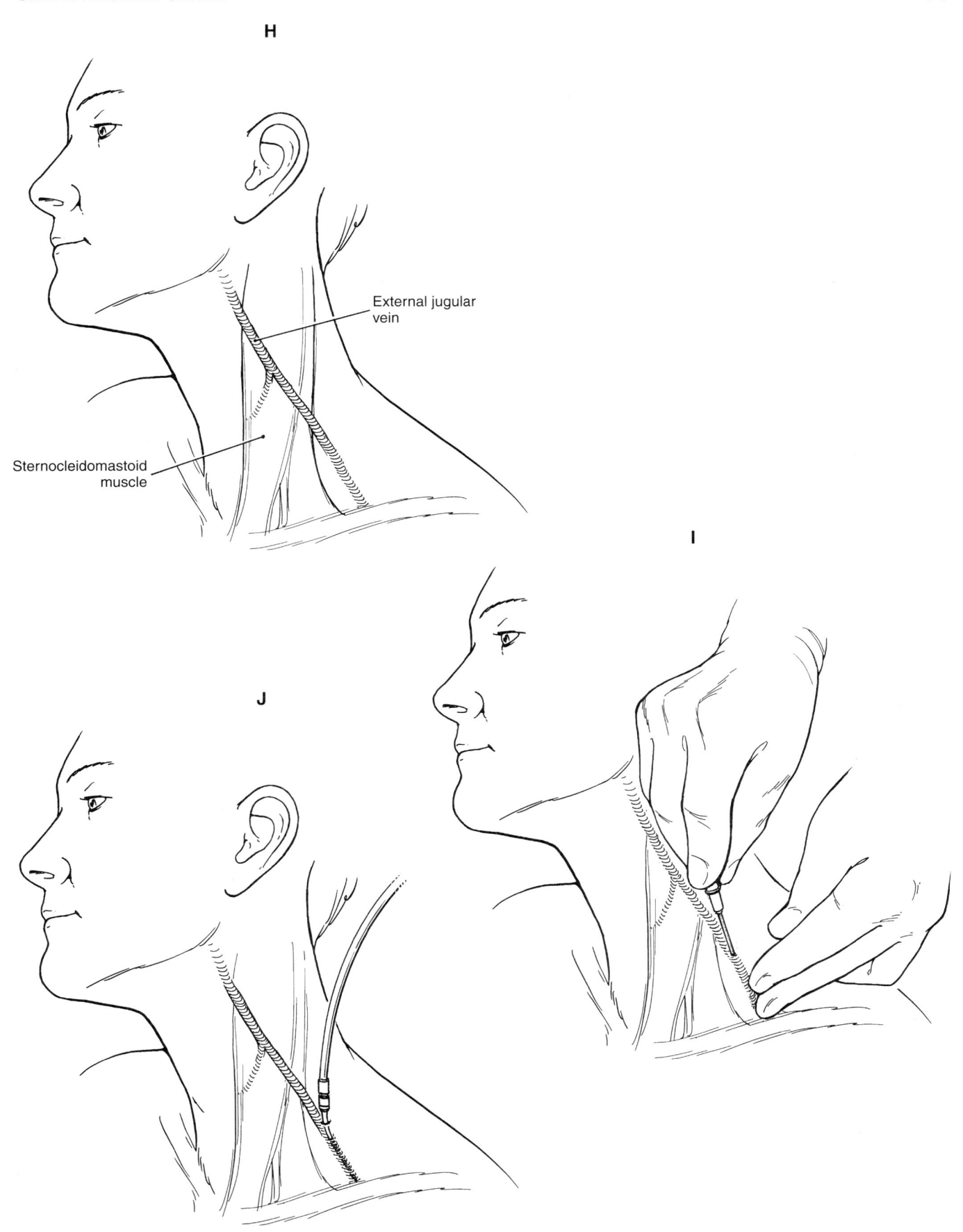

J

Scalp Vein for Infants

1. Prepare the IV fluid bag with the IV tubing set, and have the line flushed and ready to use.
2. Place a small rubberband around the head just above the ears to facilitate venous dilation.
3. Prepare the site in sterile fashion *(K)*.
4. Use your nondominant hand to pull the skin taut and stabilize the vein.
5. Using sterile technique, puncture the skin with a 25-gauge or smaller steel butterfly needle, keeping the bevel up and entering at a 30° angle from the surface. The skin should be punctured a few millimeters distal to the intended vein site.
6. Once the vein is entered, blood will appear in the tubing of the butterfly needle.
7. Attach the IV line. Fluids should flow freely.
8. Apply a sterile dressing, and tape the needle into place on the scalp *(L)*.

Complications

- Extravasation of fluid
- Hematoma
- Phlebitis
- Cellulitis
- Thrombosis

Discussion

- For more elective placement of large-bore catheters, lidocaine placed subcutaneously with a 27-gauge needle can be considered for anesthesia.
- Large, straight veins with bifurcations tend to be more easily accessed.

Bibliography

Lawrence DW, Lauro AJ: Complications from IV therapy: results from field started and emergency department started IVs compared, *Ann Emerg Med* 17:314-317, 1988.

Littenberg B, Thompson L: Gauze vs. plastic for peripheral IV dressings: testing a new technology, *J Gen Intern Med* 2:411-414, 1987.

Maki DG, Rigner M: Evaluation of dressing regimens for prevention of infection with peripheral intravenous catheters, *JAMA* 258:2396-2403, 1987.

Superficial temporal vein

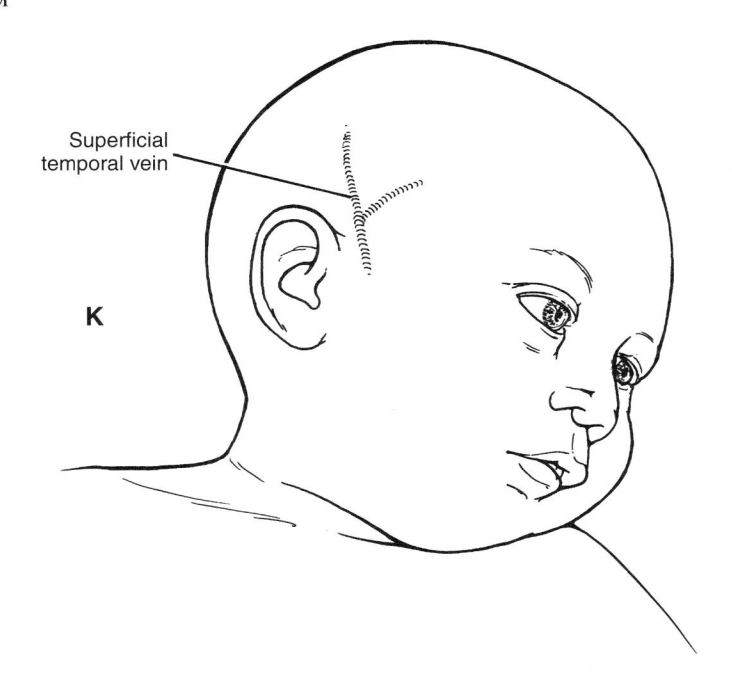

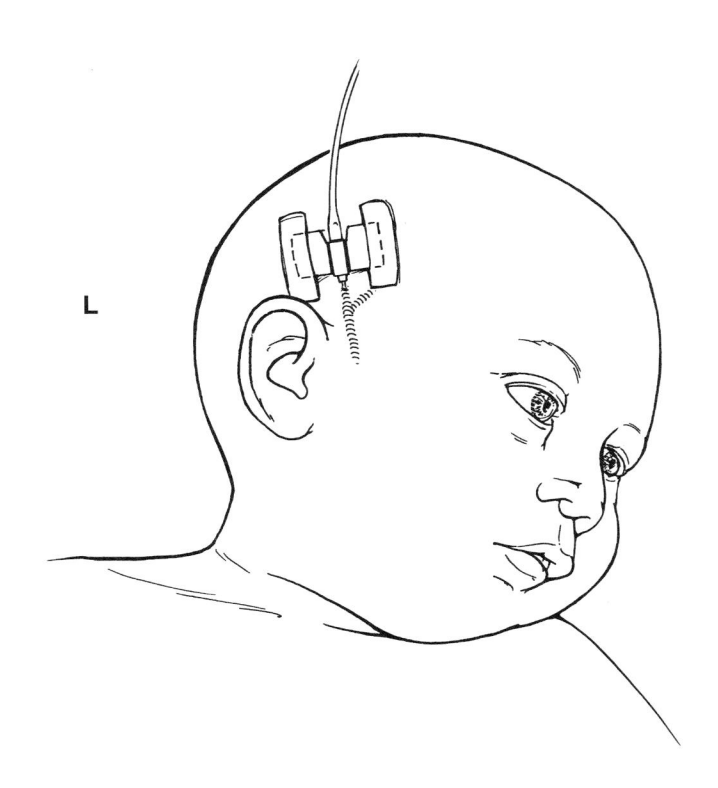

K

L

Central Venous Access

GENERAL APPROACH TO CENTRAL VENOUS ACCESS (SELDINGER GUIDEWIRE TECHNIQUE)
PHILLIP M. HARTER AND SIDNEY I. LEE

The Seldinger wire-guided technique provides the benefit of obtaining central venous access with a large-bore catheter without the inherent risks of using a large-bore needle. The general technique is described below and is applicable to the sites discussed in the following sections (subclavian, internal jugular, and femoral vein access).

Indications
- Emergency vascular access for fluid or drug therapy
- Inability to obtain peripheral IV access
- Administration of concentrated solution or total parenteral nutrition
- Measurement of central venous pressure
- Emergency IV access (medical or trauma resuscitation)
- Access for transvenous pacer or pulmonary artery catheter
- Placement of temporary hemodialysis catheter

Contraindications
- No absolute contraindications
- Relative contraindications:
  - Coagulopathy
  - Trauma, prior surgery, or radiation therapy in area of cannulation
  - Uncooperative patient
  - Overlying skin or soft tissue infection
  - Marked obesity
  - Vasculitis
  - Sclerotherapy
  - Multiple previous catheterizations at site

Equipment
- Preassembled central venous access kit, or the following:
  - Anesthetic agent (1% lidocaine), syringe, and needles
  - Introducer needle (thin-walled 18-gauge 2.5-inch size)
  - Guidewire and holder assembly
  - Catheter or sheath introducer
  - Dilator (semirigid thick-walled catheter)
  - Betadine antiseptic solution
  - Sterile drapes and gloves
  - Mask and gown
  - Gauze pads
  - Scalpel with No. 11 blade
  - 5- and 10-ml Luer-Lok syringes
  - Nonabsorbable suture (4-0 or thicker)
  - Antibiotic ointment for dressing
  - IV fluid setup
  - Additional larger syringes for drawing blood if necessary

Procedure

1. Identify anatomic landmarks according to the vessel to be cannulated (see sections on subclavian, internal jugular, and femoral central venous access).
2. Prepare and drape the area in sterile fashion
3. Use a 25- or 27-gauge needle to inject the skin and subcutaneous tissue with approximately 5 ml lidocaine for anesthesia. Anesthetize a generous area of skin to allow suturing of the catheter once in place. A larger needle or the introducer needle can be used to anesthetize deeper tissues *(A)*.
4. Locate the vessel, and insert the introducer needle attached to a syringe. Gently aspirate the entire time while inserting the introducer needle *(B)*. If redirecting the needle is necessary, always withdraw to the level of the skin before readvancing.
5. Once the needle tip enters the vessel lumen, venous blood should flow freely into the syringe. It may be helpful to aspirate blood while rotating the needle 180° to ensure that the needle is entirely through the vessel wall.
6. Remove the syringe from the needle, being careful to stabilize and keep the needle in its place. Once the syringe is removed, the hub of the needle should be capped with the thumb to prevent venous air embolism.
7. With your nondominant hand stabilizing the needle, use your dominant hand to pass the flexible guidewire through the needle *(C)*. The wire should pass easily through the needle into the vessel and should never be forced if resistance is encountered. Be sure to hold the distal end of the wire (usually covered by a plastic sheath) at all times, and do not insert this end of the wire through the needle.
8. Once most of the guidewire has been inserted through the needle, remove the needle over the wire *(D)*. Enough wire length should be left outside the body to allow passage of the full length of the catheter over the wire. Always keep hold of the guidewire during this process.

Cardiovascular System

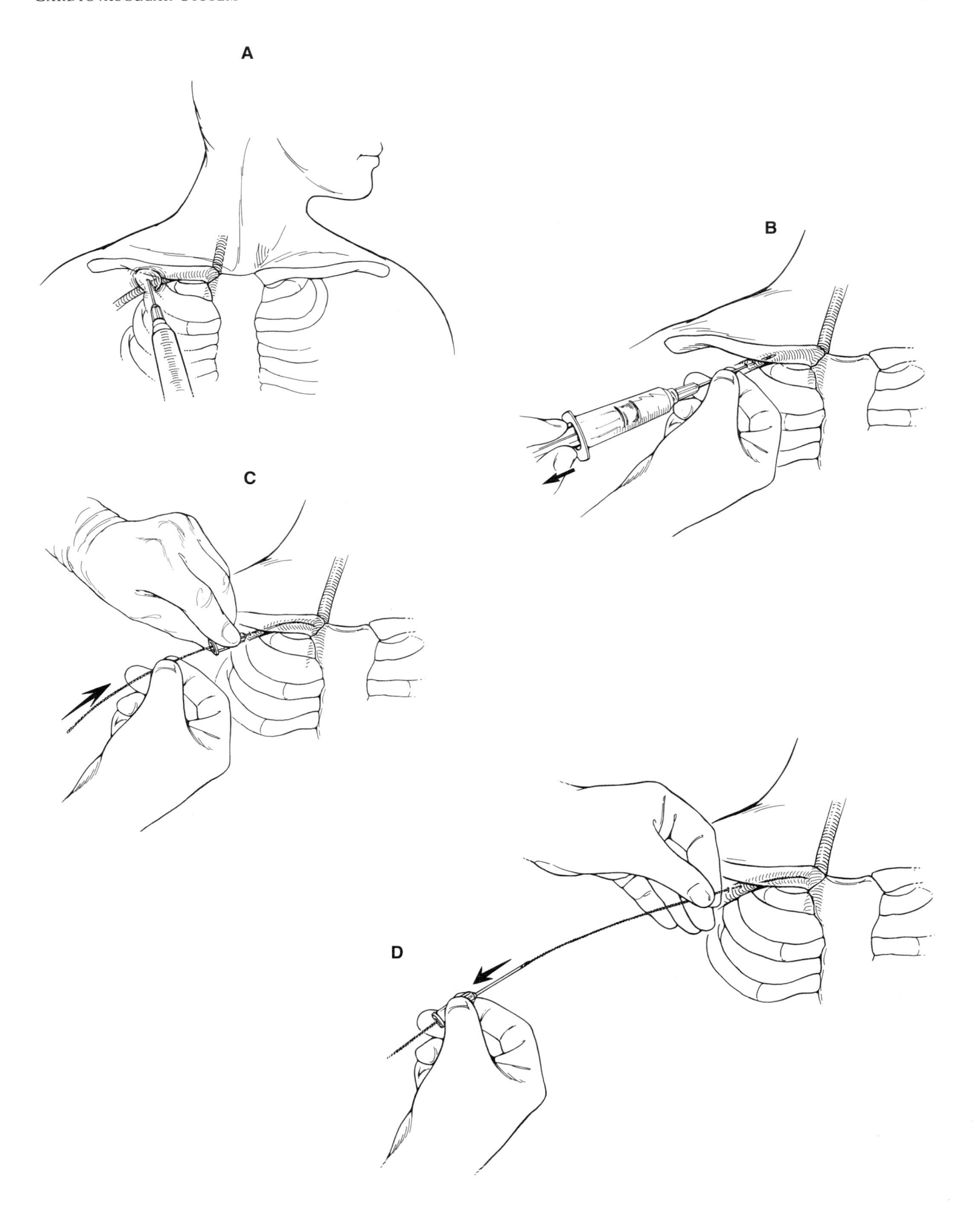

A

B

C

D

9. Make a small superficial skin incision with the scalpel at the site of the guidewire *(E)*.
10. Pass the dilator over the guidewire. Grasp the proximal end of the wire once it is through the dilator.
11. Advance the dilator over the wire with a slow, firm, twisting motion through the skin into the vessel lumen. The dilator may be passed over the wire twice to ensure easy passage of the catheter *(F_1)*.
12. Remove the dilator over the guidewire, leaving the wire in place. Always keep hold of the guidewire during this process *(F_2)*.
13. Pass the catheter over the guidewire into the vessel in a fashion similar to the dilator *(G)*.
14. Remove the guidewire through the catheter, leaving the catheter in place *(H)*.
15. Attach the catheter to the IV fluid setup, and suture the catheter in place *(I)*.

Complications

- Hematoma
- Air embolism
- Misdirected cannula
- Vein thrombosis
- Catheter embolism
- Catheter malposition
- Infection
- Arterial puncture or cannulation
- Vessel laceration or dissection
- Nerve laceration
- Knotted guidewire
- Lost guidewire
- Guidewire breakage

Discussion

- Make sure the guidewire is an appropriate length for the catheter and the vessel to be cannulated. The wire should be long enough that, once the wire is in the vessel, sufficient wire remains outside the skin so that the entire catheter can be passed over the wire without the catheter's penetrating the skin. This will allow the operator to maintain a hold on the wire (proximal or distal to the catheter) at all times.
- The type of guidewire selected may facilitate its passage. If the vessel to be catheterized has a generally straight course, a straight guidewire may be used. If the vessel course is tortuous, a J-wire will facilitate passage.
- Force should not be used if resistance is encountered when passing the wire through the needle. Resistance may indicate that the needle has been dislodged from the vessel, the wire is caught at the bend in the vessel, or the wire is abutting the wall of the vessel. Forcing the wire may result in vessel damage or thrombosis. To overcome resistance, the operator can withdraw the wire and rotate it before reattempting passage, adjust the location or angle of the needle entry into the vessel, or remove the wire completely and reaspirate through the needle to ensure that the needle is still in the vessel.
- If a sheath introducer is required rather than a catheter, place the sheath over the dilator and advance the sheath and dilator as a single unit over the guidewire. Once the unit is positioned, the dilator and wire are removed, leaving the sheath in place.
- This technique has limited use in the field because of the time needed to perform the procedure, but it is in the scope of practice of flight physicians, nurses, and some paramedics.

Bibliography

Dailey RH: Use of wire-guided (Seldinger-type) catheters in the emergency department, *Ann Emerg Med* 12:489-492, 1983.

Gibson RN et al: Major complications of central venous catheterization: a report of five cases and a brief review of the literature, *Clin Radiol* 36:205-208, 1985.

Schug CB et al: Subclavian vein catheterization in the emergency department: a comparison of guidewire and nonguidewire techniques, *Ann Emerg Med* 15:769-773, 1986.

Schwartz AJ et al: Guide wires—a caution, *Crit Care Med* 9(4):347-348, 1981.

Seldinger SI: Catheter replacement of the needle in percutaneous arteriography, *Acta Radiol* 39:368-376, 1953.

CARDIOVASCULAR SYSTEM 77

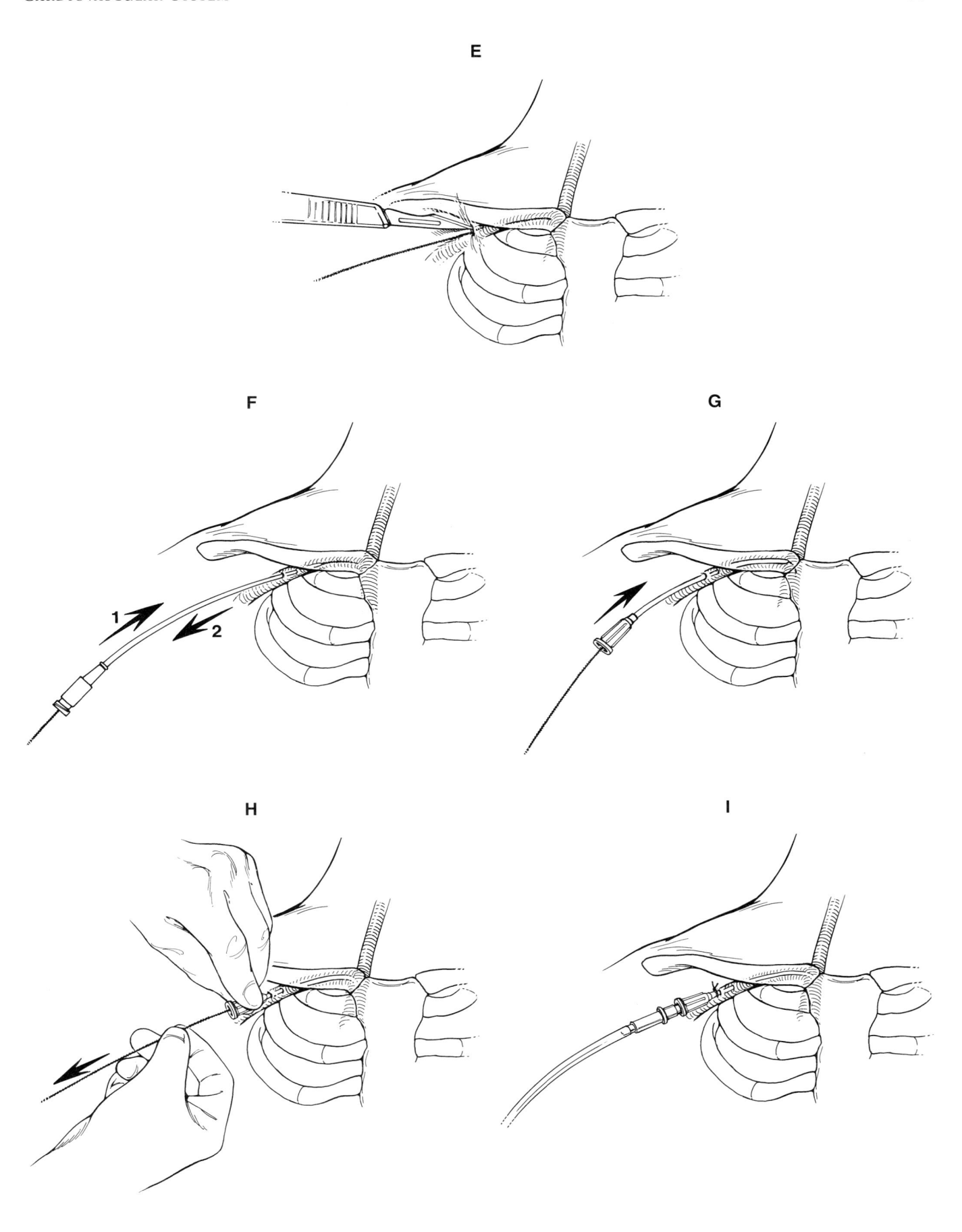

E

F

1 → ← 2

G

H

I

Subclavian Central Venous Access — Matthew David Sztajnkrycer

This section describes the specific approach to subclavian vein access. Also refer to the section on general central venous access.

Indications

- Emergency vascular access for fluid or drug therapy
- Inability to obtain peripheral IV access
- Administration of concentrated solution or total parenteral nutrition
- Measurement of central venous pressure
- Emergency IV access (medical or trauma resuscitation)
- Access for transvenous pacer or pulmonary artery catheter
- Placement of temporary hemodialysis catheter

Contraindications

- Contraindications as listed in section on central venous access
- Distorted anatomy or chest wall deformities
- Suspected vascular injury
- Previous surgery or trauma of clavicle, 1st rib, or subclavian vessels
- Subclavian vein thrombosis
- Side contralateral to pneumothorax (may be performed on ipsilateral side)
- Relative contraindications:
  - Coagulopathy
  - Uncooperative patient
  - Chronic obstructive pulmonary disease or asthma
  - Left bundle-branch block
  - Age less than 2 years

Equipment

- Preassembled central venous access kit, or the following:
  - Local anesthetic (1% lidocaine), syringe, and needles
  - Introducer needle (thin-walled, 14- to 18-gauge, 2.5-inch size)
  - Guidewire and holder assembly—J-wire
  - Catheter or sheath introducer
  - Dilator (semirigid thick-walled catheter)
  - Betadine antiseptic solution
  - Sterile drapes and gloves
  - Mask and gown
  - Gauze pads
  - Scalpel with No. 11 blade
  - 5- and 10-ml Luer-Lok syringes
  - Nonabsorbable suture (4-0 or thicker)
  - Antibiotic ointment for dressing
  - IV fluid setup
  - Additional larger syringes to draw blood if necessary

Procedure

1. Place patient in Trendelenburg position (10° to 15°).
2. Prepare the area including the clavicle, sternum, and ipsilateral neck to the angle of the mandible in sterile fashion *(A)*. A towel roll may be placed between the shoulder blades under the patient to accentuate the sternoclavicular joint.
3. Using the measurement marks along the length of the catheter, estimate the length required to position the tip of the catheter into the superior vena cava.
4. Infraclavicular approach:
   a. Anesthetize the skin overlying and just inferior to the junction of the lateral and middle thirds of the clavicle.
   b. Advance the needle to anesthetize the clavicle at the junction of the medial and middle thirds of the clavicle.
   c. Insert the introducer needle just inferior to the junction of the lateral and middle thirds of the clavicle. The bevel of the needle should be oriented inferomedially.
   d. Direct the needle medially and slightly cephalad, aiming for either the sternoclavicular junction or the suprasternal notch *(B)*.
   e. Using a shallow angle to the skin, advance the needle just posterior to the bone of the clavicle at the junction of the medial and middle thirds. With your nondominant hand, orient the suprasternal notch and apply posteriorly directed pressure on the needle to direct it just under the clavicle. Use your dominant hand to aspirate continuously while advancing the needle.
   f. Free-flowing venous blood should be aspirated once the vessel is entered.

Cardiovascular System

A

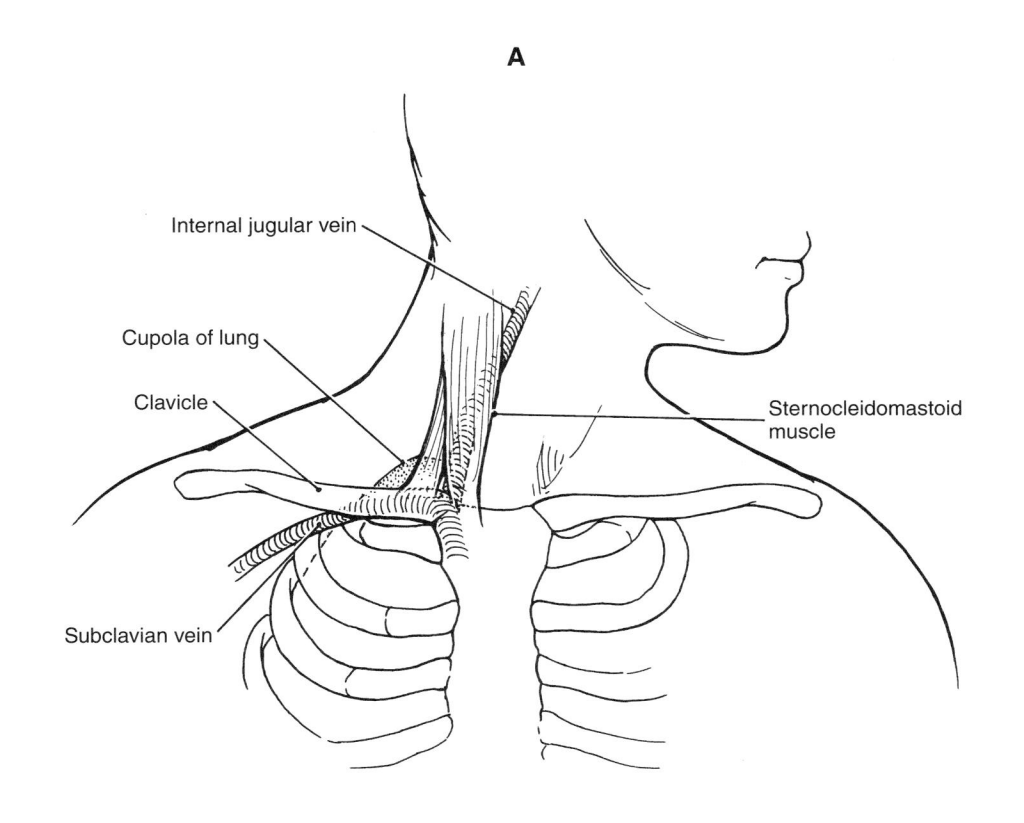

- Internal jugular vein
- Cupola of lung
- Clavicle
- Subclavian vein
- Sternocleidomastoid muscle

B

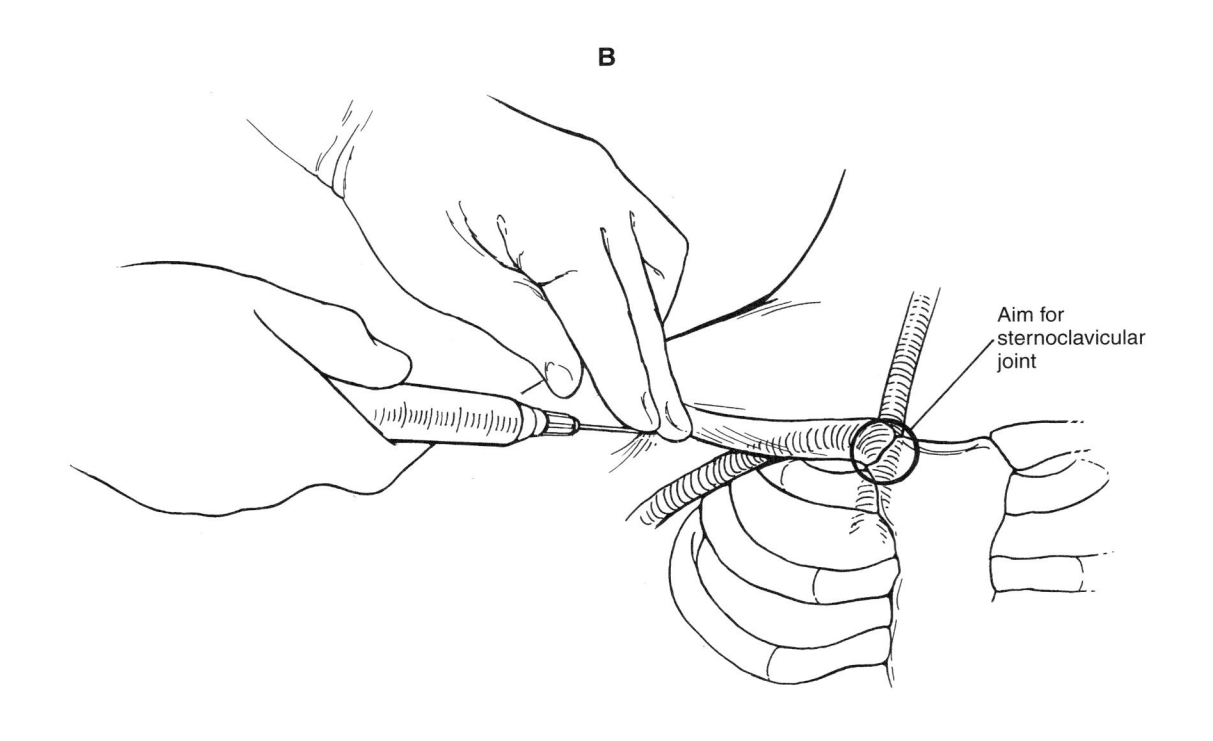

- Aim for sternoclavicular joint

5. Supraclavicular approach:
   a. Anesthetize the skin overlying the clavicle approximately 1 cm superior to the clavicle and 1 cm lateral to the clavicular head of the sternocleidomastoid.
   b. Insert the introducer at this position (1 cm superior to the clavicle and 1 cm lateral to the sternocleidomastoid clavicular head), aiming toward either the suprasternal notch or the contralateral nipple *(C)*.
   c. Direct the needle approximately 10° to 15° upward from the horizontal plane, just posterior to the clavicle.
   d. Advance the needle while aspirating continuously with the dominant hand. Use the nondominant hand to identify and refer to the suprasternal junction.
   e. Free-flowing venous blood should be aspirated once the vessel is entered.
6. Once the vessel has been located by either the infraclavicular or the supraclavicular approach, insert the guidewire, dilator, and catheter by the Seldinger guidewire technique as described in the section on central venous access.
7. The catheter should be inserted to the predetermined level to place the tip into the superior vena cava.
8. Obtain a chest radiograph to verify correct catheter position and the presence or absence of complications.

Complications

- See complications in the section on central venous access.
- Complications specific to subclavian vein access:
  - Pneumothorax
  - Tracheal puncture
  - Endotracheal tube cuff puncture
  - Neck hematoma, tracheal compression
  - Internal jugular vein injury
  - Phrenic nerve injury
  - Brachial plexus injury
  - Thoracic duct injury (procedure performed on left side)
  - Dysrhythmias

Discussion

- See the section on central venous access. In a situation of full arrest, subclavian vein access provides a rapid alternative to other lines without interfering with airway management.
- Unlike the femoral or internal jugular veins, the subclavian veins are noncompressible. Thus bleeding from a subclavian vein or inadvertent arterial puncture can be difficult to control.
- This technique may be used for patients with pneumothorax, but only on the ipsilateral side because of the risk of bilateral pneumothoraces.
- Insertion of the guidewire may irritate the right ventricle, resulting in a right bundle-branch block or ventricular dysrhythmia. If this occurs, the wire should be withdrawn until the dysrhythmia resolves.
- When the clavicular region is being prepped, it may be useful to prep the neck as well so that internal jugular cannulation can be attempted if subclavian cannulation is unsuccessful.

Bibliography

Dronen SC et al: Subclavian vein catheterization during cardiopulmonary resuscitation, *JAMA* 247:3227-3230, 1982.

Muhm M et al: Supraclavicular approach to the subclavian/innominate vein for large-bore central venous catheters, *Am J Kidney Dis* 30:802-808, 1997.

Sterner S et al: A comparison of the supraclavicular approach and the infraclavicular approach for subclavian vein catheterization, *Ann Emerg Med* 15:421-424, 1986.

Tripathi M, Tripathi M: Subclavian vein cannulation: an approach with definite landmarks, *Ann Thorac Surg* 61:238-240, 1996.

Yoffa D: Supraclavicular subclavian venipuncture and catheterization, *Lancet* 2:614-617, 1965.

Cardiovascular System

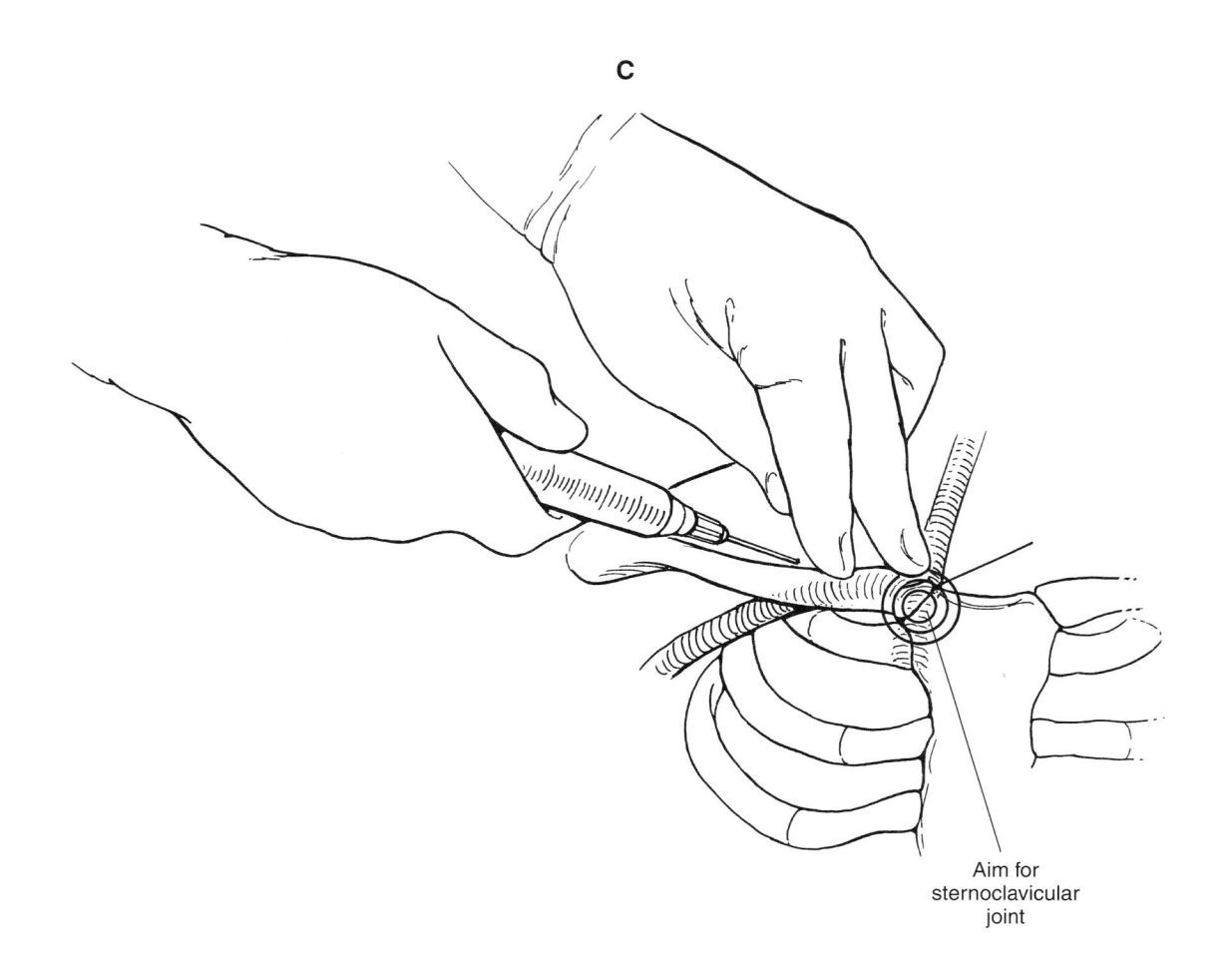

C

Aim for sternoclavicular joint

Internal Jugular Central Venous Access   Joseph E. Clinton

This section describes the specific approach to internal jugular vein access. Also refer to the section on general central venous access.

Indications

- Emergency vascular access for fluid or drug therapy
- Inability to obtain peripheral IV access
- Administration of concentrated solution or total parenteral nutrition
- Measurement of central venous pressure
- Emergency IV access (medical or trauma resuscitation)
- Access for transvenous pacer or pulmonary artery catheter
- Placement of temporary hemodialysis catheter

Contraindications

- Relative contraindications as listed in section on central venous access
- Other relative contraindications:
  - Cervical spine fracture or suspected fracture
  - Neck wound
  - Kyphosis
  - Neck hematoma

Equipment

- Preassembled central venous access kit, or the following:
  - Local anesthetic (1% lidocaine), syringe, and needles
  - Introducer needle (thin-walled, 14- to 18-gauge, 2.5-inch size)
  - Guidewire and holder assembly—J-wire
  - Catheter or sheath introducer
  - Dilator (semirigid thick-walled catheter)
  - Betadine antiseptic solution
  - Sterile drapes and gloves
  - Mask and gown
  - Gauze pads
  - Scalpel with No. 11 blade
  - 5- and 10-ml Luer-Lok syringes
  - Nonabsorbable suture (4-0 or thicker)
  - Antibiotic ointment for dressing
  - IV fluid setup
  - Additional larger syringes to draw blood if necessary

Procedure

1. Place patient in Trendelenburg position (10° to 15°) with head turned to face contralateral side.
2. Prepare and drape the area including the clavicle, sternum, and ipsilateral neck from the angle of the mandible to the upper chest in sterile fashion.
3. Using the measurement marks along the length of the catheter, estimate the length required to position the tip of the catheter into the superior vena cava.
4. Middle approach:
   a. Identify the sternocleidomastoid triangle formed by the clavicle and the sternal and clavicular heads of the sternocleidomastoid muscle. The internal jugular veins runs in this triangle, lateral to the carotid artery
   b. Anesthetize the skin and soft tissue overlying the apex of the triangle (where the sternal and clavicular heads join).
   c. Insert the introducer needle at the apex at a 30° to 45° angle to the skin, and aim the needle toward the ipsilateral nipple, intending to encounter the vein in the lateral aspect of the triangle at a needle depth of 1 to 3 cm *(A, B)*.
   d. Aspirate while advancing the needle. Free flow of venous blood into the syringe indicates entry into the internal jugular vein.

Cardiovascular System

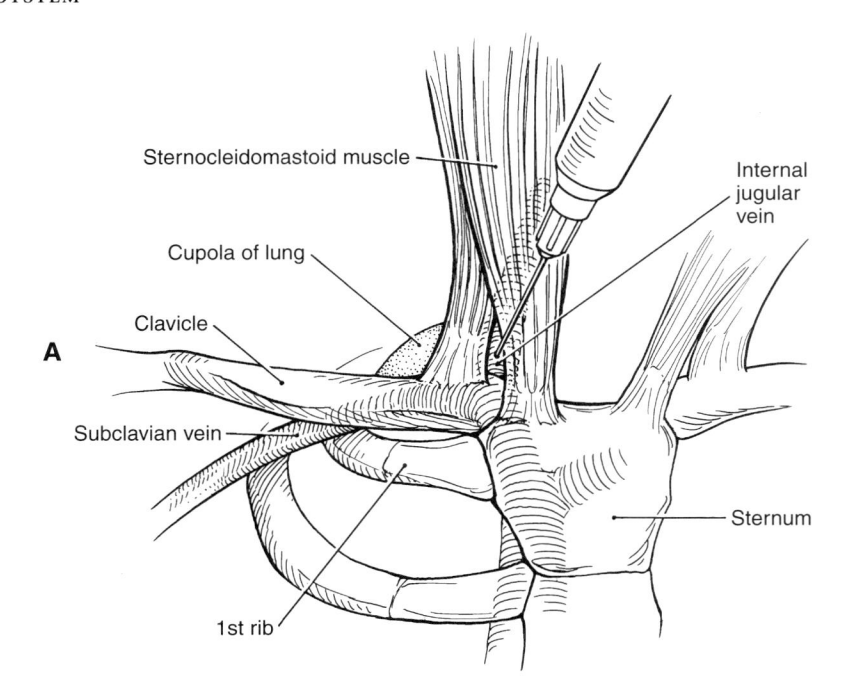

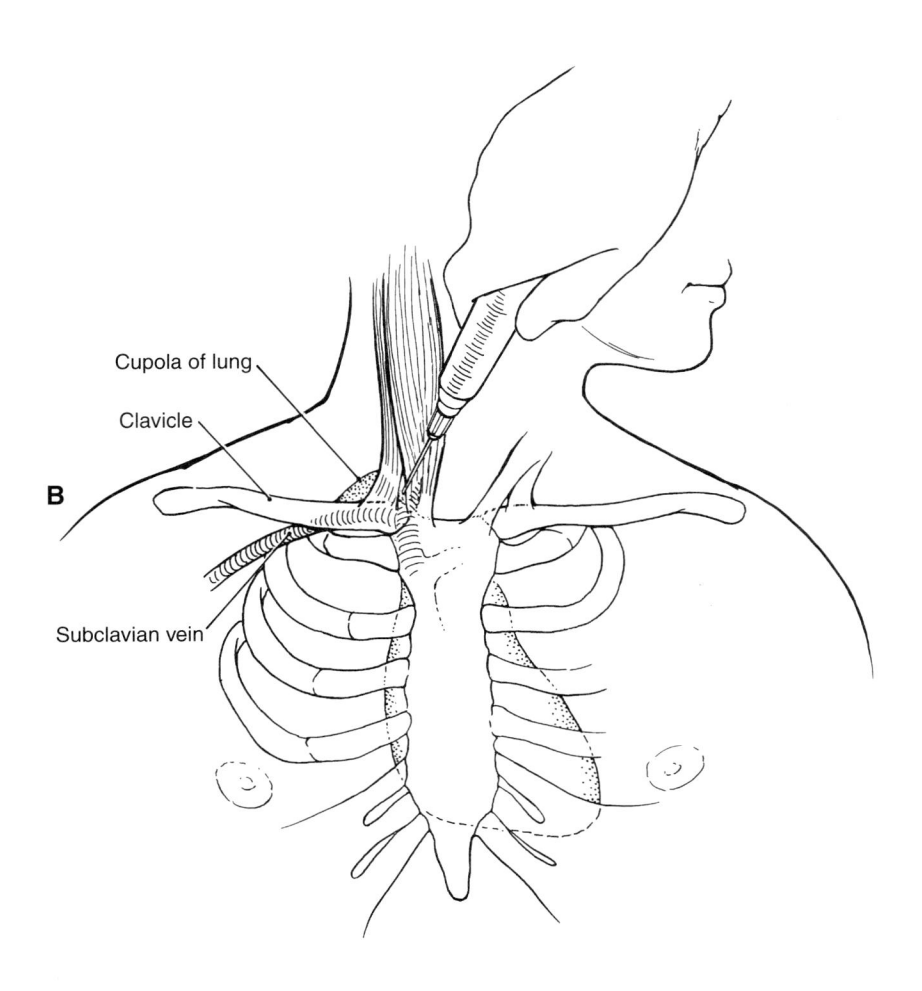

A
- Sternocleidomastoid muscle
- Cupola of lung
- Clavicle
- Subclavian vein
- 1st rib
- Internal jugular vein
- Sternum

B
- Cupola of lung
- Clavicle
- Subclavian vein

5. Posterior approach:
   a. Identify the posterior (or lateral) side of the sternocleidomastoid muscle.
   b. Anesthetize the skin and soft tissue around the posterior aspect of the muscle *(C)*.
   c. Insert the introducer needle along the posterior muscle edge at a level one third the distance from the clavicle to the mastoid, just superior to where the external jugular crosses the muscle.
   d. Direct the needle underneath the muscle toward the jugular notch of the sternum.
   e. Aspirate while advancing the needle. Free flow of venous blood into the syringe indicates entry into the internal jugular vein.
6. Anterior approach:
   a. Identify the anterior (or medial side) of the sternocleidomastoid muscle. Palpate the carotid artery. The internal jugular runs anterolateral to the artery.
   b. Anesthetize the skin and soft tissue around the medial aspect of the muscle.
   c. Insert the introducer needle along the anterior edge at a level half the distance from the clavicle to the mastoid, taking care to avoid the carotid artery. The needle should be inserted at a 45° angle to the skin.
   d. Direct the needle toward the ipsilateral nipple.
   e. Aspirate while advancing the needle. Free flow of venous blood into the syringe indicates entry into the internal jugular vein.
7. Once the vessel has been located by the introducer needle, insert the guidewire, dilator, and catheter by the Seldinger guidewire technique as described in the section on central venous access.
8. The catheter should be inserted to the predetermined level to place the tip into the superior vena cava.
9. Obtain a chest radiograph to verify correct catheter position and the presence or absence of complications.

Complications

- See complications in the section on central venous access.
- Complications specific to internal jugular vein access:
  - Pneumothorax
  - Carotid artery puncture
  - Neck hematoma or tracheal compression
  - Dysrhythmias

Discussion

- Internal jugular cannulation is often preferred over subclavian cannulation for patients at high risk for pneumothorax, obese patients, those with chronic obstructive pulmonary disease, infants, and patients with anatomic challenges, such as scoliosis. The neck has the additional advantage that the vessels in this location are compressible and any resultant bleeding can potentially be controlled.
- In critically ill patients requiring airway management, other sites of central venous access, such as the subclavian or femoral vein, are preferable to the internal jugular vein. It has been suggested that the internal jugular vein can be cannulated with the head in a neutral rather than a turned position.
- The middle approach is preferred over the anterior or posterior approach because the anatomic landmarks are consistent and reliable and the risk of carotid puncture is low.
- When possible, the right side of the neck is often preferred over the left because of the straighter course to the superior vena cava and the absence of risk to the thoracic duct.
- Ultrasound can be used to guide needle placement and distinguish anatomic landmarks and arterial and venous structures.

Bibliography

Daily PA et al: Percutaneous internal jugular vein cannulation, *Arch Surg* 101:534, 1970.

Defalque RH: Percutaneous catheterization of the internal jugular vein, *Anesth Analg* 53:116, 1974.

Denys BG et al: Ultrasound-assisted cannulation of the internal jugular vein: a prospective comparison to the external landmark-guided technique, *Circulation* 87:1557-1562, 1993.

Willeford KL, Reitan JA: Neutral head position for placement of internal jugular vein catheters [see comments], *Anaesthesia* 49:202-204, 1994.

C

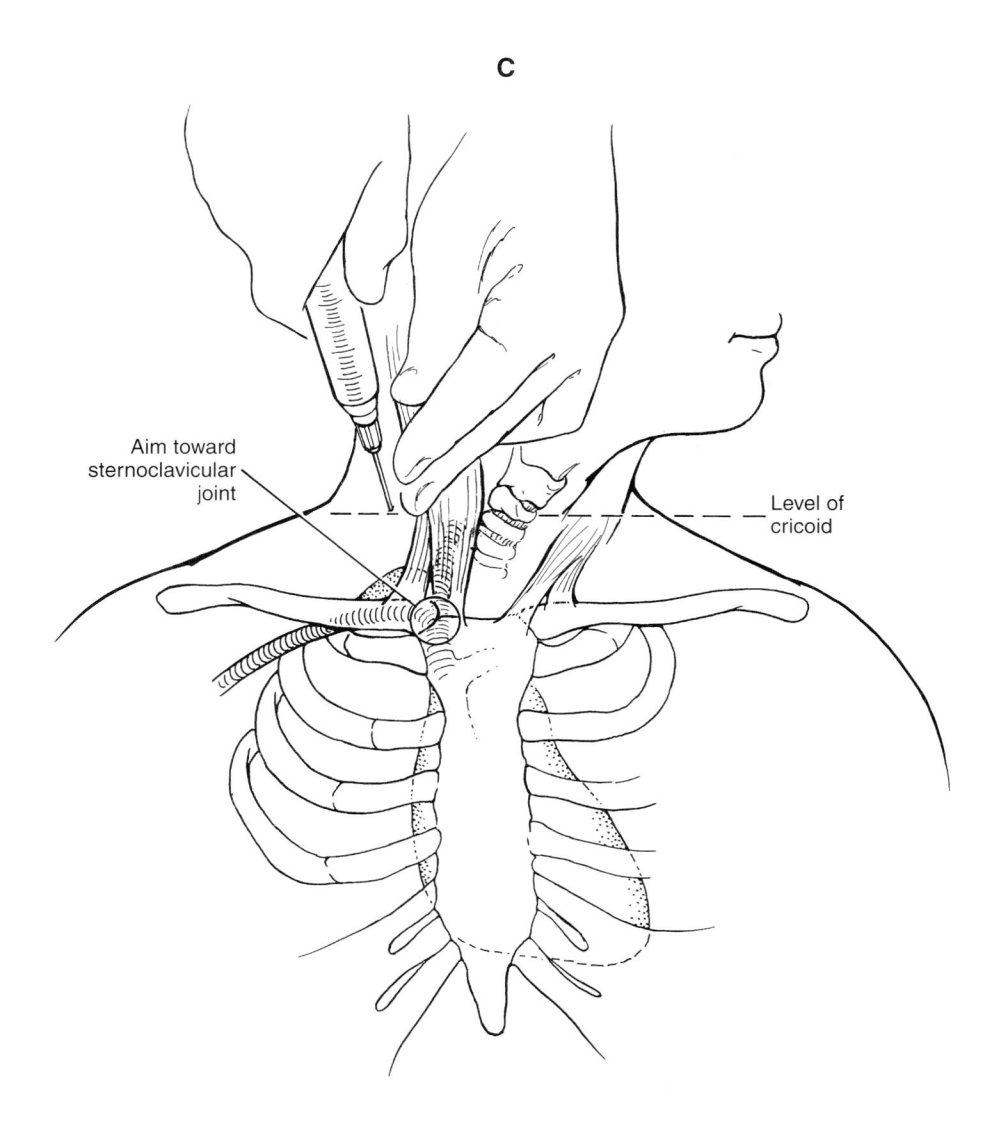

Aim toward sternoclavicular joint

Level of cricoid

FEMORAL CENTRAL VENOUS ACCESS   DONALD DEMETRIUS ZUKIN

This section describes the specific approach to femoral vein access. Also refer to the section on general central venous access.

Indications
- Emergency vascular access for fluid or drug therapy
- Inability to obtain peripheral IV access
- Administration of concentrated solution or total parenteral nutrition
- Measurement of central venous pressure
- Emergency IV access (medical or trauma resuscitation)
- Access for transvenous pacer
- Placement of temporary hemodialysis catheter
- Central access when other sites are contraindicated (i.e., ongoing airway management or chest compressions)

Contraindications
- Contraindications as listed in central venous access section
- Other relative contraindications:
  - Injury to inferior vena cava
  - Hypercoagulable states (increased incidence of thrombophlebitis)

Equipment
- Preassembled central venous access kit, or the following:
  - Local anesthetic (1% lidocaine), syringe, and needles
  - Introducer needle (thin-walled, 14- to 18-gauge, 2.5-inch size)
  - Guidewire and holder assembly
  - Catheter or sheath introducer
  - Dilator (semirigid thick-walled catheter)
- Betadine antiseptic solution
- Sterile drapes and gloves
- Mask and gown
- Gauze pads
- Scalpel with No. 11-blade
- 10-ml Luer-Lok syringe
- Nonabsorbable suture (4-0 or thicker)
- Antibiotic ointment for dressing
- IV fluid setup
- Additional larger syringes to draw blood if necessary

Procedure

1. Place the patient in supine position with the ipsilateral hip in slight external rotation.
2. Prepare and drape the inguinal and femoral regions in sterile fashion.
3. Identify the approximate location of the femoral vein.
   a. Palpate the femoral artery, which is located approximately midway along a line drawn from the anterior superior iliac spine to the pubic tubercle.
   b. The femoral vein lies medial to the femoral artery in the region of the inguinal crease. Anatomically, the structures underlying the inguinal ligament, from lateral to medial, are the femoral **N**erve, femoral **A**rtery, femoral **V**ein, and **L**ymphatics (mnemonic NAV or NAVL) *(A)*.

Anterior superior iliac spine
Inguinal ligament
Femoral nerve
Femoral artery
Femoral vein
Pubic tubercle

A

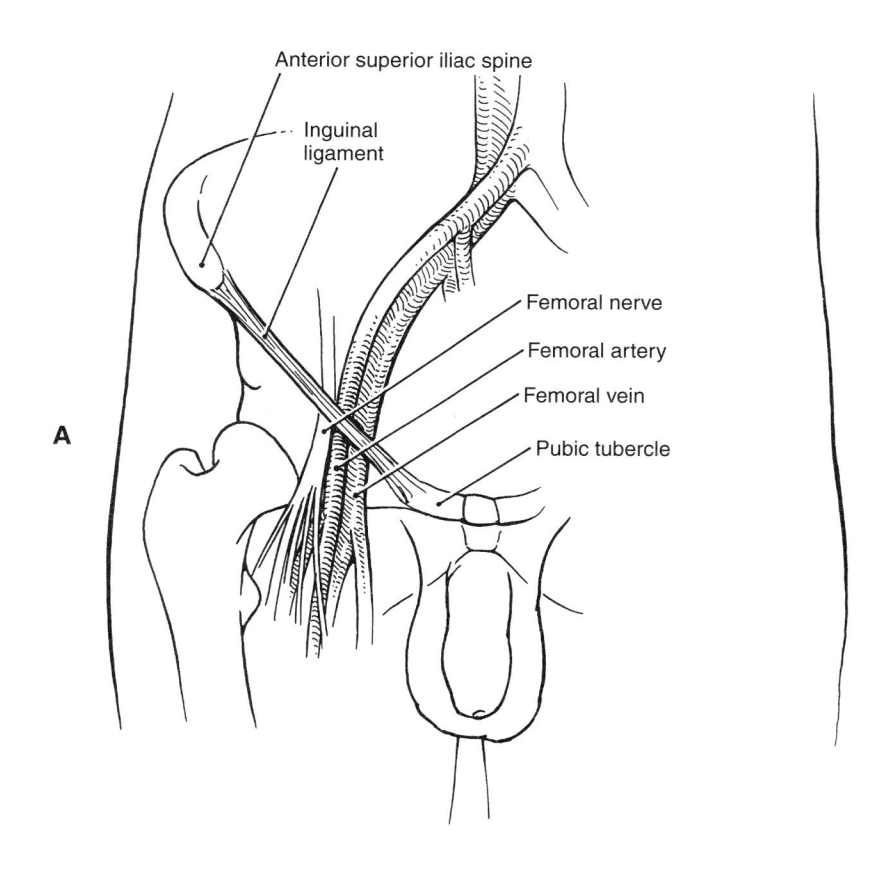

4. Insert the introducer needle with bevel up approximately 1 to 2 fingerbreadths below (distal to) the inguinal crease and immediately medial to the femoral pulse *(B)*.
5. Direct the needle cephalad at a 45° angle to the plane of the thigh, aspirating with the syringe while advancing the needle.
6. Venous blood should flow into the syringe when the femoral vein is entered.
7. Drop the angle of the needle to 20° (almost parallel to the vein), and advance the needle an additional 2 to 3 mm to ensure that the entire bevel of the needle is within the femoral vein.
8. Insert the guidewire, dilator, and catheter by the Seldinger guidewire technique as described in the section on central venous access.

Complications

- See complications in the section on central venous access.
- Hematoma
- Air embolism
- Misdirected cannula
- Vein thrombosis
- Catheter embolism
- Catheter malposition
- Infection
- Arterial puncture or cannulation
- Vessel laceration or dissection
- Nerve laceration
- Knotted guidewire
- Lost guidewire
- Guidewire breakage

Discussion

- During chest compressions the palpable pulse at the groin may be retrograde down the vein and not from the artery. Therefore, if unsuccessful when entering medial to the pulse, attempt cannulation by entering the skin directly over the palpable pulse.
- The femoral vein can be cannulated with a sheath-over-needle IV catheter rather than the Seldinger wire-guided technique. In this case the catheter needle is inserted into the femoral vein as described above, after which the catheter sheath is passed over the needle into the vein and the needle is removed.

Bibliography

Agee KR, Balk RA: Central venous catheterization in the critically ill patient, *Crit Care Clin* 8(4):677-686, 1992.

Macnab AJ, Macnab M: Teaching pediatric procedures: the Vancouver model for instructing Seldinger central venous access via the femoral vein, *Pediatrics* 103(1):E8, 1999.

Cardiovascular System

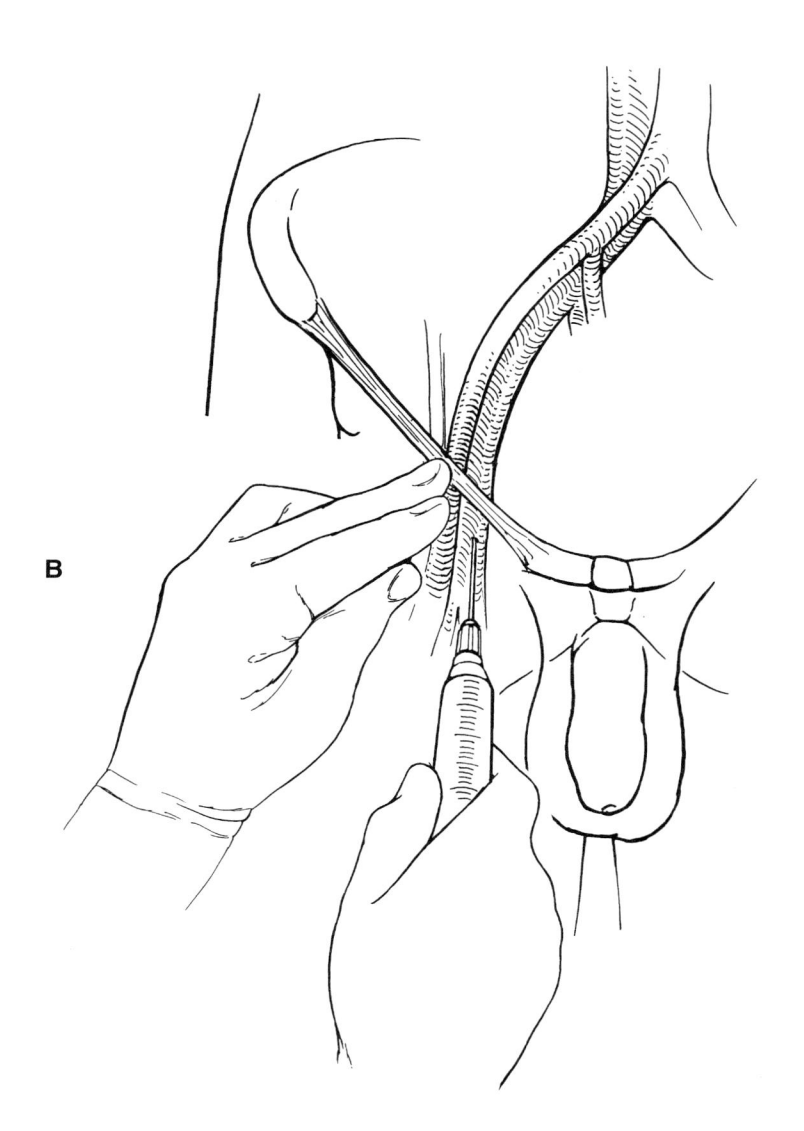

B

Alternative Venous Access

GREATER SAPHENOUS VENOUS CUTDOWN   GEORGE STERNBACH

Indications
- Need for emergency venous access when no good site for peripheral transcutaneous cannulation is available

Contraindications
- Known injury to the venous system proximal to the cutdown site.
- Major blunt or penetrating trauma to the leg on which the procedure is to be performed

Equipment
- Betadine antiseptic solution
- Sterile gloves and drapes
- Local anesthetic (1% lidocaine), syringe, and needles
- Scalpels with No. 10, 11, and 15 blades
- Curved Kelly and mosquito hemostats
- Vein pick
- 3-0 absorbable suture ligaments
- 4-0 nylon suture
- IV cannula
- 4 × 4 sterile gauze sponges

Procedure

1. Prepare the skin over the medial ankle site in sterile fashion.
2. Make a transverse incision at the level of the medial malleolus between the apex of the malleolus and the anterior tibialis tendon *(A)*.
3. Dissect through the subcutaneous tissue by spreading the tissue with a curved mosquito hemostat.
4. Insert the hemostat on the medial side of the incision, and pass the tip to the tibial periosteum.
5. Turn the tip of the hemostat, and exit at the lateral side of the incision. The vein will lie within the tissue atop the hemostat *(B)*.
6. Clear the vein of adventitious tissue by blunt dissection. Pass a 3-0 absorbable suture tie beneath the vein by grasping it with the hemostat *(C)*.
7. Cut the suture at its midpoint, creating two sutures *(D)*. Clamp the sutures, and position them at proximal and distal points on the exposed vein.

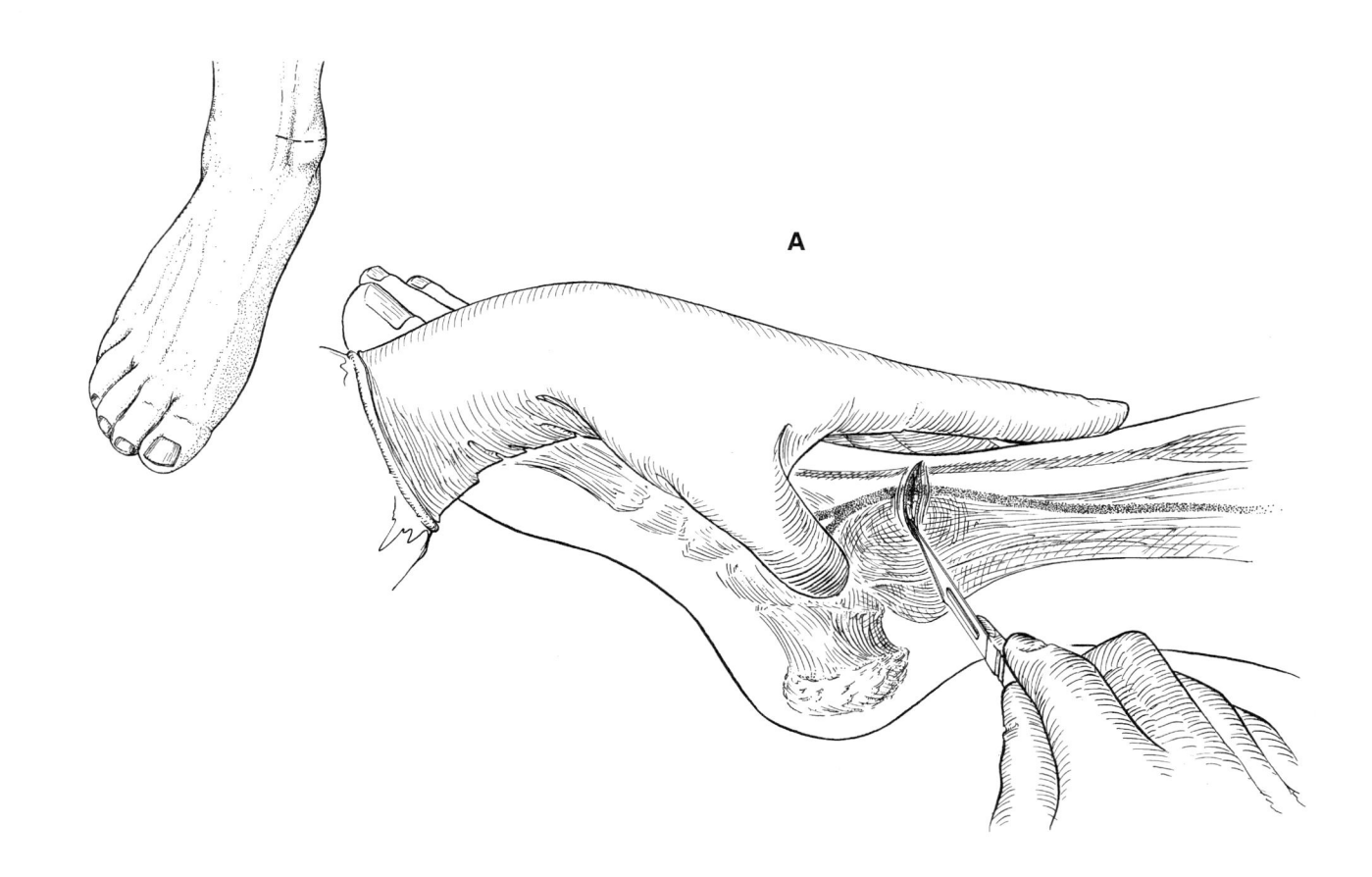

A

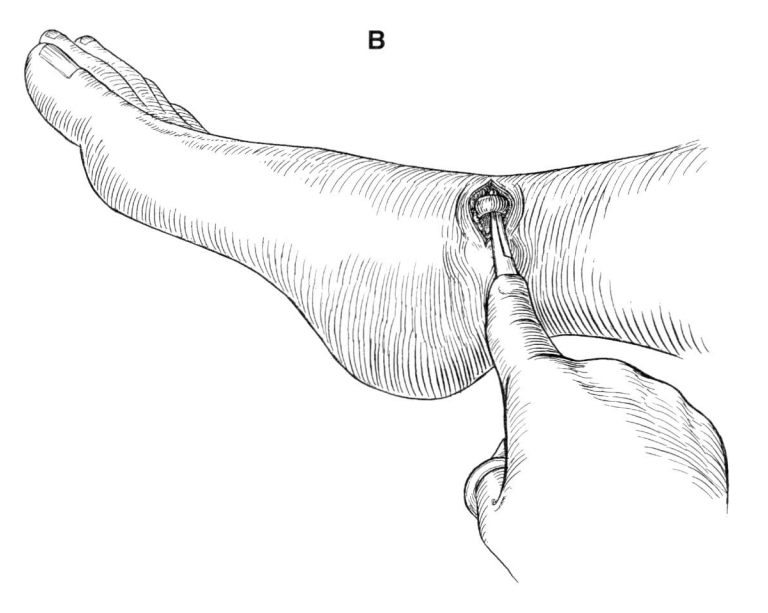

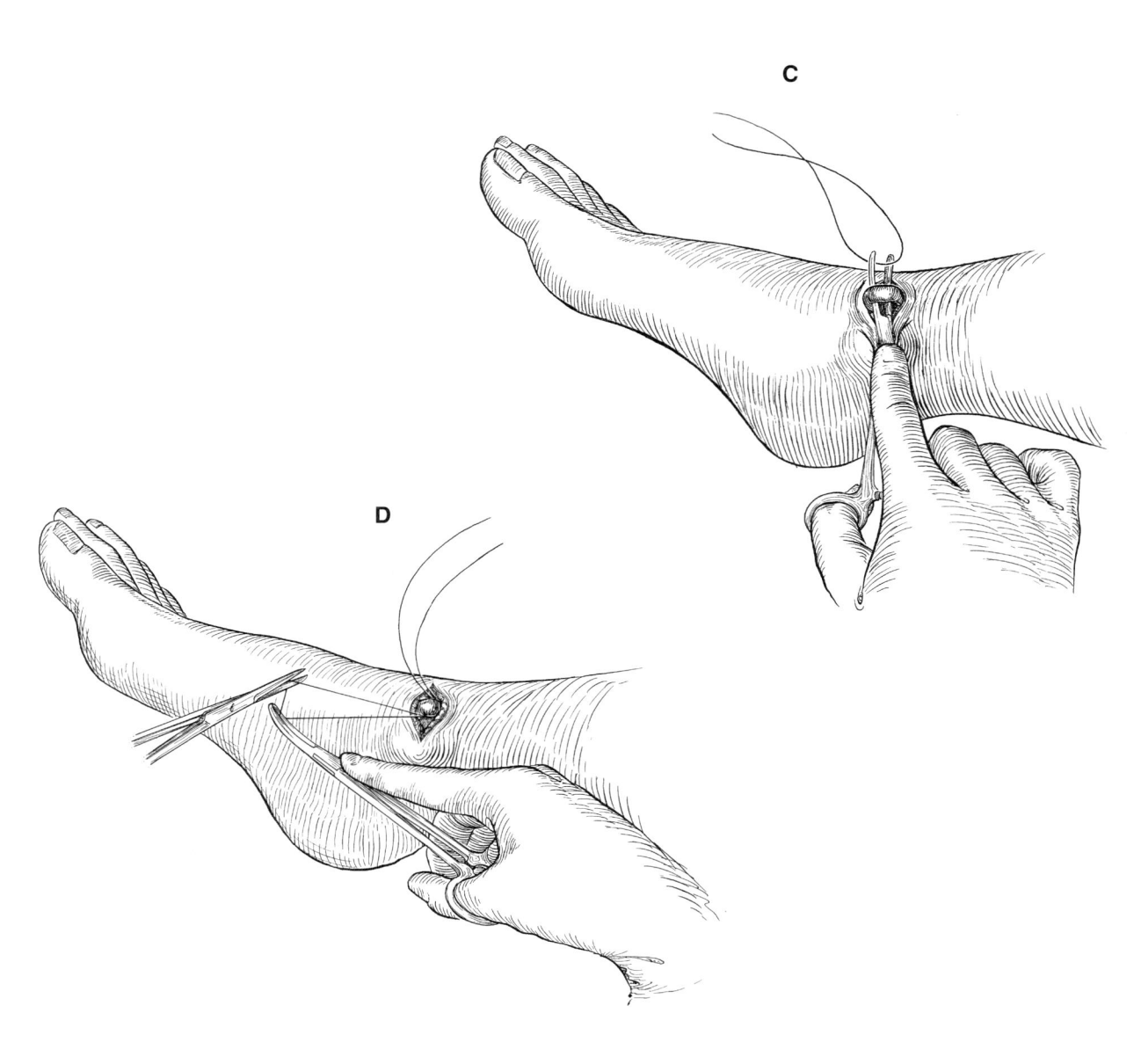

Cardiovascular System

B

C

D

8. Tie the distal suture, thereby ligating the vessel distally *(E)*.
9. Raising the vein by applying traction to the sutures, make a flap incision on the anterior wall of the vessel with a No. 11 scalpel blade *(F, G)*.
10. Insert a vein pick to elevate the flap in the vein.
11. Pulling the vein taut by applying traction on the proximal suture, advance a catheter into the vessel by using the vein pick *(H)*.
12. Flush the catheter with a small amount of sterile saline solution, and attach an IV line.
13. Tie the proximal suture around the portion of the vein containing the catheter *(I)*.
14. Cut the ends of the proximal and distal ligatures.
15. Suture the catheter to the skin, and close the incision with 4-0 nylon suture.
16. Cover the incision site with a dressing. Tape the IV tubing in place, looping it around the big toe.

Complications

- Hematoma formation
- Thrombophlebitis
- Injury to adjacent structures, including tibialis anterior tendon and saphenous nerve
- Transection of vein without ability to cannulate

Discussion

- An alternative technique involves passing a needle subcutaneously beginning at the incision site and exiting through the skin several centimeters distally. Pass the catheter through the needle. Remove the needle and pass the catheter into the vein as described above. The advantage of this method is that the IV catheter exits the skin outside the cutdown incision. However, a through-the-needle catheter must be used, and this may be too small for rapid infusion.
- When the procedure is performed on a child or adult with a small vessel, injection of a small amount of lidocaine into the vein helps to overcome vascular spasm.

Bibliography

Hansbrough J et al: Placement of 10-gauge catheter by cutdown for rapid fluid replacement, *J Trauma* 23:231-234, 1983.

Posner MC, Moore EE: Distal saphenous vein cutdown—technique of choice for rapid volume resuscitation, *J Emerg Med* 3:395-399, 1985.

Rhee K et al: Rapid venous access using saphenous vein cutdown at the ankle, *Am J Emerg Med* 7:262-266, 1989.

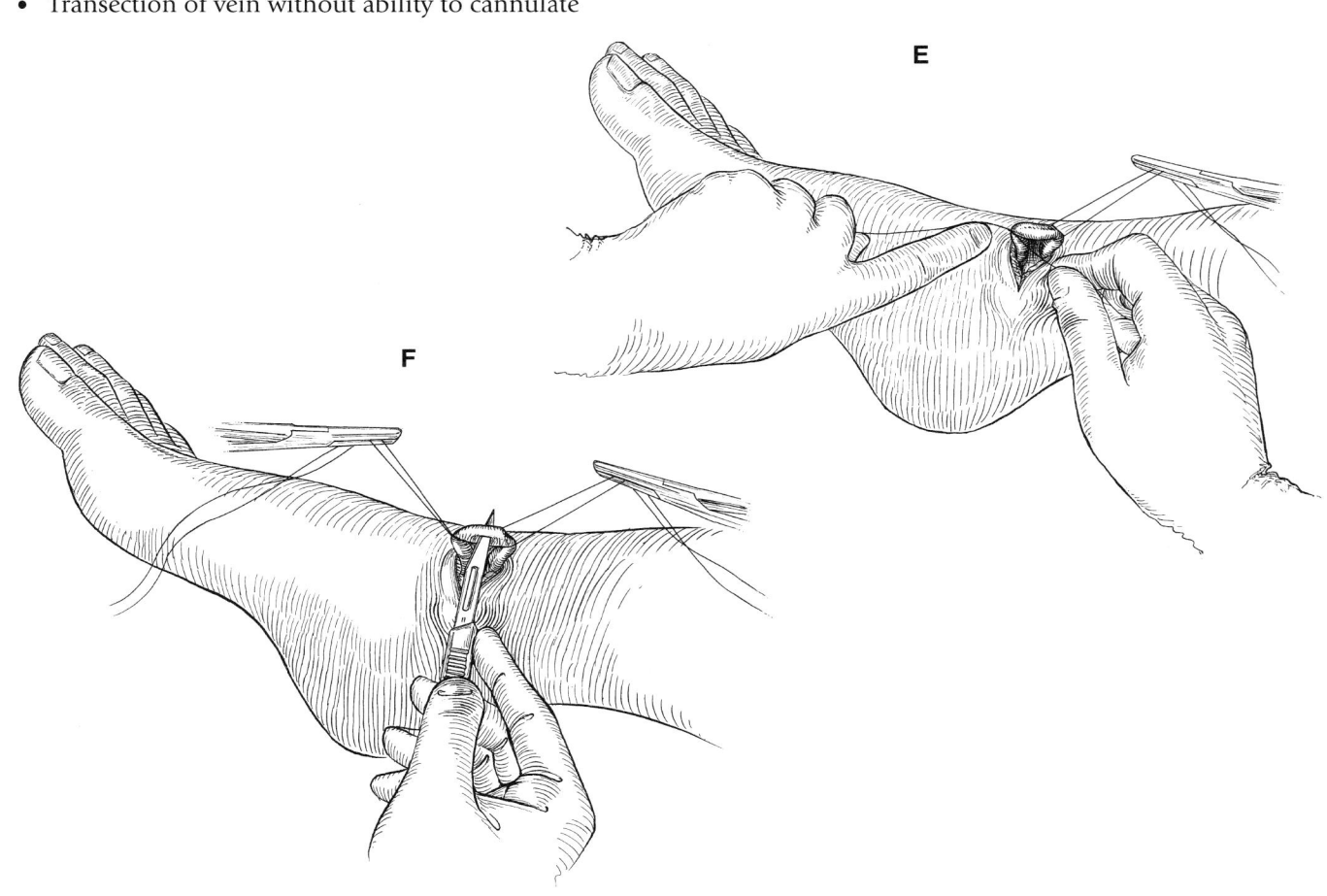

CARDIOVASCULAR SYSTEM 93

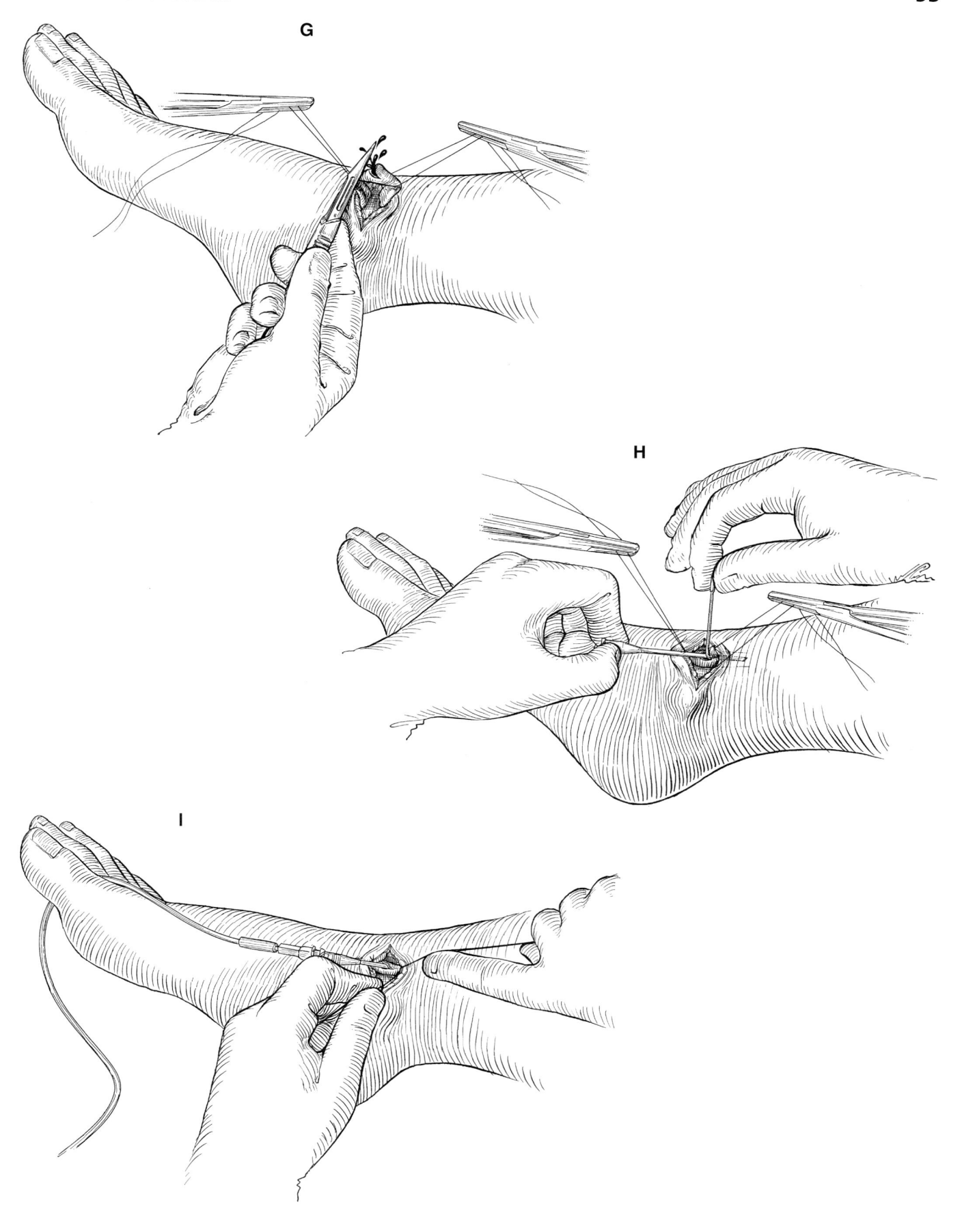

G

H

I

Saphenofemoral Venous Cutdown GEORGE STERNBACH

Indications
- Need for emergency venous access when no good site for peripheral transcutaneous cannulation is available

Contraindications
- Known injury to the venous system proximal to the cutdown site
- Major blunt or penetrating trauma to the groin or region of abdomen on which the procedure is to be performed

Equipment
- Betadine antiseptic solution
- Sterile gloves and drapes
- Local anesthetic (1% lidocaine), syringe, and needles
- Scalpels with No. 10 and 11 blades
- Curved Kelly and mosquito hemostats
- 3-0 absorbable suture
- 4-0 nylon suture
- Large-bore IV cannula, sterile IV tubing, or pediatric feeding tube
- 4 × 4 sterile gauze sponges

Procedure

1. Prepare the groin area in sterile fashion.
2. Make an incision 1 cm below the inguinal ligament and 1 cm medial to the pulsation of the femoral artery *(A)*. The incision should be about 6 cm long.
3. In the absence of a femoral pulsation, make the incision midway between the symphysis pubis and the iliac crest.
4. Carry the incision down through the subcutaneous tissue and Scarpa's fascia *(B)*. The vein lies immediately below this fascia. Use a combination of blunt and sharp dissection to dissect it free of its investing fascia *(C)*. (Subsequent steps are shown in illustrations C to I on pp. 91 to 93.)
5. Pass a hemostat beneath the vein. Pass two 3-0 absorbable suture ties beneath the vein, and clamp each with a hemostat.
6. Identify and ligate nearby branches of the saphenous vein. Free the vein of its investing adventitious tissue.
7. Tie the distal suture.
8. Incise the vein with a No. 11 scalpel blade.
9. Pass a large-bore IV cannula, the beveled end of standard IV tube, or a pediatric feeding tube into the vein.
10. Tie the proximal suture around the portion of the vein containing the catheter.
11. Flush the catheter with a small amount of sterile saline solution. Attach an IV line.
12. Close the fascia with 3-0 absorbable suture and the incision with 4-0 nylon suture.
13. Anchor the catheter to the skin with one or several 4-0 nylon sutures.
14. Cover the incision site with a dressing, and tape the IV tube in place.

Complications

- Hematoma formation
- Thrombophlebitis
- Hemorrhage
- Injury to adjacent structures, including the femoral artery or nerve
- Transection of vein without ability to cannulate

Discussion

- The saphenofemoral cutdown is technically more difficult than cutdown in other sites. The saphenous vein is joined by multiple branches before it enters the femoral vein, and these may require identification and ligation before cannulation is attempted.

Bibliography
Dronen SC et al: Proximal saphenous vein cutdown, *Ann Emerg Med* 10:328-330, 1981.
McIntosh BB, Dulchavsky SA: Peripheral vascular cutdown, *Crit Care Clin* 8:807-818, 1992.
Rogers FB: Technical note: a quick and simple method of obtaining venous access in traumatic exsanguination, *J Trauma* 34:142-143, 1993.

Cardiovascular System

A

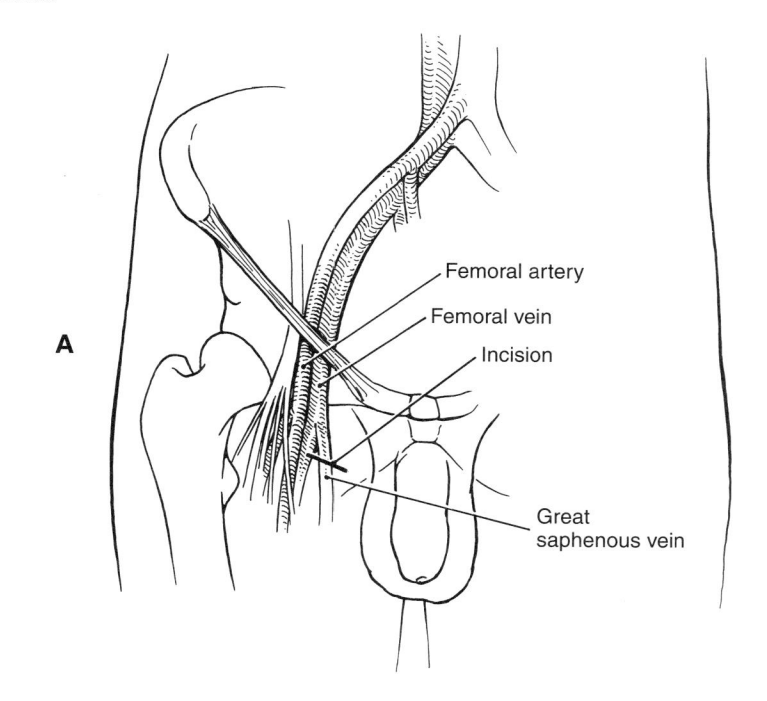

- Femoral artery
- Femoral vein
- Incision
- Great saphenous vein

B

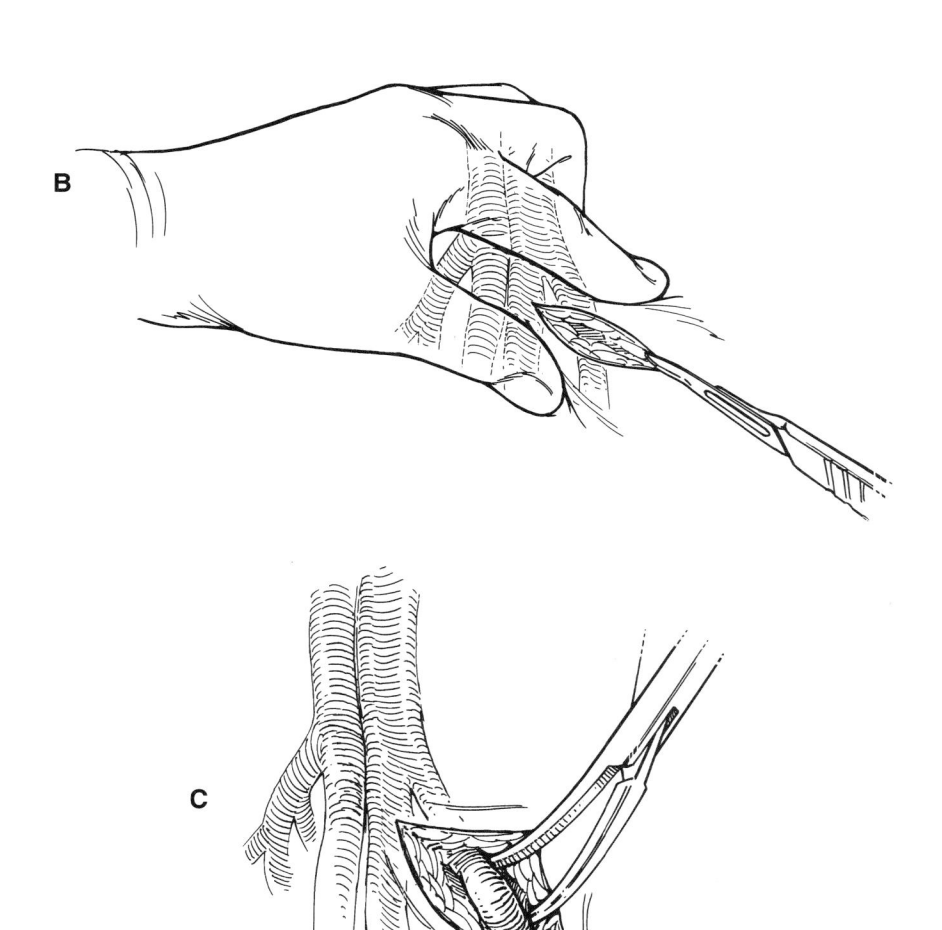

C

Upper Extremity Venous Cutdown — George Sternbach

Indications
- Need for emergency venous access in a patient without a good site for peripheral transcutaneous cannulation

Contraindications
- Known injury to the venous system proximal to the cutdown site

Equipment
- Betadine antiseptic solution
- Sterile drapes and gloves
- Local anesthetic (1% lidocaine), syringe, and needles
- Scalpels with No. 10 and 11 blades
- Curved Kelly and mosquito hemostats
- 3-0 absorbable suture
- 4-0 nylon suture
- IV cannula
- Vein pick
- 4 × 4 sterile gauze sponges

Procedure

1. Prepare site on the arm in sterile fashion. Administer local anesthetic into subcutaneous tissue of the selected site.
2. Locate the vessel.
   a. *Basilic vein cutdown:* The basilic vein is often encountered about 2 cm lateral to the medial epicondyle of the humerus on the anterior surface of the arm. A transverse incision over the medial portion of the arm 2 cm proximal and 2 to 3 cm lateral to the medial epicondyle will reveal this vessel *(A)*.
   b. *Cephalic vein cutdown:* The cephalic vein is located over the lateral portion of the distal arm. The incision is made transversely approximately 2 cm proximal to the antecubital crease, halfway between the lateral epicondyle and the biceps tendon *(A)*.
3. Dissect through the subcutaneous tissue by spreading the tissue with a curved mosquito hemostat.
4. Insert the hemostat on the medial side of the incision, and pass the tip under the vein.
5. Turn the tip of the hemostat, and exit at the lateral side of the incision. The vein will lie within the tissue atop the hemostat. (Subsequent steps are shown in illustrations *C* to *I* on pp. 91 to 93.)
6. Clear the vein of adventitious tissue by blunt dissection. Pass a 3-0 absorbable suture tie beneath the vein by grasping it with the hemostat.
7. Cut the suture at its midpoint, creating two sutures. Clamp the sutures, and position them at proximal and distal points on the exposed vein.
8. Tie the distal suture, thereby ligating the vessel distally.
9. Raising the vein by applying traction to the sutures, make a flap incision on the anterior wall of the vessel with a No. 11 scalpel blade.
10. Insert a vein pick to elevate the flap in the vein.
11. Pulling the vein taut by applying traction on the proximal suture, advance a catheter into the vessel by using the vein pick.
12. Flush the catheter with a small amount of sterile saline solution, and attach an IV line.
13. Tie the proximal suture around the portion of the vein containing the catheter.
14. Cut the ends of the proximal and distal ligatures.
15. Suture the catheter to the skin, and close the incision with 4-0 nylon suture.
16. Cover the incision site with a dressing. Tape the IV tubing in place.

Complications
- Hematoma formation
- Thrombophlebitis
- Injury to adjacent structures
- Transection of vein without ability to cannulate

Discussion
- The venous pattern of the upper extremity is more variable than that of the leg, and the location of a vein cannot be predicted with the same degree of certainty as the greater saphenous vein at the ankle.
- When the procedure is performed on a child or adult with a small vessel, injection of a small amount of lidocaine into the vein helps to overcome vascular spasm.

Bibliography
Simon RR et al: Modified new approaches for rapid intravenous access, *Ann Emerg Med* 16:44-49, 1987.

Wax PM, Talan DA: Advances in cutdown techniques, *Emerg Med Clin North Am* 7:65-82, 1989.

A

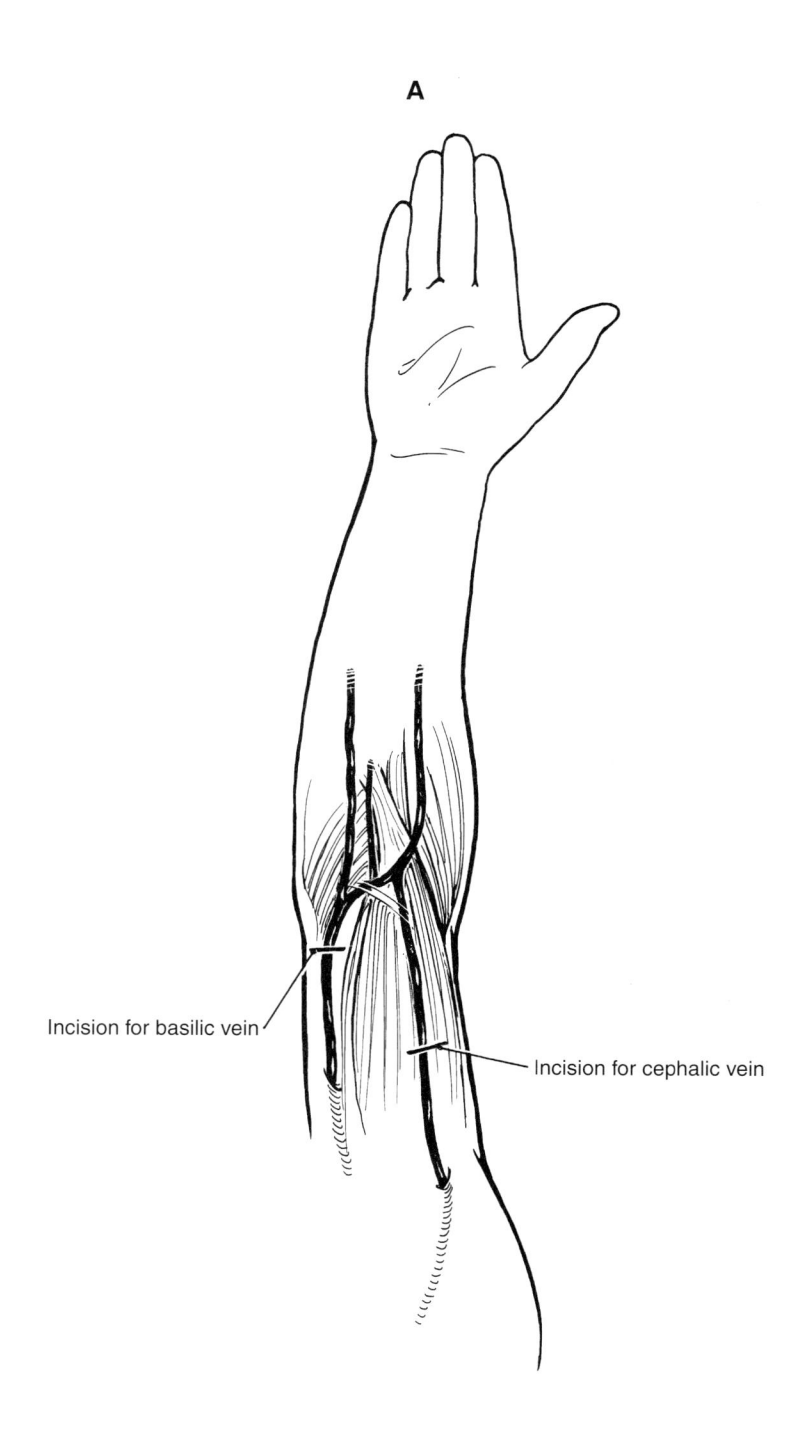

Incision for basilic vein

Incision for cephalic vein

Intraosseous Infusion EDWARD A. WALTON

Indications
- Inability to obtain emergency peripheral IV access
- Young child in full cardiopulmonary arrest

Contraindications
- Fractured or previously penetrated bone
- Cellulitis or burn at site of insertion
- History of osteogenesis imperfecta or osteoporosis

Equipment
- Sterile drapes and gloves
- Mask, gown, and goggles
- Sandbag or towel roll for support
- Povidine-iodine preparation
- Local anesthetic (1% lidocaine), syringe, and needles
- 15- or 18-gauge Jamshidi or similar needle with central trocar
- IV bag with IV tubing
- Pressure infusion pump
- Tape, 4 × 4 gauze pads, clear medicine cup

Procedure

1. Identify the insertion site on the proximal tibia, 1 to 2 cm below the tibial tuberosity on the medial surface, and prepare in sterile fashion *(A)*.
2. For a responsive patient, instill lidocaine through the skin to the periosteum at the insertion site.
3. Support the leg from behind with a sandbag or towel roll, and stabilize it with one hand while the other hand places the trocar.
4. Angle the needle slightly away from the joint, but nearly perpendicular to the bone.
5. Hold the needle approximately 1 cm from the tip for control to prevent penetration of both cortices of the bone.
6. Use a back-and-forth rotary motion with steady pressure until you feel a sensation of "giving way," which signals that the bone has been penetrated *(B)*.
7. The needle should then stand on its own.
8. Remove the trocar *(C)*, and confirm its position by the presence of pinkish marrow fluid in the needle when aspirated or by easy injection of a small amount of saline solution without evidence of extravasation. Strong resistance implies improper placement.
9. Attach the IV tubing with fluid, and reexamine the site for signs of extravasation. The fluid may have to be infused under pressure *(D)*.
10. Secure the needle with split 4 × 4 gauze pads and tape, and protect it with a clear medicine cup taped over the site.

Complications
- Extravasation or subcutaneous fluid infiltration
- Tibial fracture
- Compartment syndrome
- Osteomyelitis
- Cellulitis
- Fatty embolism

Discussion
- This procedure has been used successfully in the prehospital setting.
- Alternative sites in older children include the distal tibia in the midline, the junction of the medial maleollus, and the shaft of the tibia. In infants the distal femur in the midline 1 to 2 cm above the patella has also been used.
- Not all successful placements will have marrow returned on aspiration. If the site infuses well without evidence of extravasation, placement is considered correct.
- Medications that can be used in an intraosseous infusion include adenosine, antibiotics, atrocurium, atropine, calcium chloride, calcium gluconate, dexamethasone, diazepam, diazoxide, digoxin, dobutamine, dopamine, epinephrine, heparin, isoproterenol, levarterenol, lidocaine, lorazepam, phenytoin, propranolol, sodium bicarbonate, pentothal, succinylcholine, thiopental, normal saline, lactated Ringer's solution, dextrose, whole and packed red blood cells, and colloid.

Bibliography

Glaeser PW et al: Five-year experience in prehospital intraosseous infusions in children and adults, *Ann Emerg Med* 22:1119-1124, 1993.
Orlowski JP: Emergency alternatives to intravenous access, *Pediatr Clin North Am* 41:1183-1199, 1994.
Sawyer RW et al: The current status of intraosseous infusion, *J Am Coll Surg* 179:353-360, 1994.
Smith RJ et al: Intraosseous infusions by prehospital personnel in critically ill pediatric patients, *Ann Emerg Med* 17:491-495, 1988.
Spivey WH: Intraosseous infusions, *J Pediatr* 111:639-643, 1987.

Cardiovascular System

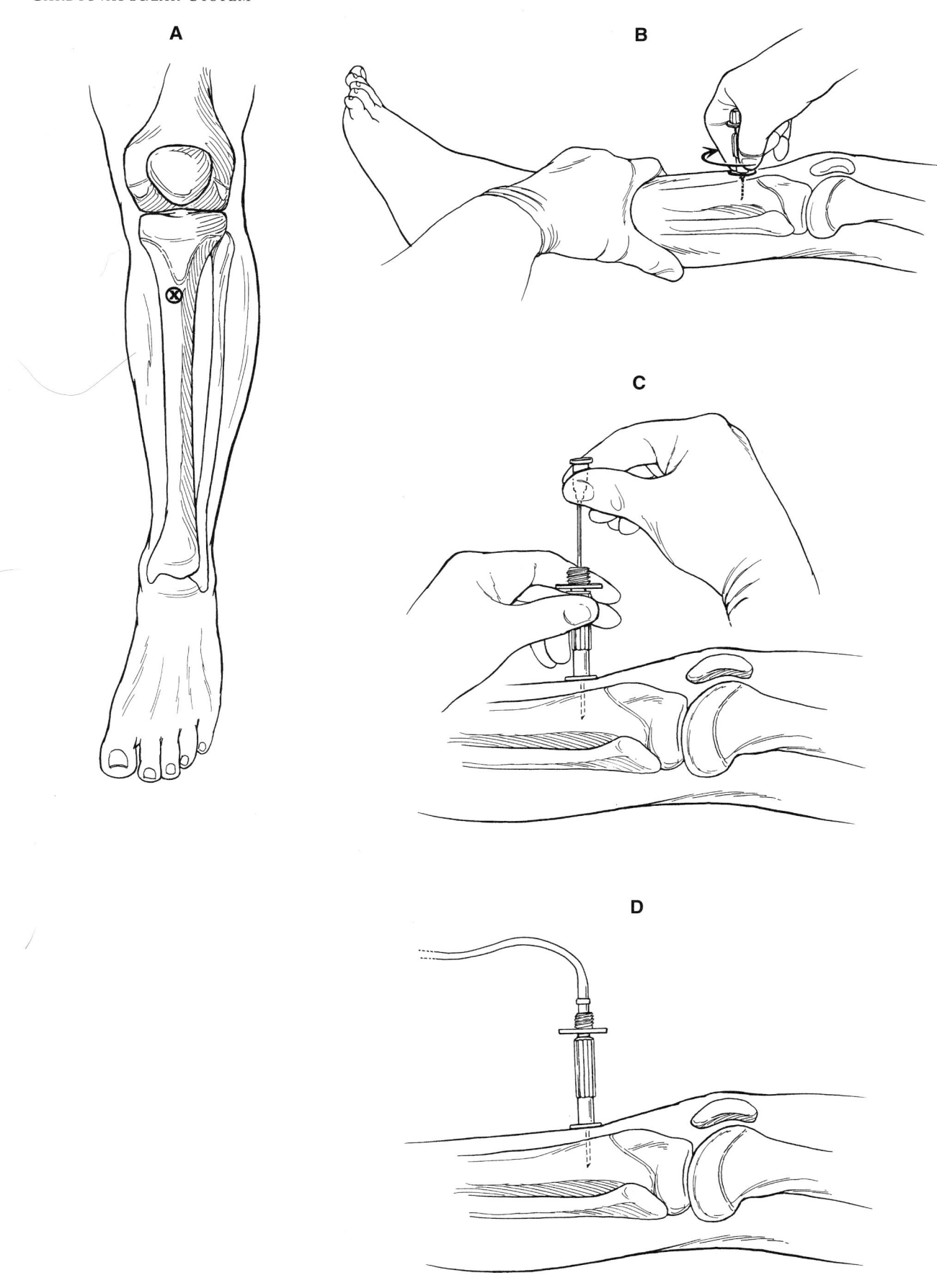

A

B

C

D

Umbilical Venous Catheter — Edward A. Walton

Indications
- Fluid or pharmacologic support of a severely depressed neonate

Contraindications
- Neonate with umbilical stump too dried to be cannulated

Equipment
- Sterile gloves and drapes
- Radiant warmer
- Umbilical tape or 3-0 silk suture
- Betadine antiseptic solution
- Sterile towels or clear sterile drape if wavailable
- Scalpel with No. 15 blade
- Mosquito hemostats
- 3.5 and 5.0 Fr umbilical catheters, 3.0 Fr feeding tube, or 18-gauge IV catheter flushed with heparinized saline
- Three-way stopcock, syringes, and fluid for IV infusion

Procedure
1. Place the infant supine under a radiant warmer with the extremities restrained.
2. Prepare the area around the umbilicus in sterile fashion.
3. Drape the patient with towels or the clear sterile drape, which allows better assessment of the neonate's status.
4. Place umbilical tape or suture around the base of the umbilicus, and tie it loosely.
5. Cut the umbilicus 1 to 2 cm from the abdomen *(A)*.
6. Three vessels—two thick-walled arteries and one thin-walled collapsible vein—should be seen.
7. To stabilize the edges of the umbilicus, grasp them with the hemostats.
8. Apply umbilical stump traction toward the feet, straightening the umbilical vein.
9. Place the flushed catheter, attached to a three-way stopcock and syringe, into the umbilical vein.
10. Advance the catheter to just below the skin, and tie it into place with the umbilical tape *(B)*.

Complications
- Infection
- Hepatic necrosis

Discussion
- In a resuscitation the catheter should be advanced to just below the skin, to the point where blood can be aspirated easily. More experienced operators may attempt to advance the catheter past the liver, approximately 7 to 12 cm, but this increases the risk of infusion directly into the liver. This deeper placement should be confirmed by x-ray examination before fluids or medications are infused. All medications required for neonatal resuscitation can be given via an umbilical vein catheter.

Bibliography
Balagtas R et al: Risk of local and systemic infections associated with umbilical vein catheterization: a prospective study in 86 newborn patients, *Pediatrics* 48:359-367, 1971.

Bloom R, Cropley C: Lesson 6. Medications. In American Academy of Pediatrics and American Heart Association: *Textbook of neonatal resuscitation,* Dallas, 1996, The Academy and The Association, pp 6-1-6-46.

Emergency Cardiac Care Committee and Subcommittees of the American Heart Association: Guidelines for cardiopulmonary resuscitation and emergency cardiac care, *JAMA* 268:2276-2281, 1992.

McAneney C: Umbilical vessel catheterization. In Deickman RA et al, eds: *Pediatric emergency and critical care procedures,* St Louis, 1997, Mosby, pp 503-505.

Pediatric Working Group of the International Liaison Committee on Resuscitation: ILCOR advisory statements: pediatric resuscitation, *Circulation* 95:2185-2195, 1997.

A

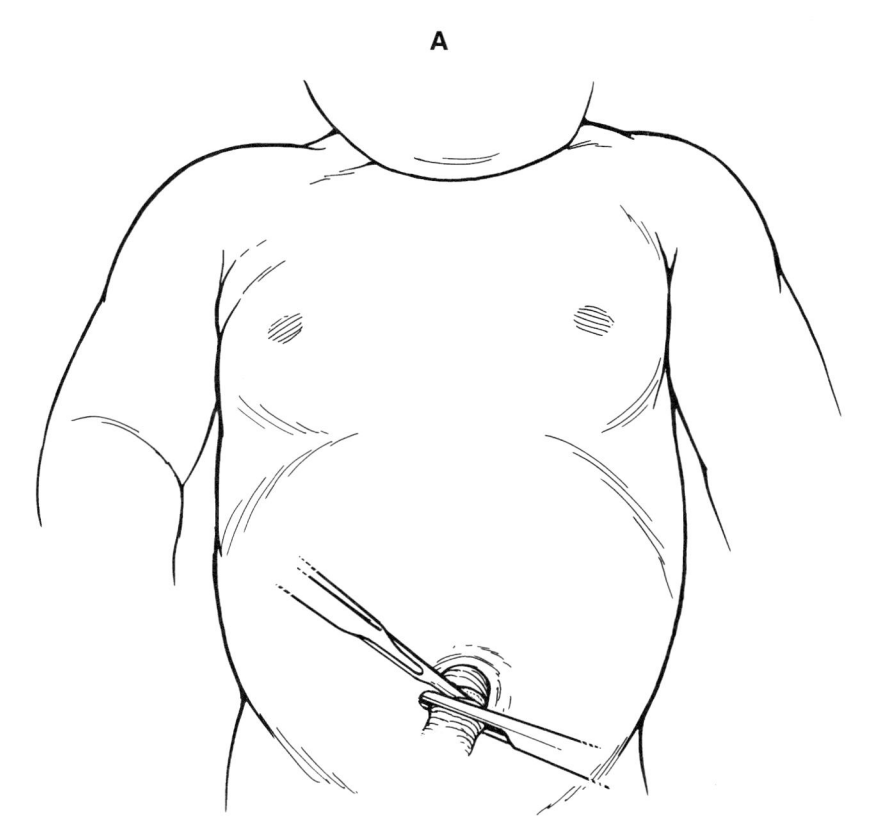

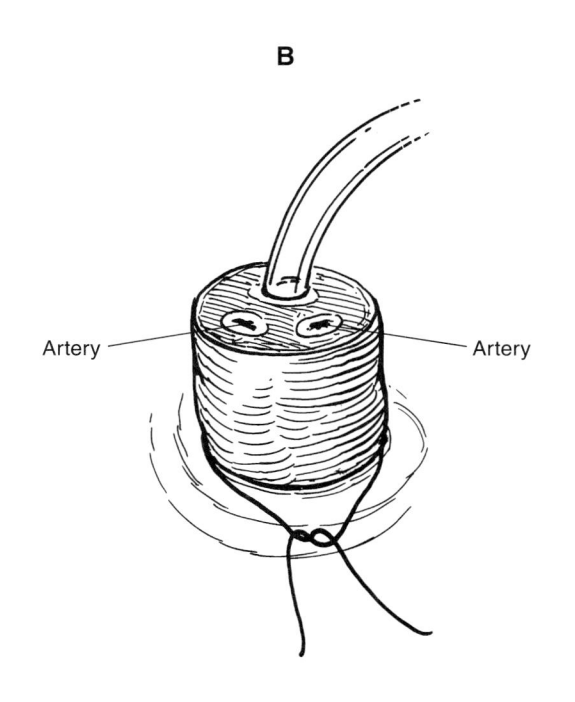

B

Artery — — Artery

CHAPTER 4

ABDOMEN

Nasogastric Intubation ■ JOHN MARX

Indications

- Diagnostic indications:
  - Visualization of diaphragmatic hernia
  - Insertion of air to assess for intraperitoneal perforation
  - Ascertainment of presence, volume, and rapidity of an upper gastrointestinal hemorrhage
  - Laboratory analysis of intragastric contents
- Therapeutic indications:
  - Administration of medication (e.g., charcoal)
  - Treatment of recurrent vomiting
  - Relief of bowel obstruction
  - Preoperative gastric decompression

Contraindications

- Absolute contraindications:
  - Cribriform plate injury or midface fractures because of high risk of intracranial intubation (orogastric tube placement may be considered)
- Relative contraindications:
  - Esophageal stricture or weakening (e.g., recent alkali exposure)
  - Coagulopathy
  - Recent nasal surgery or obstruction

Equipment

- Gloves, gown, and mask
- Nasogastric (NG) tube (Levin, Salem sump)
- Topical vasoconstrictor spray or liquid
- Topical anesthetic jelly or ointment (viscous lidocaine jelly)
- Lubricant jelly
- Topical anesthetic agent (e.g., benzocaine)
- Tongue blade
- Water and flexible drinking straw
- 50- to 60-ml syringe
- Affixing tape
- Magill forceps

Procedure

1. Use universal precautions, and gown the patient appropriately.
2. Position the patient sitting upright against bed or backrest to prevent the patient from withdrawing during the procedure.
3. Select tube type and size. A Levin tube has a single lumen used for diagnostic aspiration or instillation of material; a Salem sump contains a second lumen that permits venting during continuous suctioning. Standard adults require 16 Fr size, but larger tubes are preferred for lavage or when viscous or particulate matter is anticipated.
4. Estimate tube insertion depth by adding the distance from the tip of the nose to the earlobe plus the distance from the earlobe to the xiphoid. Add 6 to 8 inches to this distance for the portion of the tube that will be exterior to the nares.
5. Check the nares for patency by occluding each nostril separately and asking the patient to inhale.
6. Administer topical vasoconstrictor liquid or spray to the naris selected for insertion. A topical anesthetic agent may be sprayed into the oropharynx to diminish gagging.
7. Anesthetize and lubricate the naris by administering 5 to 10 ml of topical jelly or ointment via syringe and massaging it into the naris with the little finger.
8. Lubricate the distal 6 cm of the NG tube with the lubricant jelly (anesthetic lubricant here is unnecessary and ineffective).
9. Insert the tip of the tube into the inferior portion of the naris. The tube should be directed at a 90° angle to the patient's face so that the tube will slide along the nasal floor beneath the inferior turbinate. Mild resistance will be met as the tube reaches the posterior nasopharynx.
10. Apply gentle pressure to help the tube turn the corner, and proceed in a caudad direction. Have the patient sip water through the straw to facilitate passage of the tube through the esophagus and into the stomach *(A,B)*.

Abdomen

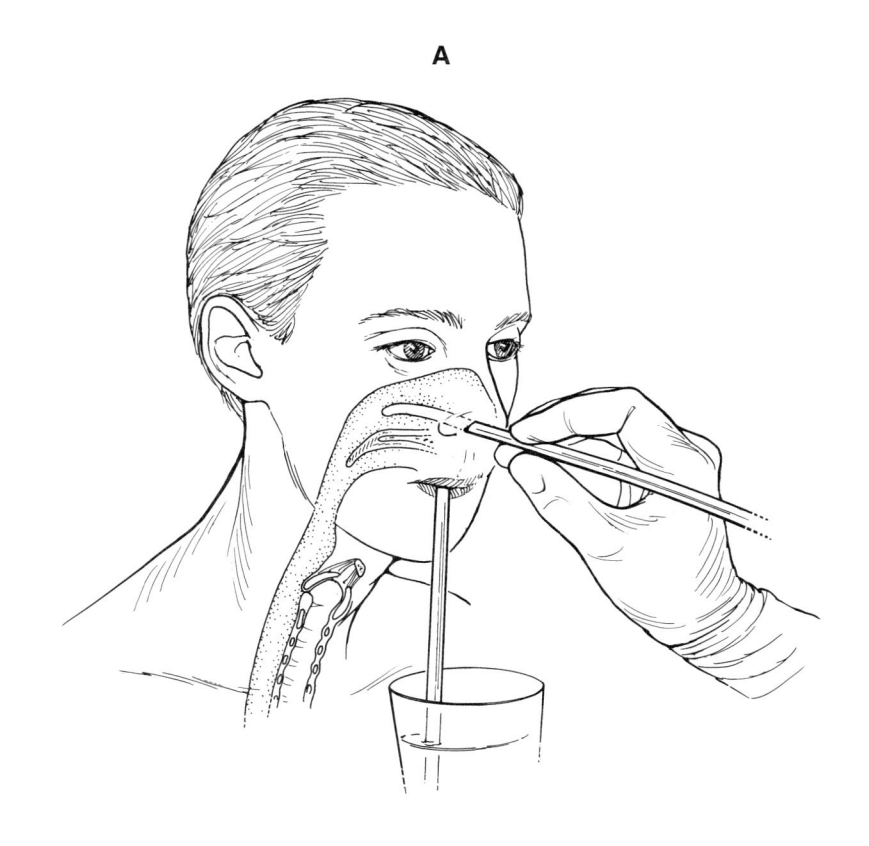

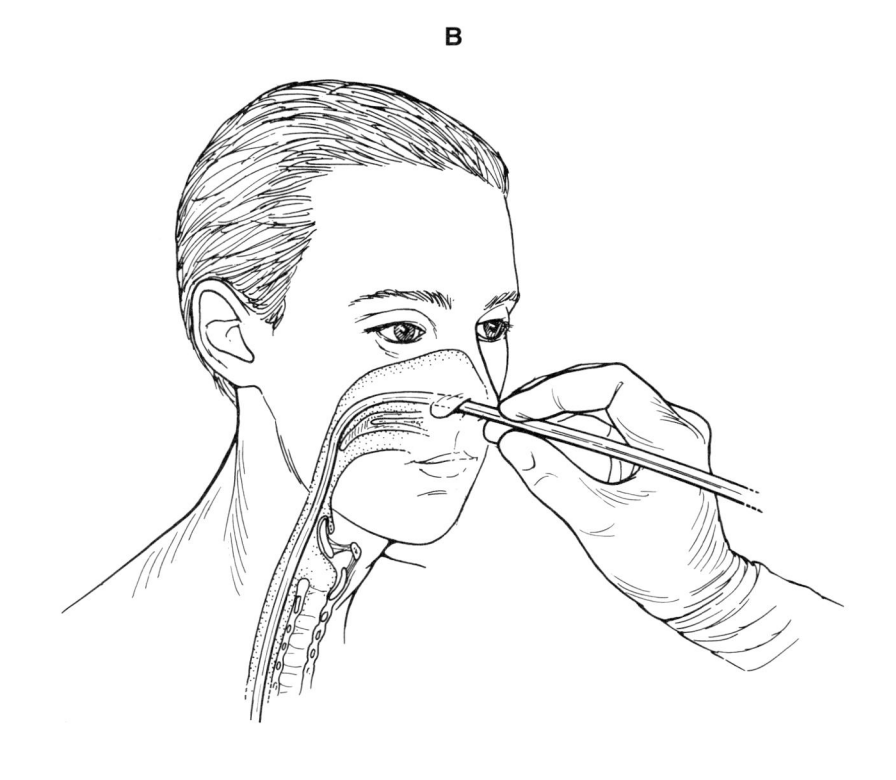

A

B

11. Confirm NG tube placement by instilling 50 to 60 cc of air into it while auscultating the gastric area for air sounds *(C)*. Another means of confirmation relies on pH testing of aspirated material. A pH less than 4 strongly indicates gastric contents.
12. Secure the tube by wrapping adhesive tape around it and securing it to each side of the nose. Also affix the tube to some part of the patient's clothing with a safety pin to prevent inadvertent removal.

Complications

- Oropharyngeal coiling
- Endotracheal intubation
- Nasopharyngeal injury (epistaxis, erosion)
- Pulmonary placement
- Pneumothorax
- Pneumomediastinum
- Mediastinitis
- Intracranial placement
- Pulmonary aspiration
- Increased intracranial pressure
- Sinusitis and otitis media

Discussion

- Only mild force should be used when inserting the tube to avoid injuring the naris, oropharynx, or esophagus. The use of a nasal trumpet may be more acceptable to patients as a first step before NG tube insertion.
- Intubation of the trachea is a common occurrence and is heralded by profound coughing, inability to speak, and misting of the NG tube. The tube should be removed immediately and the procedure reattempted. Mild neck flexion and gentle grasping and lifting of the thyroid cartilage can displace the larynx forward and assist in the correct placement of the tube.
- NG tubes may be difficult to insert in patients who are endotracheally intubated. This problem can be overcome by quickly deflating the endotracheal balloon, passing the NG tube, and reinflating the balloon.
- Oropharyngeal coiling can be prevented by cooling the NG tube in ice water (to make it stiffer) or using a larger bore tube. The operator can also manually (or by use of Magill forceps) guide the tube away from the oropharynx and down into the esophagus.
- If NG tube placement is unsuccessful or contraindicated, orogastric tube placement should be considered. In addition, esophagoscopy can be used when standard placement is unsuccessful or contraindicated or when direct visualization will help prevent complications.

Bibliography

Day AC et al: Diagnostic peritoneal lavage: integration with clinical information to improve diagnostic performance, *J Trauma* 32:52, 1992.

Engrav LH et al: Diagnostic peritoneal lavage in blunt abdominal trauma, *J Trauma* 15:854, 1975.

Goff JS: Gastroesophageal varices: pathogenesis and therapy of acute bleeding, *Gastroenterol Clin North Am* 22:779, 1993.

Prall JA et al: Early definitive abdominal evaluation in the triage of unconscious normotensive blunt trauma patients, *J Trauma* 37:792, 1994.

Ritter DM et al: Placement of nasogastric tubes and esophageal stethoscopes in patients with documented esophageal varices, *Anesth Analg* 67:283, 1988.

ABDOMEN	107

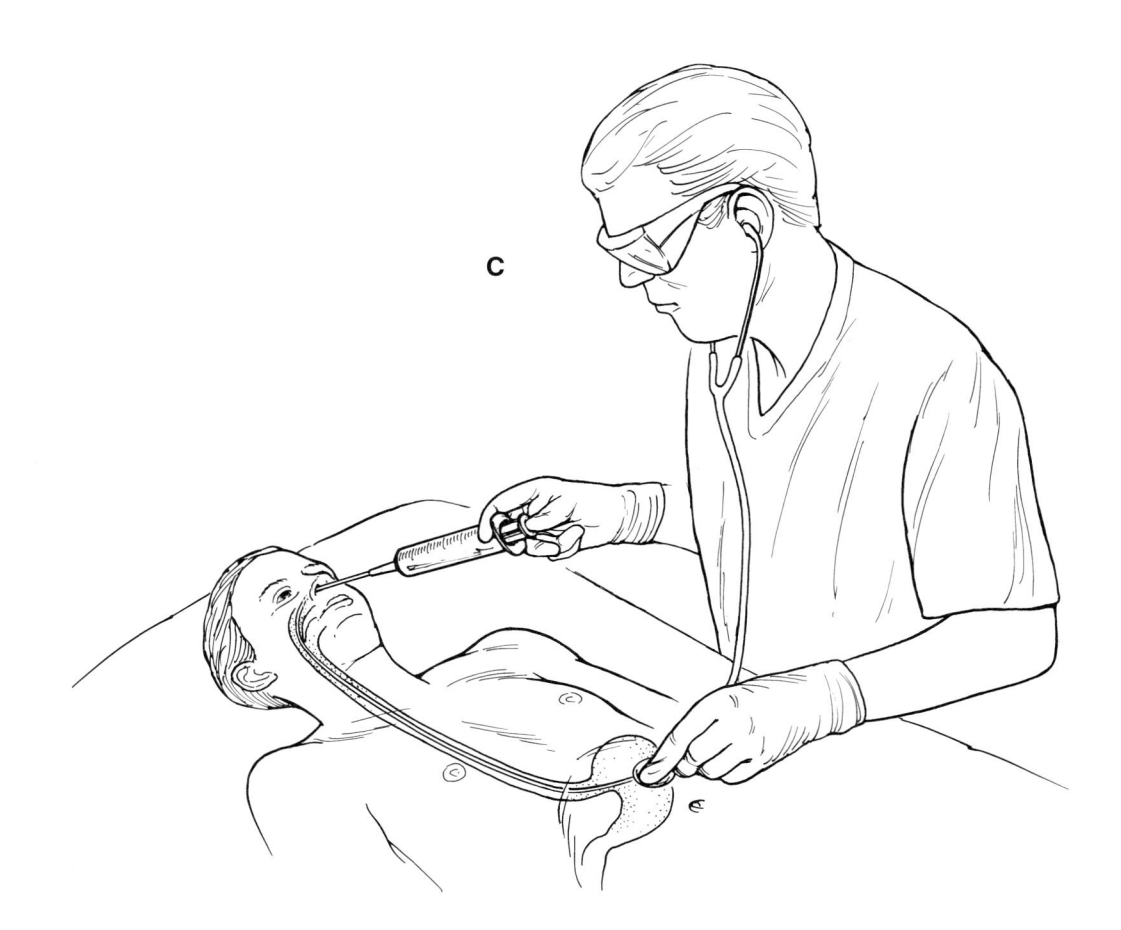

C

Semiopen Diagnostic Peritoneal Lavage • JOHN MARX

Indications
- In cases of trauma, rapid determination of the presence of intraperitoneal hemorrhage (peritoneal aspirate) or of solid and hollow organ injury or diaphragmatic injury (peritoneal lavage)
- Treatment of hypothermia by lavage of the peritoneal cavity with warmed fluids
- Diagnosis of various conditions by discovery of blood or infection

Contraindications
- Absolute contraindications:
  - Clinical mandate for laparotomy
- Relative contraindications:
  - Midline abdominal surgery
  - Obesity
  - Coagulopathy
  - Abdominal wall infection
  - Second or third trimester of pregnancy
  - Pelvic fracture (lavage interpretation only)

Equipment
- Sterile gloves and drapes
- Betadine antiseptic solution
- Local anesthetic (1% lidocaine without epinephrine), syringe, and needles
- Scalpel with No. 11 blade
- Small curved clamps
- Four towel clips
- Lavage catheter with trocar
- Right-angle adaptor and IV tubing
- 1-L bag of normal saline solution
- 10-ml non-Luer-Lok syringe

Procedure
1. Ideally this procedure is performed with an assistant.
2. Use universal precautions, and assemble equipment.
3. Decompress the stomach and bladder (with nasogastric tube and urinary catheter).
4. Prepare the field over the midline abdomen in sterile fashion.
5. Identify the diagnostic peritoneal lavage (DPL) site: the midline infraumbilical ring region approximately 2 cm below the umbilicus.
6. Anesthetize the DPL site with 1% lidocaine without epinephrine.
7. Make a 4- to 6-cm vertical midline infraumbilical incision with a No. 11 blade *(A)*.
8. Use towel clamps to lift tissue, and the No. 11 blade to cut down to the rectus fascia *(B, C)*. A second set of towel clamps can be used to get deeper grasp of the tissue *(D)*.
9. Using the curved clamp or handle of the scalpel, bluntly dissect (curved clamp) to better expose the rectus fascia through the incision.
10. Apply a towel clip to each side of the rectus fascia, and gently lift the rectus fascia.
11. Make a 3-mm incision through the rectus fascia in the midline (linea alba) with a No. 11 scalpel *(E)*.

Abdomen

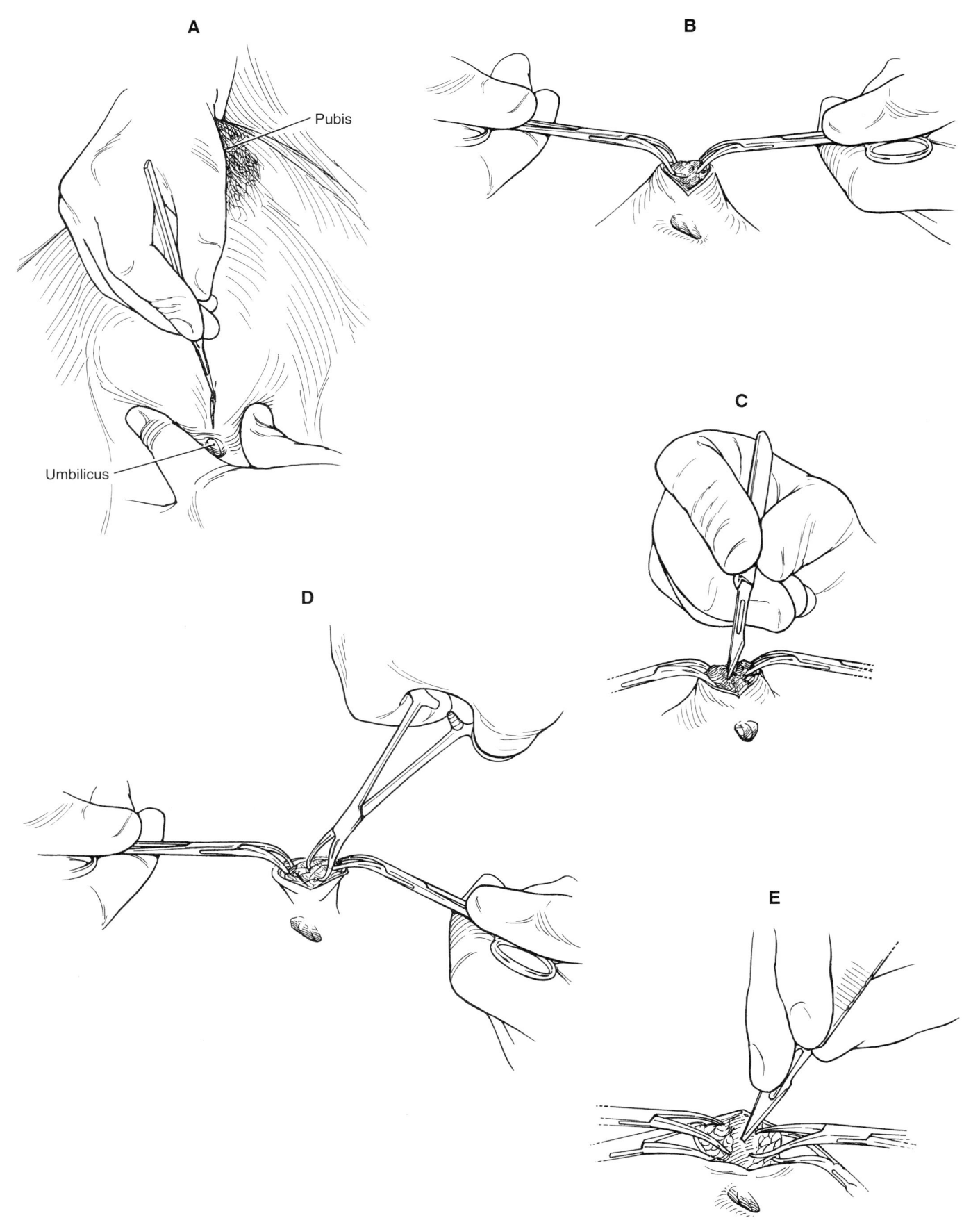

A

Pubis

Umbilicus

B

C

D

E

12. Insert a catheter with trocar at 45° caudad through the rectus fascia and peritoneum *(F)*. A slight resistance should be felt that gives way when the peritoneum is penetrated. Have one hand on the catheter-trocar at its distal end so that after entry through the fascia the trocar can be prevented from excessive penetration through the peritoneum.
13. Once the catheter-trocar assembly has been advanced 0.5 to 1 cm, remove the trocar and advance the catheter caudad toward the pelvis, gently entering the right or left pelvic gutter. Do not use excessive force. A gentle twisting motion during advancement of the catheter may minimize visceral or omental injury.
14. Attach the right-angle adaptor and extension tubing *(G)*.
15. Attempt peritoneal aspiration with the 10-ml non-Luer-Lok syringe (recovery of 10 ml blood terminates the procedure).
16. Perform DPL by removing the syringe and attaching a 1-L bag of normal saline solution to extension tubing. Elevate the bag so that fluid runs into the peritoneal cavity through the catheter. Generally, 15 ml/kg (1 L for an adult) of normal saline should be infused into the peritoneal cavity.
17. After the normal saline lavage fluid has been infused, place the IV bag below the abdomen (e.g., on the floor) and allow fluid to return by gravity drainage. Ideally at least 700 ml of the 1 L will return *(H)*.
18. Submit effluent fluid samples for laboratory analysis.
19. Close the rectus fascia (single-layer absorbable suture) if laparotomy is not needed (i.e., DPL results are negative).
20. Close the subcutaneous tissue and skin (single-layer nonabsorbable suture) if laparatomy is not indicated.

Complications

- Infection
- Hematoma
- Wound separation or dehiscence
- Systemic infection
- Hollow visceral injury
- Vascular penetration
- Preperitoneal placement
- Diaphragmatic tear

Discussion

- The semiopen procedure has traditionally been considered the safest and most accurate. However, a Seldinger wire-guided approach has been described and may be an acceptable alternative. The fully open technique should be used when the semiopen or closed technique is unsuccessful. The open technique is identical to the semiopen except that the peritoneal cavity is opened under direct supervision.
- The preferred site for DPL is midline at the infraumbilical ring. Alternative sites may be considered, including the midline supraumbilical region (pelvic fracture, pregnancy) or left lower quadrant (dense midline scarring). In these cases a fully open technique should be used.
- In a patient whose condition is unstable, the attempted peritoneal aspiration of blood is the critical portion of the procedure. This can generally be accomplished in less than 5 minutes. The introduction and recovery of lavage effluent may require 20 to 30 minutes, but decision making concerning these patients can be delayed for that period of time without problem.
- A number of complications may prevent adequate return of lavage effluent, including preperitoneal catheter placement, obstruction of lavage catheter by air, peritoneum, or omentum, compartmentalization of fluid by adhesions, and diaphragmatic tear. The operator should aspirate air in the IV line or bag as needed. Gentle movement and twisting of the catheter while in place may dislodge any obstruction at the catheter tip. Gentle palpation of the subject's abdomen may also increase lavage effluent.

Bibliography

Henneman PL et al: Diagnostic peritoneal lavage: accuracy in predicting necessary laparotomy following blunt and penetrating trauma, *J Trauma* 30:1345-1355, 1990.

Lopez-Viego MA et al: Open versus closed diagnostic peritoneal lavage in the evaluation of abdominal trauma, *Am J Surg* 160:594-597, 1990.

Marx JA: Diagnostic peritoneal lavage. In Ivatury RR, Cayten CG (eds): *The textbook of penetrating trauma*, Baltimore, 1996, Williams & Wilkins, pp 335-343.

Moore G et al: Is closed diagnostic peritoneal lavage contraindicated in patients with previous abdominal surgery? *Acad Emerg Med* 4:287, 1997.

Root HD et al: Diagnostic peritoneal lavage, *Surgery* 57:633-637, 1965.

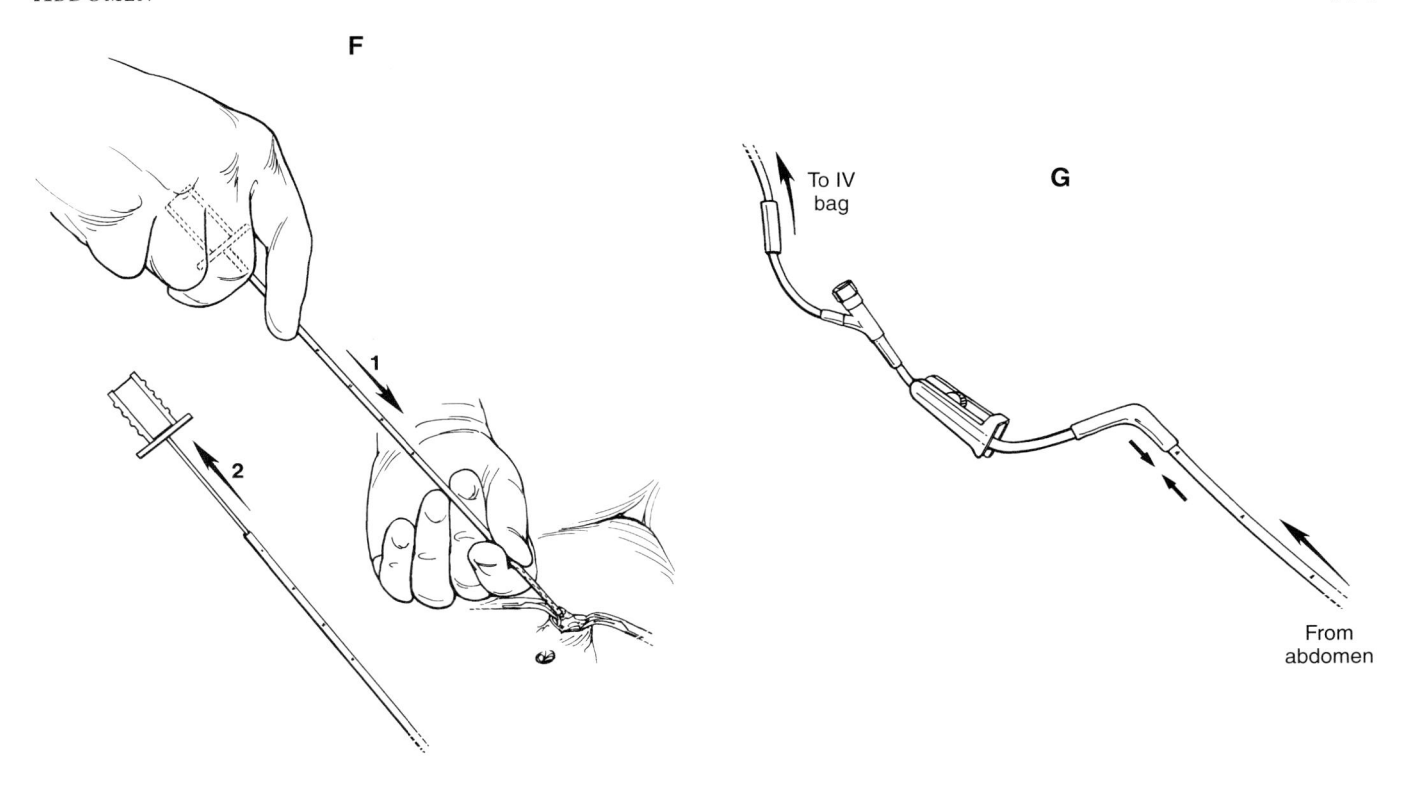

ABDOMEN

F

G To IV bag

From abdomen

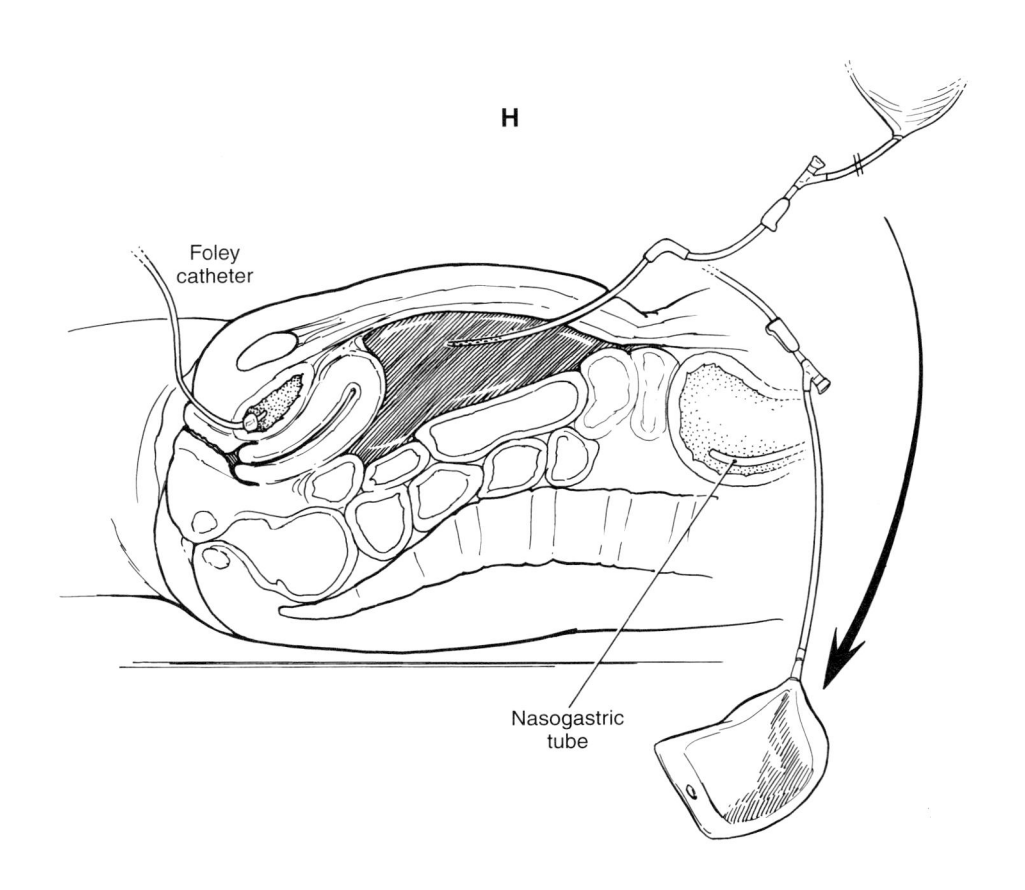

H

Foley catheter

Nasogastric tube

Paracentesis ■ THEODORE C. CHAN

Indications
- Determination of etiology of ascites
- Suspected bacterial peritonitis
- Therapeutic large-volume tap in presence of tense ascites

Contraindications
- Coagulopathy
- Thrombocytopenia
- Infection overlying site
- Pregnancy (relative contraindication)

Equipment
- Sterile gloves and drapes
- Betadine antiseptic solution
- Local anesthetic (1% lidocaine with epinephrine), syringe, and needles
- 50-ml or larger syringe
- 18-gauge angiocatheter
- IV connection tubing and vacuum containers (for large-volume therapeutic paracentesis)

Procedure

1. Have the patient empty the bladder.
2. Place the patient in a supine semirecumbent position with the head of the bed elevated so that dependent ascites fluid collects in the lower abdomen.
3. Identify the appropriate site for paracentesis. Select either lower quadrant just lateral to the rectus muscle (avoiding the epigastric vessels) or midline a few centimeters below the umbilicus where dependent ascites fluid is clinically detected *(A)*.
4. Prepare and drape site in sterile fashion.
5. Inject a small wheal of local anesthetic at the site *(B)*.
6. Attach the angiocatheter to the larger syringe. Direct the angiocatheter into the site at a 70° to 90° angle to the skin *(C)*. Apply slight traction on the skin at the site when first entering the skin. This will form a Z-track through the skin and subcutaneous tissue that will help seal the needle tract and prevent leakage once the angiocatheter is removed *(D)*.
7. When advancing the angiocatheter, draw back on the plunger at all times. Once peritoneal fluid returns into the syringe, stop advancing the angiocatheter.
8. For diagnostic paracentesis:
   a. Remove as much fluid as needed (usually 20 to 50 ml).
   b. Withdraw the angiocatheter with inner needle completely and dress the site.
9. For therapeutic paracentesis:
   a. Advance the catheter over the needle into the peritoneal space
   b. Withdraw the inner needle, leaving the catheter in place. Place a finger over the hub of the catheter.
   c. Attach one end of the IV tubing to the hub of the catheter. Attach the other end of the tubing by needle to a vacuum container bottle.
   d. Drain the desired amount of fluid (usually 1 to 2 L).
   e. Withdraw the catheter completely and dress the site.

Complications
- Site infection
- Bleeding
- Hematoma
- Bacterial peritonitis
- Bowel or bladder perforation
- Vascular or nerve injury
- Peritoneal foreign body
- Ascitic fluid leakage

Discussion
- Large-volume paracentesis can be safely performed in the emergency department. Commercially available kits that include a catheter, trocar, tubing, and collection containers can be used for such procedures.
- Ascites fluid can be loculated because of mesenteric attachments, prior surgery, and adhesions. Ultrasound guidance is often useful in identifying pockets of fluid for paracentesis. Ultrasound guidance, as well as a supraumbilical approach, is strongly suggested for pregnant patients.
- The site should not be over a surgical scar because of the presence of intraabdominal adhesions and increased risk of bowel perforation. Sites with overlying visible collateral venous channels on the abdominal wall, commonly seen in patients with liver disease, should also be avoided. In patients with liver disease, clotting and platelet abnormalities may need to be corrected before the procedure to prevent significant bleeding.

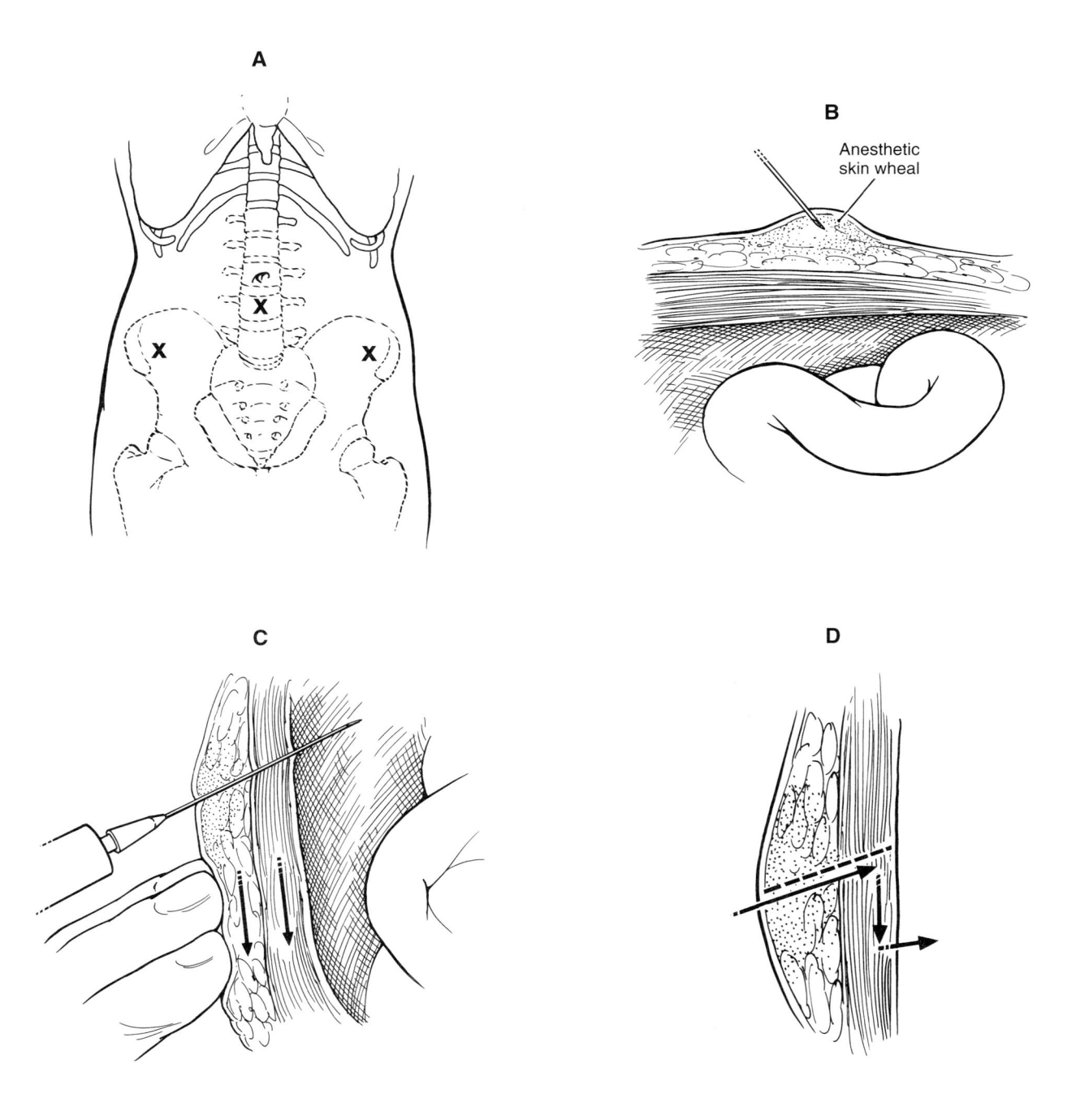

- If initial fluid flow stops, the needle or catheter may be gently advanced, rotated, or angulated. In addition, the patient may be rolled to the lateral decubitus position in order to direct fluid toward the needle site. Palpation and pressure over other parts of the abdomen may also move fluid toward the needle site.

Bibliography

Arroyo V et al: Treatment of ascites in cirrhosis: diuretics, peritoneovenous shunt, and large-volume paracentesis, *Gastroenterol Clin North Am* 21(1):237-255, 1992.

Hudson PPA, Promes SB: Abdominal ultrasonography, *Emerg Med Clin North Am* 15(4):825-848, 1997.

Neighbor ML: Ascites, *Emerg Med Clin North Am* 7(3):683-697, 1989.

Anoscopy • STEVEN LARSON

Indications
- Evaluate rectal discomfort or pain with defecation, bright red blood per rectum, anorectal drainage, perirectal infections, fistulas, tears, foreign bodies, or internal hemorrhoids

Contraindications
- Imperforate anus
- Anal stenosis and severe pain (relative contraindications)

Equipment
- Anoscope with removable obturator
- Internal or external light source
- Topical anesthetic (2% lidocaine gel)
- Lubricants
- Swabs
- Forceps
- Culture media

Procedure
1. Administer appropriate sedative or analgesic.
2. Place the patient in the lateral (Sims') position (A) or the knee-chest position (A on p. 117).
3. Administer anesthetic.
4. Apply lubricant.
5. Perform digital examination to locate the pain and assess for fecal impaction, mass, stricture, and prostate disease.
6. Insert a well-lubricated anoscope with a fully inserted obturator while the patient gently bears down (B).
7. Advance the anoscope until the outer flange rests against the anal verge, and remove the obturator (C, D).
8. As you visualize the mucosa, slowly withdraw the anoscope, rotating it to facilitate complete inspection (E).

Complications
- Bleeding from local irritation (most common complication)

Discussion
- The operator's thumb should be kept on the obturator during insertion. The obturator should not be reinserted until the anoscope is completely removed.
- Anorectal emergencies are associated with increased pain and anxiety. Liberal use of sedation and analgesia is recommended if these symptoms do not allow adequate visualization with topical anesthetic.

Bibliography
Abcarian H et al: Benign anorectal disease: definition, characterization, and analysis of treatment, *Am J Gastroenterol* 89(suppl):S182-S193, 1994.

Coates W: Disorders of the anorectum. In Rosen P, Barkin R (eds): *Emergency medicine: concepts and clinical practice*, ed 4, St Louis, 1998, Mosby, pp 2037-2052.

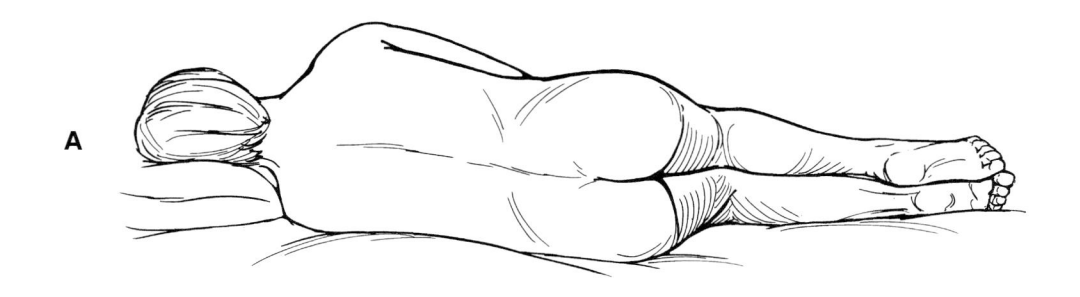

A

B

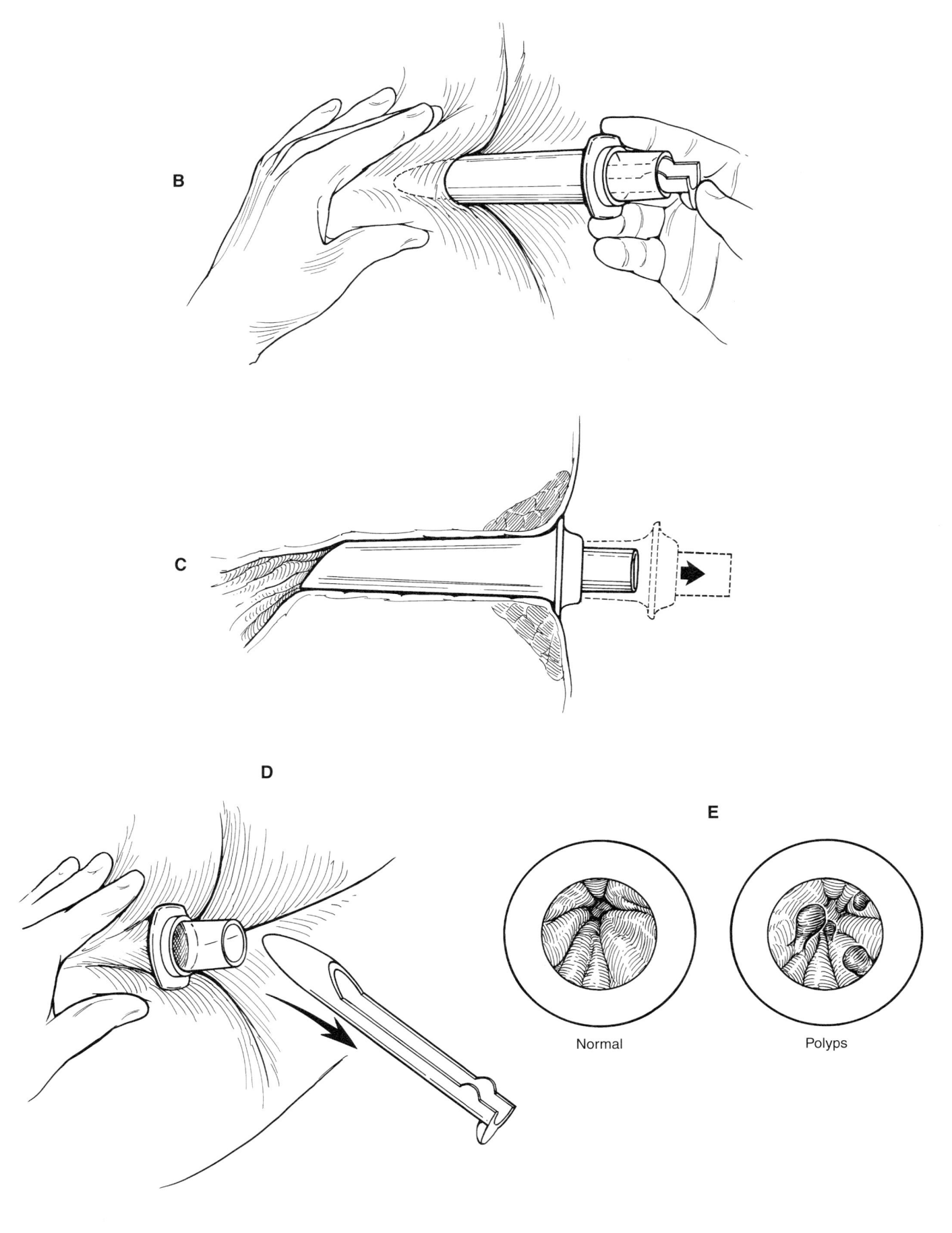

C

D

E

Normal   Polyps

Excision of Thrombosed External Hemorrhoid ▪ STEVEN LARSON

Indications
- Within 48 hours of symptom onset for large, painful, thrombosed external hemorrhoids that appear clinically as firm, tender, engorged perianal veins with a bluish discoloration

Contraindications
- Prolapsed internal hemorrhoids
- Nonthrombosed venous plexus
- Bleeding disorders
- Pediatric patients
- Pregnant women
- Immunocompromised patients

Equipment
- Local anesthetic (lidocaine), syringe, and needles
- Betadine antiseptic solution
- Tincture of benzoin
- Sterile drapes
- Tape
- Standard laceration repair kit
- Scalpel with No. 11 blade
- 4 × 4 gauze pads

Procedure

1. Place patient in prone position on proctoscopic table or in knee-chest (Skinner's) position *(A)*.
2. Apply tincture of benzoin along the buttocks.
3. Tape the buttocks open to expose the anal region *(B)*.
4. Prepare the area in sterile fashion.
5. Administer local anesthetic beneath the skin at the site, but not into the hemorrhoid *(C, D_1)*.
6. Elevate the skin with forceps, and make an elliptical incision directed radially from the anal orifice *(D_2)*.
7. Excise the flap of skin to expose the clot *(D_3)*.
8. Remove underlying clot with forceps or digital pressure *(D_4)*.
9. If minor bleeding persists, apply direct pressure.
10. Place gauze or a perineal pad in the gluteal cleft, with the buttocks taped together until bleeding stops.
11. Prescribe oral analgesics and stool softeners, and give the patient instructions regarding local wound care and sitz baths every 6 hours.

Complications

- Bleeding (in occasional cases)
- Infection (rarely)

Discussion

- Use of a linear incision should be avoided because this can result in incomplete evacuation of the clot.
- Small thrombosed hemorrhoids can be managed conservatively with stool softener, sitz baths, and topical ointments.
- Antibiotics are not clinically indicated.
- Liberal use of sedation and analgesia is recommended to facilitate examination and the procedure.

Bibliography

Abcarian H et al: Benign anorectal disease: definition, characterization, and analysis of treatment, *Am J Gastroenterol* 89:S182-S193, 1994.

Coates W: Disorders of the anorectum. In Rosen P, Barkin R (eds): *Emergency medicine: concepts and clinical practice*, ed 4, St Louis, 1998, Mosby, pp 2037-2052.

Smith L: Hemorrhoids: a review of current techniques and management, *Gastroenterol Clin North Am* 16(1):79-91, 1987.

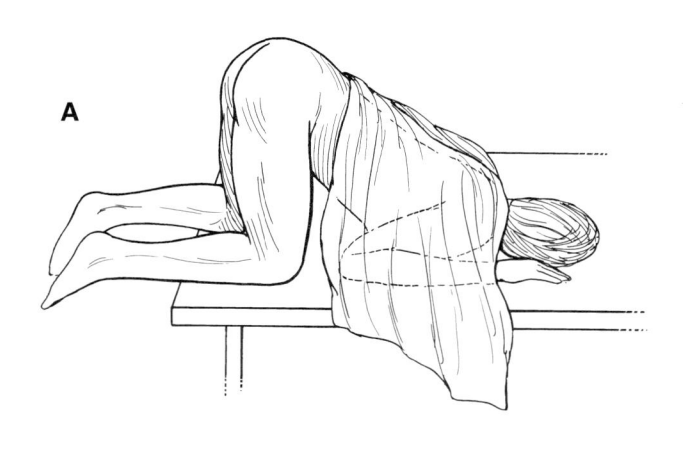

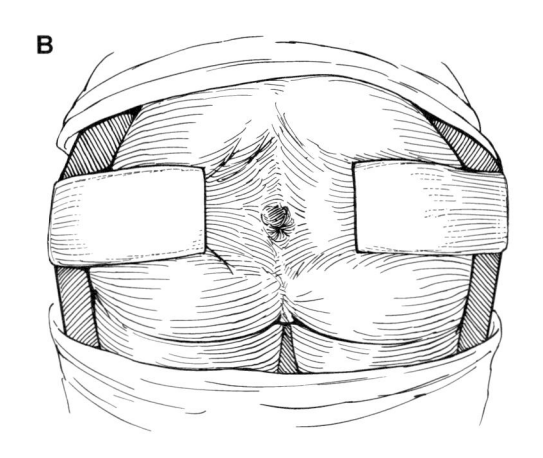

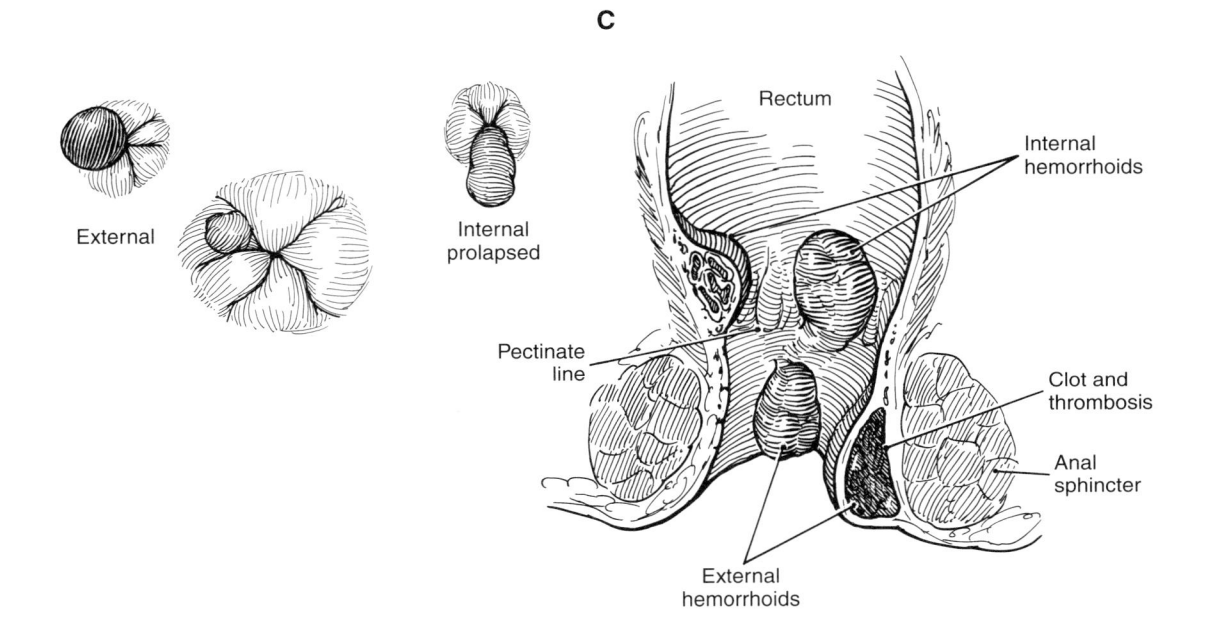

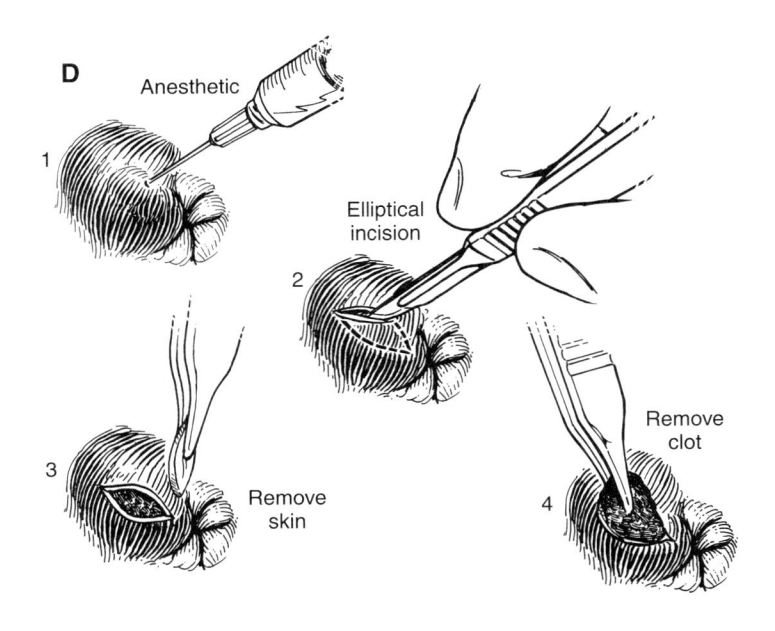

Abdomen

A

B

C

Rectum

Internal hemorrhoids

External

Internal prolapsed

Pectinate line

Clot and thrombosis

Anal sphincter

External hemorrhoids

D

1. Anesthetic
2. Elliptical incision
3. Remove skin
4. Remove clot

Pilonidal Abscess Drainage • STEVEN LARSON

Indications
- Swelling, tenderness, and induration in the sacrococcygeal region without systemic symptoms

Contraindications
- Deep infections, which need more definitive treatment

Equipment
- Local anesthetic (lidocaine), syringe, and needles
- Betadine antiseptic solution
- Gloves and drapes
- Tape
- Normal saline solution and syringe for irrigation
- 4 × 4 gauze pads
- ¼-inch iodoform gauze packing
- Standard laceration repair kit with hemostats and forceps
- Scalpel with No. 11 blade
- Yankauer suction setup (optional)

Procedure
1. Place the patient in the lateral Sims' position *(A)*.
2. Prepare and drape the site in sterile fashion.
3. Inject the anesthetic agent into the subcutaneous tissue over the site.
4. Cut down on the point of maximal swelling with the scalpel *(B)*.
5. Find the origin point of the pilonidal abscess, insert the hemostat into the wound, and spread.
6. Remove pus and debris from the wound *(C)*.
7. Irrigate the wound with normal saline solution.
8. Pack the wound with ¼-inch iodoform gauze wick, being careful not to overpack *(D)*.
9. Apply bulk dressing such as a perineal pad.
10. The patient should be given oral analgesics, as well as instructions regarding wound care and daily sitz baths. The wound should be checked in 48 to 72 hours.

Complications
- Recurrence (commonly occurs unless the sinus tract is completely excised)

Discussion
- Copious foul-smelling drainage should be expected. An abundance of 4 × 4 gauze pads should be available to contain drainage, or a sterile Yankauer suction can be used to remove debris and drainage material from the surgical field.
- Liberal use of analgesia and sedation is recommended to facilitate the examination and procedure.

Bibliography
Lord P: Pilonidal sinus: a simple treatment, *Br J Surg* 52:298-300, 1965.
Walter I: Total excision versus non-resectional methods in the treatment of acute and chronic pilonidal disease, *Br J Surg* 82:752-753, 1995.

A

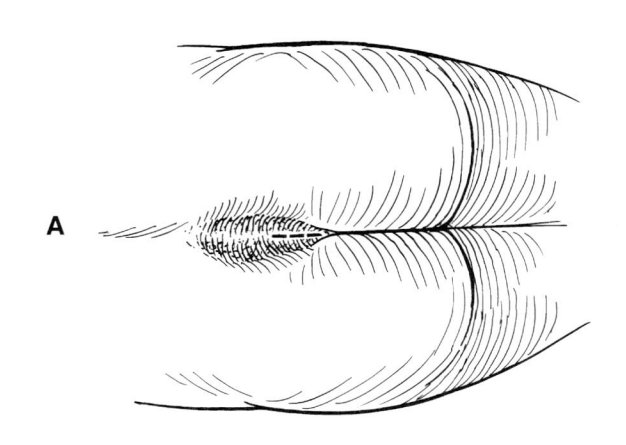

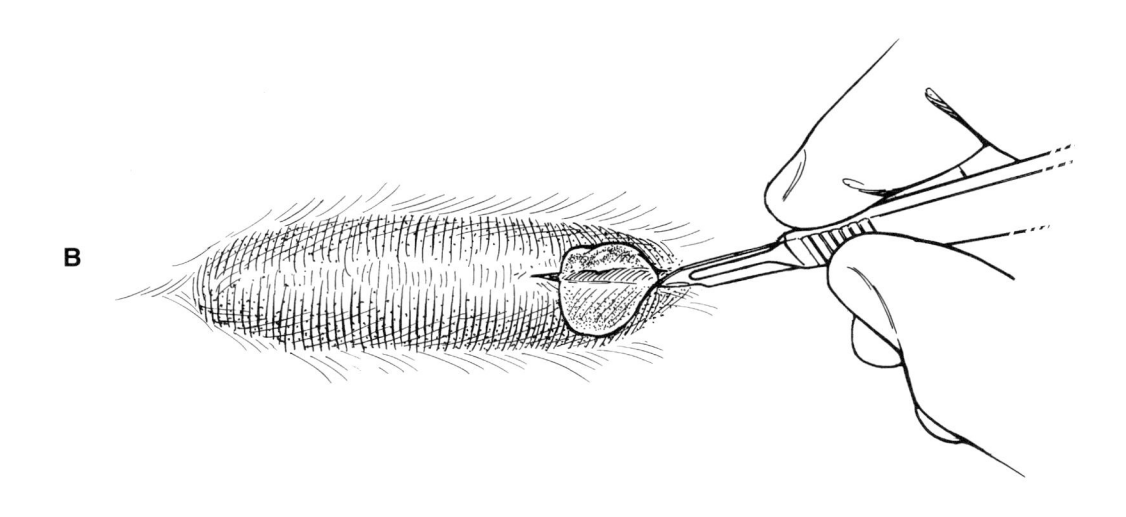

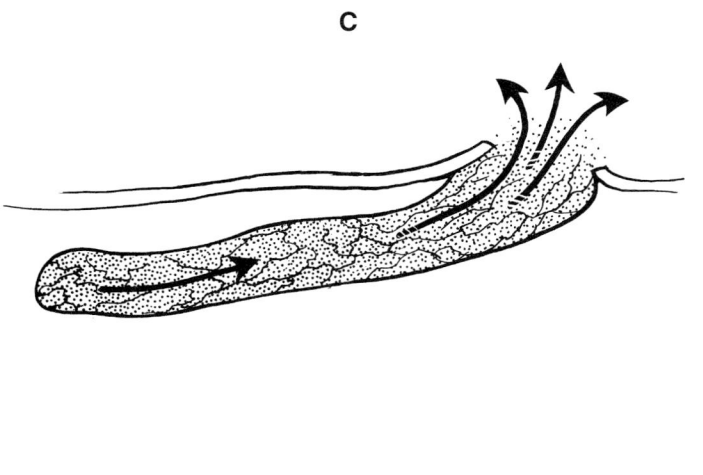

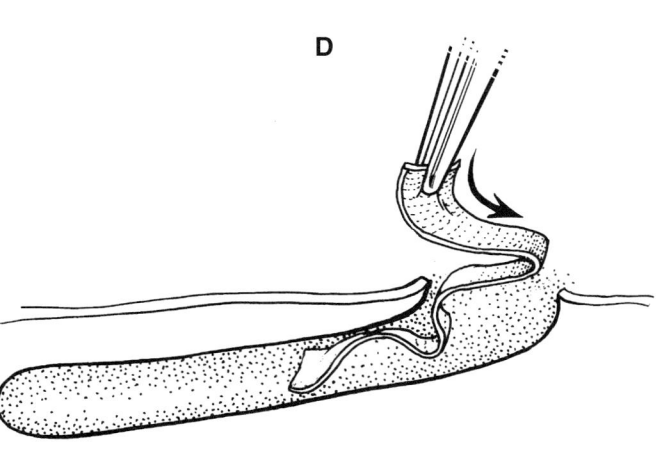

B

C

D

Perianal Abscess Drainage ▪ STEVEN LARSON

Indications
- Isolated, simple perianal abscess manifested as a tender, swollen fluctuant mass in the superficial subcutaneous tissue adjacent to the anus

Contraindications
- Presence of larger, perirectal abscess (ischiorectal or intersphincteric abscess)
- Relative contraindications:
  - Diabetes mellitus
  - Extremes of age
  - Immunocompromised host

Equipment
- Local anesthetic (lidocaine), syringe, and needles
- Betadine antiseptic solution
- Sterile gloves and drapes
- Tape
- ¼-inch iodoform gauze packing
- 4 × 4 gauze pads
- Standard laceration repair kit
- Scalpel with No. 11 blade

Procedure
1. Place the patient in the lateral Sims' position (A on p. 114) or prone knee-chest (Skinner's) position (A on p. 117) on the proctoscopic table.
2. Tape the buttocks open.
3. Prepare and drape the site in sterile fashion.
4. Administer and inject local anesthetic into the subcutaneous tissue over the site.
5. Make a linear incision over the site of maximal fluctuance *(A, B)*.
6. Drain and gently explore the wound with hemostats to break up loculations.
7. Irrigate the wound with normal saline solution.
8. Pack with gauze (do not overpack the wound) *(C)*.
9. Discharge the patient with oral analgesics and instructions regarding local wound care, follow-up check, and packing change within 48 hours.

Complications
- Incomplete drainage
- Underestimation of depth or degree of involvement in an immunocompromised patient
- Necrotizing fasciitis

Discussion
- Pain on digital examination and fluctuance proximal to the internal sphincter may indicate the presence of a perirectal abscess that requires intraoperative drainage.
- Liberal use of analgesia and sedation is recommended to facilitate the examination and procedure. If an adequate digital examination still cannot be performed, evaluation in the operating room should be considered.
- Antibiotics are indicated if an associated cellulitis is present.

Bibliography
Abcarian H et al: Benign anorectal disease: definition, characterization, and analysis of treatment, *Am J Gastroenterol* 89(suppl):S182-S193, 1994.

Coates W: Disorders of the anorectum. In Rosen P, Barkin R (eds): *Emergency medicine: concepts and clinical practice*, ed 4, St Louis, 1998, Mosby, pp 2037-2052.

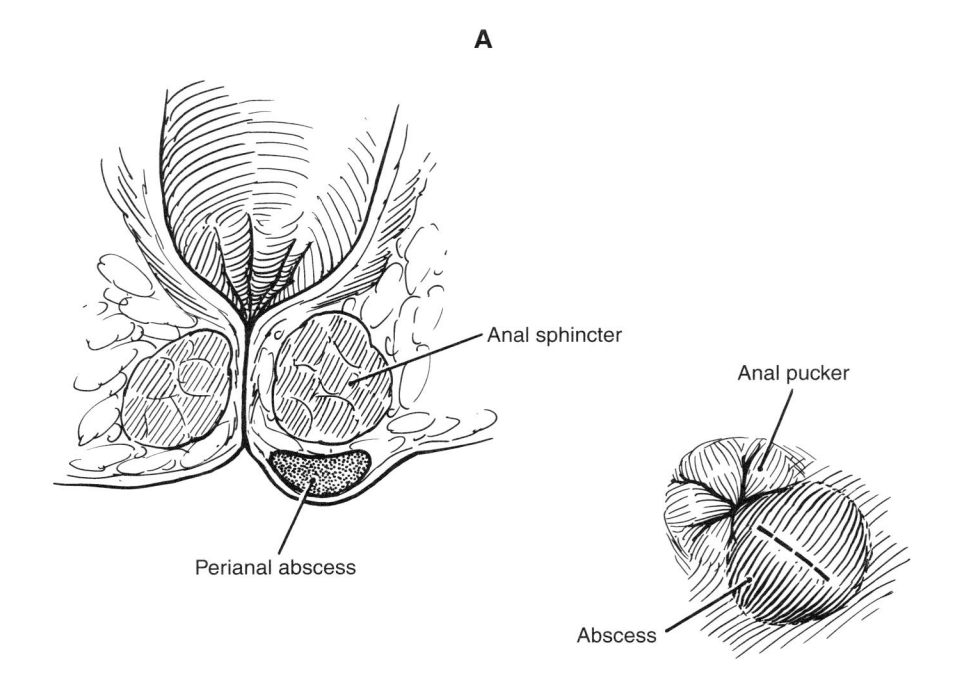

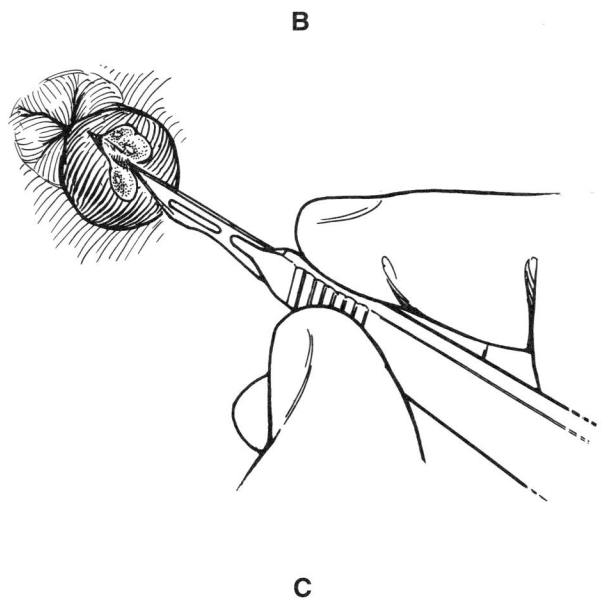

Abdomen

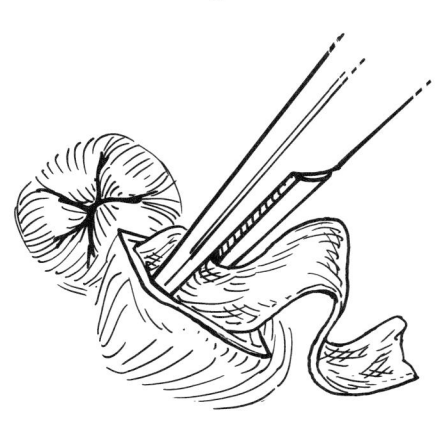

A

Anal sphincter

Anal pucker

Perianal abscess

Abscess

B

C

CHAPTER 5

GENITOURINARY SYSTEM

Urethral Catheterization ▪ GARY M. VILKE

Indications
- Acute urinary retention
- Monitoring of urine output
- Urine collection for diagnostic purposes
- Urologic evaluation of lower urinary tract
- Neurogenic bladder or mechanical inability to void

Contraindications
- No urethral meatus
- Trauma with blood at meatus, obvious penile deformity, or high-riding prostate
- Perineal hematoma

Equipment
- Commercial urinary catheter set, which should include the following:
  - Betadine antiseptic solution
  - Cotton balls
  - Pickups
  - Lubricant
  - Sterile gloves and drapes (both fenestrated and nonfenestrated)
  - 16 Fr Foley catheter
  - 10-ml syringe with sterile saline solution
  - Sterile urine collection system

Procedure

1. Place the patient in a lithotomy position *(A)*.
2. Soak cotton balls with antiseptic solution, and have lubricant available on the operational surface of the kit.

Female Patient

1. Place the fenestrated drape over the perineum and the nonfenestrated drape between the patient's legs.
2. Spread the labia with the nondominant hand, allowing good exposure to the urethra (this hand will not be sterile for the remainder of the procedure).
3. Use the pickups to hold the cotton balls. Prepare the area in sterile fashion by running the cotton balls over the meatus in an anterior to posterior direction three separate times *(B)*.
4. Cover the tip of the catheter with lubricant *(C)*.
5. Introduce the catheter into the meatus *(D)*. Quickly advance the catheter until about half is inserted *(E)*. At this point urine should flow through the catheter.
6. Inflate the catheter balloon with the 10 ml of saline solution. Pull the catheter back until the balloon is snug against the bladder *(F)*. Attach the urine collection system, and secure the catheter to the leg with tape.

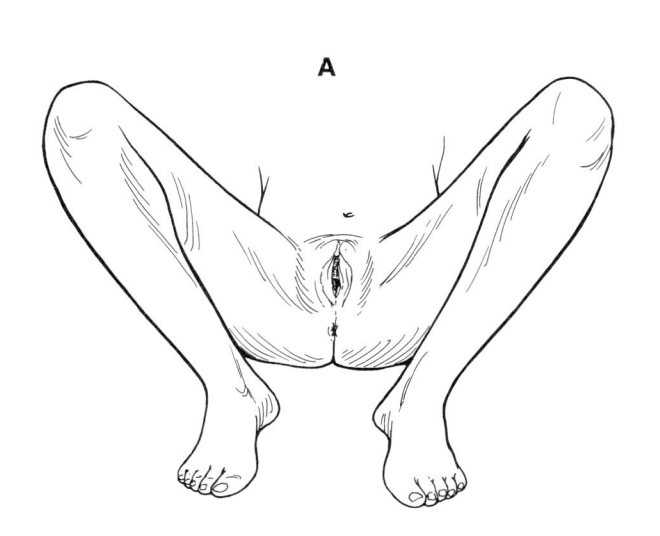

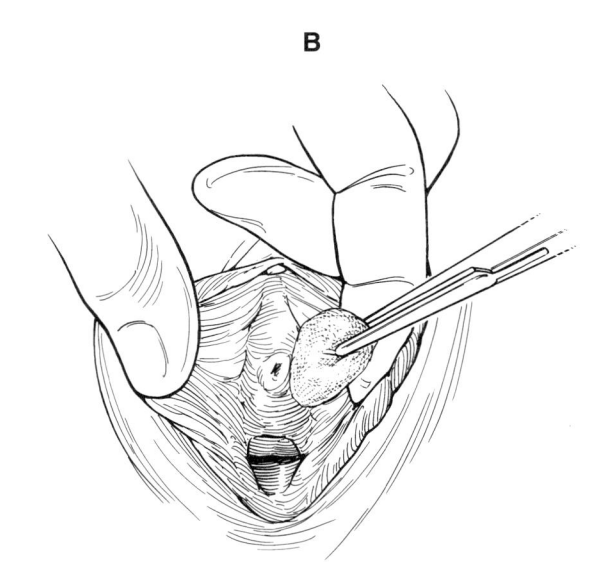

GENITOURINARY SYSTEM 125

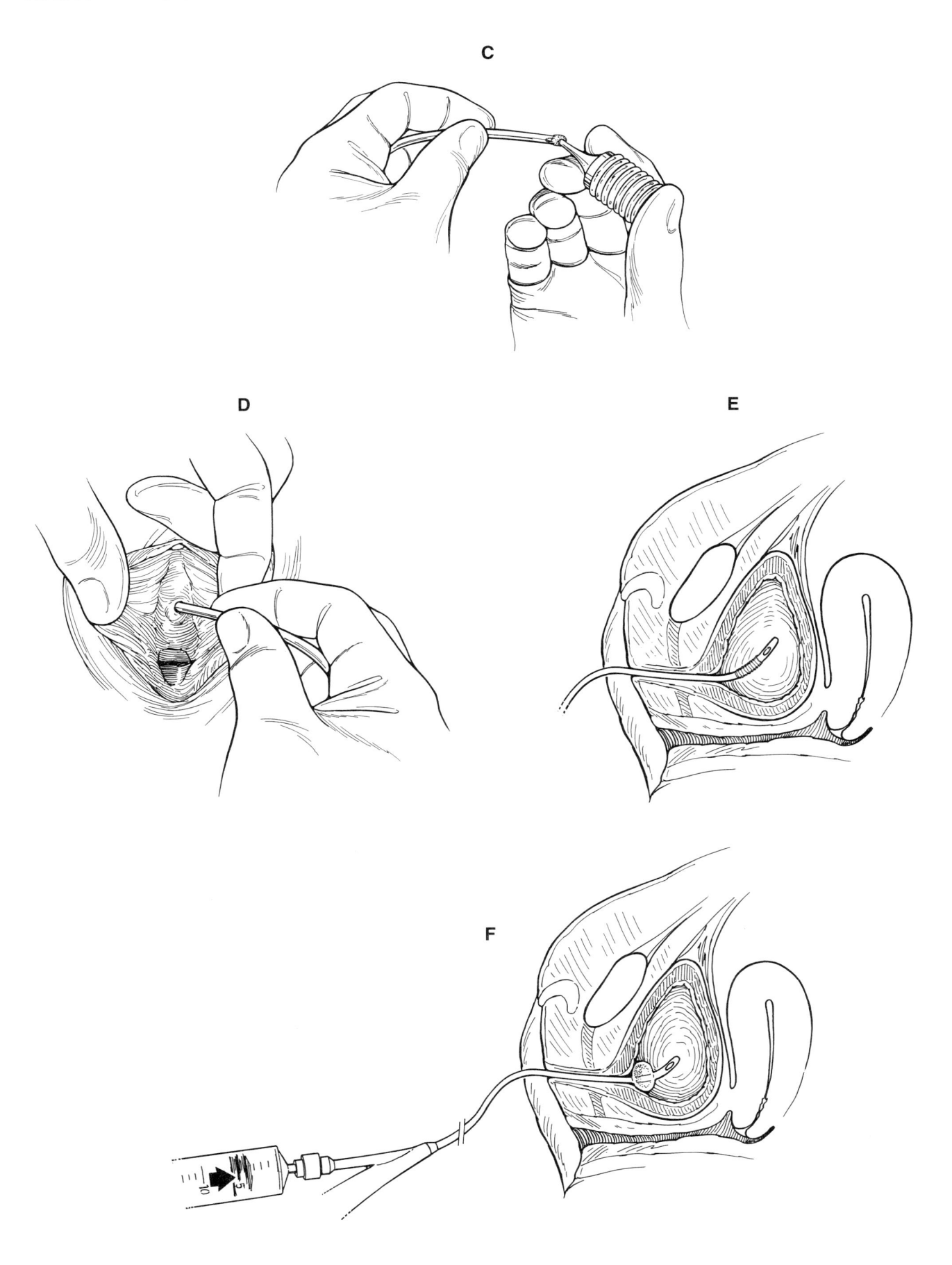

C

D   E

F

Male Patient

1. Place the fenestrated drape over the penis and the nonfenestrated drape between the patient's legs.
2. If the patient is uncircumcised, retract the foreskin. Grasp the penis with the nondominant hand (this hand will not be sterile for the remainder of the procedure). Hold the penis at length in a direction perpendicular to the perineum.
3. Use the pickups to hold the cotton balls. Prepare the area in sterile fashion by running the cotton balls over the meatus and glans three separate times *(G)*.
4. Cover the tip of the catheter with lubricant, and lubricate the urethra *(H)*.
5. Introduce the catheter into the meatus *(I)*. Quickly advance the catheter until about half is inserted *(J)*. At this point urine should flow through the catheter.
6. Inflate the catheter balloon with the 10 ml of saline solution. Pull the catheter back until the balloon is snug against the bladder. Attach the urine collection system, and secure the catheter to the leg with tape *(K)*.

Complications

- Microscopic hematuria (gross hematuria is uncommon)
- Inability to pass the catheter
- Infection
- Passage of the catheter into a blind pouch (male)

Discussion

- If lubricant is available in a tube, it can be injected directly into the urethral meatus. Lidocaine jelly can be used as a lubricant to lessen the discomfort of catheterization.
- A Coudé tip catheter may be necessary in a male patient with a large prostate that makes standard catheterization difficult *(J_1)*.
- In women the biggest error in placement is trying to catheterize the clitoris, mistaking it for the urethra. The urethra is more posterior and has a slitlike opening.

Bibliography

Neuwirth H et al: Genitourinary imaging and procedures by the emergency physician, *Emerg Med Clin North Am* 7(1):1-28, 1989.

Stine RJ et al: Diagnostic and therapeutic urologic procedures, *Emerg Med Clin North Am* 6(3):547-578, 1988.

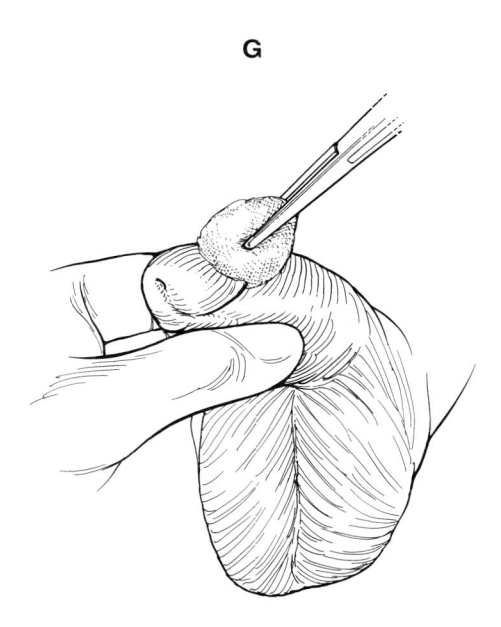

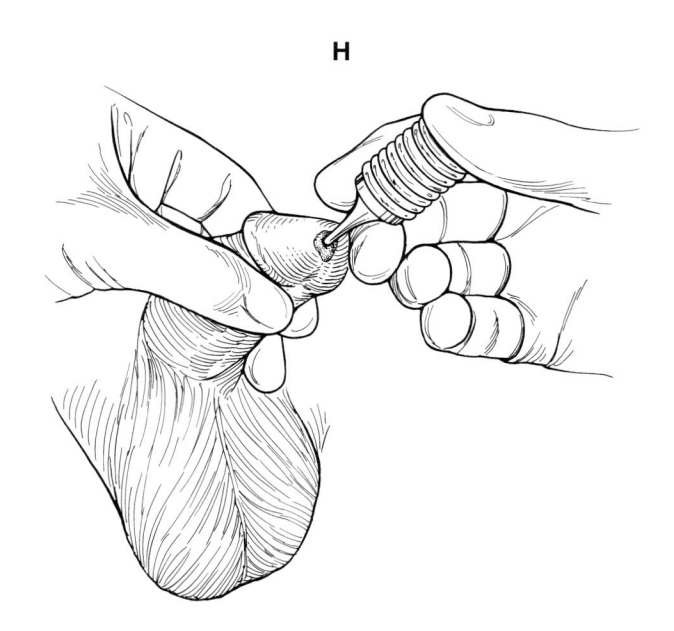

G

H

I

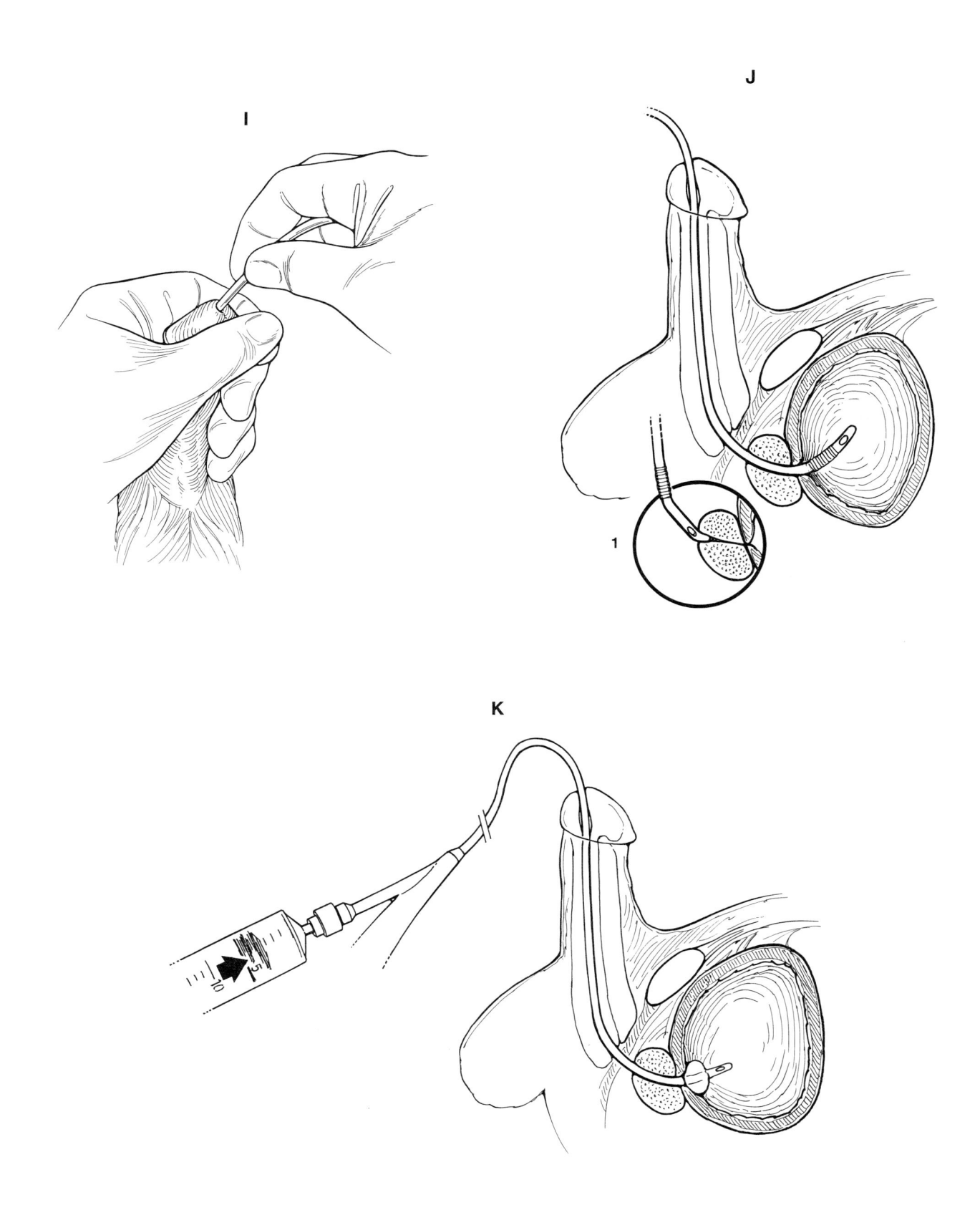

J

1

K

Cystostomy ▪ GARY M. VILKE

Indications
- Any patient who warrants a urethral catheter but cannot have it placed because of the following:
  - Phimosis in a male patient
  - Urethral foreign body
  - Complex prostatic disease
  - Urethral stricture
  - Urethral or prostatic disruption in a trauma patient

Contraindications
- Empty bladder
- Previous lower abdominal surgery with scarring
- Previous pelvic radiation with scarring
- Significant bleeding disorders (relative contraindication)

Equipment
- Betadine antiseptic solution
- Sterile gloves and drapes
- Percutaneous suprapubic cystostomy kit, which usually includes the following:
  - Local anesthetic (1% lidocaine), syringe, and needles
  - 22-gauge 3-inch spinal needle
  - 4×4 gauze pads
  - Scalpel with No. 11 blade
  - Suture material
  - J-tip guidewire
  - Dilator
  - Sheath
- 14 Fr Foley catheter
- Sterile closed system urinary drainage bag
- Tape

Procedure
1. Palpate the bladder, and identify the insertion site at midline and 2 cm cephalad to the pubic bone.
2. Prepare and drape the area in sterile fashion
3. Inject local anesthetic to raise a small wheal at the insertion site.
4. Attach the 22-gauge spinal needle to the syringe containing the local anesthetic. Introduce the needle at the insertion site at a 20° to 30° angle from the perpendicular at midline.
5. Inject approximately 5 ml of local anesthetic into the tissue while advancing the needle toward the bladder. Intermittently aspirate for urine while injecting the anesthetic. Stop advancing once urine is aspirated.
6. Keep the needle in place, remove the syringe, and advance the guidewire through the needle into the bladder *(A)*.
7. Remove the needle, leaving the wire in place *(B)*. Make a small incision with the scalpel adjacent to the wire.
8. Advance the dilator and sheath over the wire into the bladder. Remove the dilator and guidewire, leaving only the sheath in the bladder.
9. Pass the Foley catheter through the sheath, and confirm placement by return of urine. Inflate the Foley balloon, and attach it to the closed urine collection system.
10. Peel and remove the sheath, and gently pull on the catheter until the balloon is snug against the inner bladder wall *(C, D)*.
11. Dress the area with 4×4 gauze pads and sterile dressing.

Complications
- Hematuria
- Bowel perforation
- Catheter obstruction (kinking or blood)
- Extravasation around the catheter
- Ureteral injury
- Large vessel injury
- Infection or abscess formation
- Inadvertent tube removal
- Failure of procedure

Discussion
- If the operator is unable to palpate the bladder, ultrasound guidance often proves helpful. Gross hematuria is a common but usually transient occurrence. Occasionally bladder irrigation is needed to clear clots.

Bibliography
Neuwirth H et al: Genitourinary imaging and procedures by the emergency physician, *Emerg Med Clin North Am* 7(1):1-28, 1989.

Stine RJ et al: Diagnostic and therapeutic urologic procedures, *Emerg Med Clin North Am* 6(3):547-578, 1988.

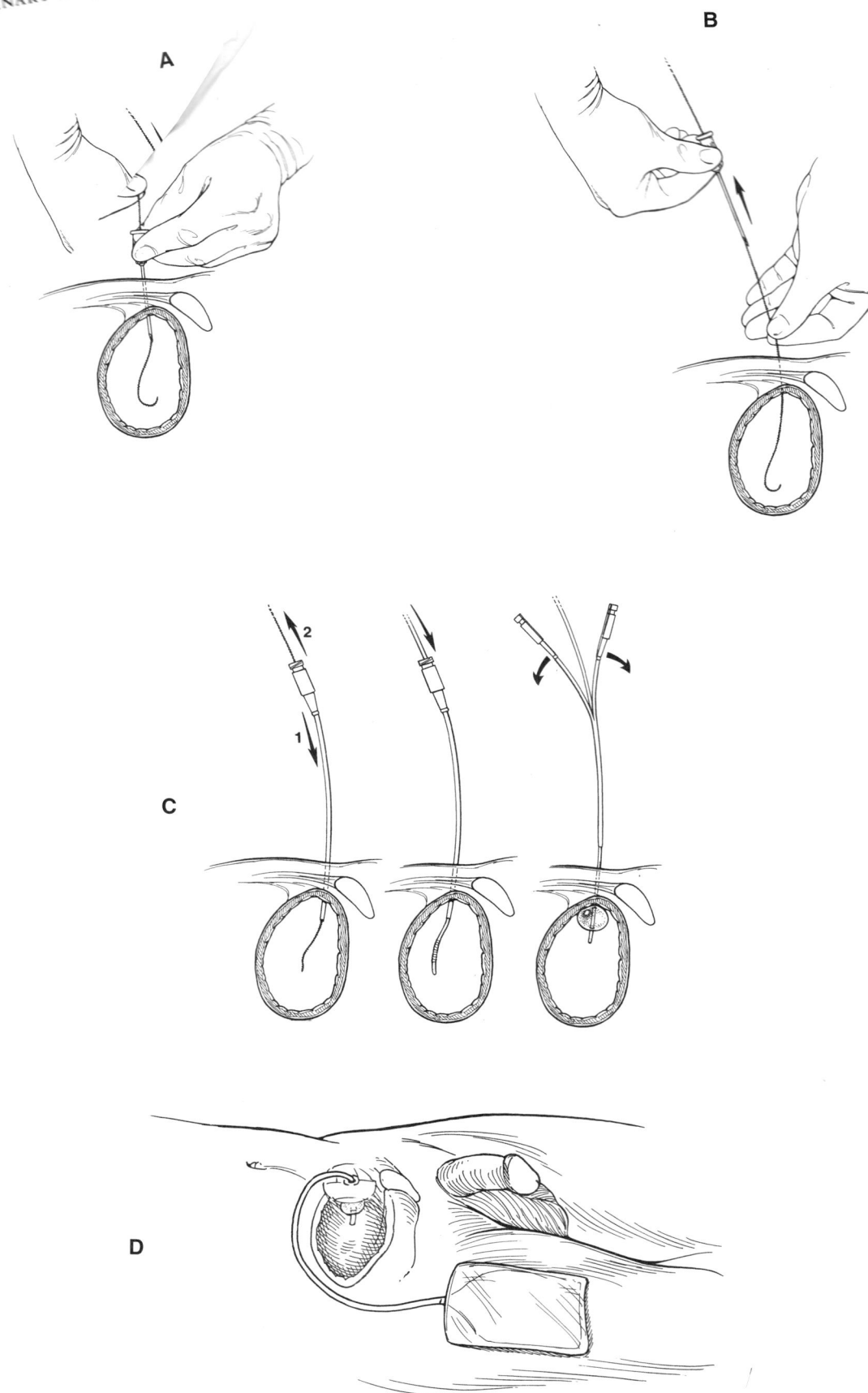

GENITOURINARY SYSTEM

A

B

C

D

Bladder Aspiration ▪ GARY M. VILKE

Indications
- Patient less than 2 years of age
- Phimosis in male patient
- Urethral stricture in male patient
- Chronic urethral infection

Contraindications
- Empty bladder (nonpalpable in adults, voiding within last hour in children)
- Previous lower abdominal surgery with scarring

Equipment
- Betadine antiseptic solution
- 22-gauge 1½-inch needle (for pediatric patient)
- 22-gauge 3-inch needle (for adult patient)
- Sterile 5- or 10-ml syringe
- Local anesthetic (1% lidocaine), syringe, and needles
- Sterile gloves

Procedure

Pediatric Patient
1. Place the child in frog-legged position.
2. Identify the insertion site at midline and 2 cm cephalad to the pubic bone.
3. Prepare the area in sterile fashion.
4. At the insertion site, introduce the 22-gauge 1½-inch needle attached to the 5-ml syringe. Direct the needle in the cephalad direction (the bladder is an abdominal organ in infants) at a 10° to 20° angle from the perpendicular at midline. Gently aspirate while introducing the needle.
5. If no urine is aspirated, withdraw the needle to the subcutaneous space and readvance it in a slightly different direction, 10° more caudad or cephalad. Do not pass the needle more than three times.
6. Once urine is obtained, remove the needle and dress the wound.

Adult Patient
1. With the patient in the supine position, palpate the bladder (A) and identify the insertion site at midline and 2 cm cephalad to the pubic bone.
2. Prepare the area in sterile fashion (B).
3. Inject local anesthetic subcutaneously at the insertion site.
4. At the insertion site, introduce the 22-gauge needle attached to the 10-ml syringe. Direct the needle caudad (the bladder is a peritoneal organ in adults) at a 10° to 20° angle from the perpendicular at midline (C). Gently aspirate while introducing the needle.
5. If no urine is aspirated, withdraw the needle to the subcutaneous space and readvance in a slightly different direction, 10° more caudad or cephalad. Do not pass the needle more than three times.
6. Once urine is obtained, remove the needle and dress the wound.

Complications
- Microscopic hematuria (gross hematuria is uncommon)
- Bowel perforation
- Failure to obtain urine

Discussion
- Ultrasound can be used as an adjunct to guide needle placement.

Bibliography

Garcia-Nieto V et al: Standards for ultrasound guidance of suprapubic bladder aspiration, *Pediatr Nephrol* 11(5):607-609, 1997.

Nystrom K et al: Suprapubic catheterization of the urinary bladder as a diagnostic procedure, *Scand J Urol Nephrol* 7:130, 1973.

Pollack CV Jr et al: Suprapubic bladder aspiration versus urethral catheterization in ill infants: success, efficiency and complication rates, *Ann Emerg Med* 23(2):225-230, 1994.

GENITOURINARY SYSTEM

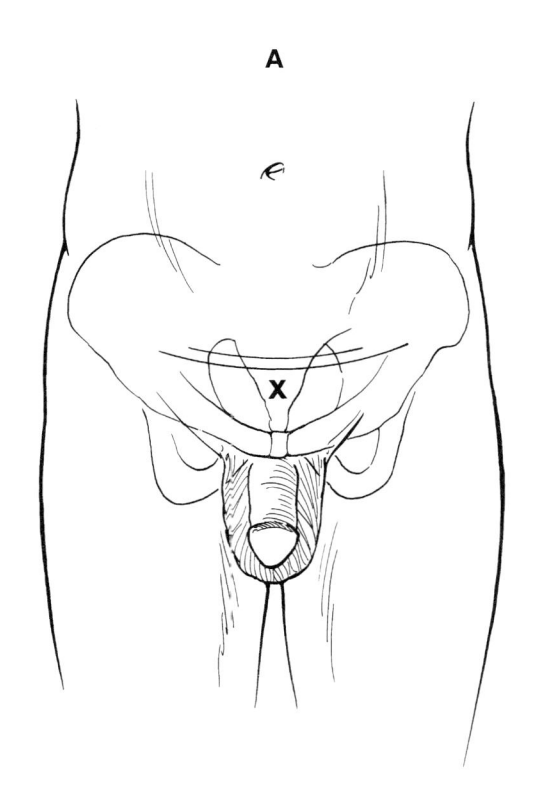

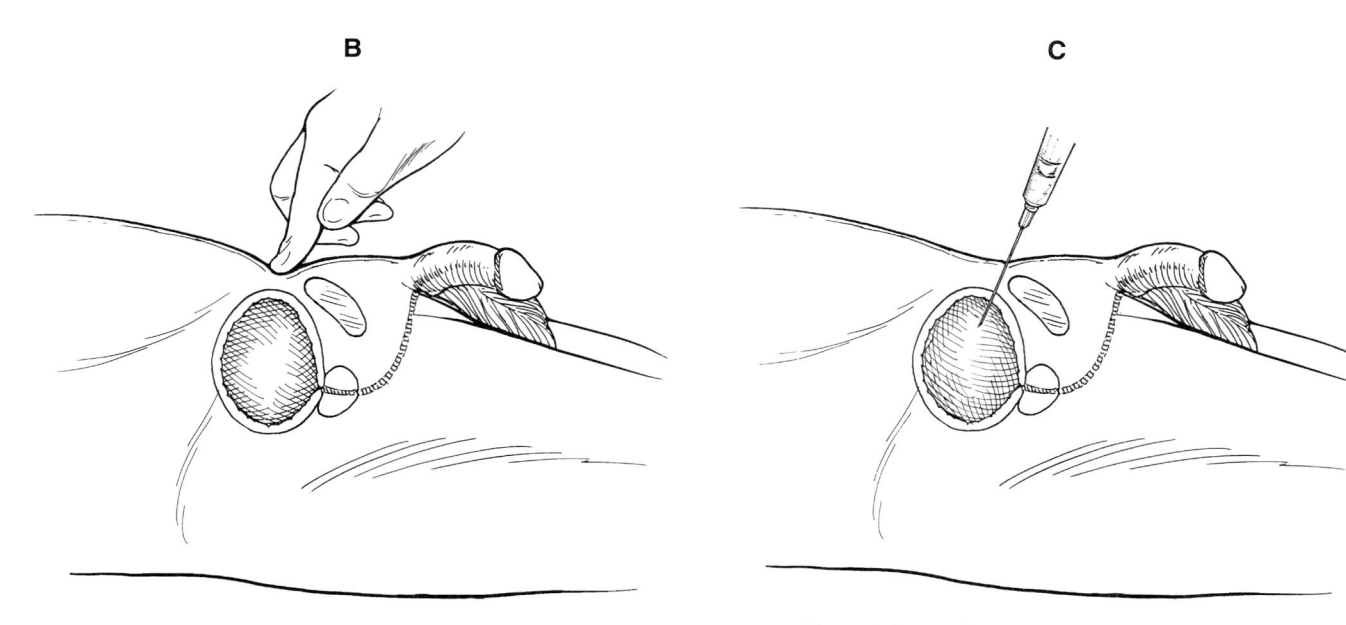

A

B

C

Young children: direct needle slightly cephalad
Older children and adults: direct needle slightly caudad

Dorsal Slit in Phimosis • GARY M. VILKE

Indications
- Phimosis with inability to void or ischemia of penis

Contraindications
- Bleeding dyscrasia (relative)

Equipment
- Sterile gloves and towels
- Betadine antiseptic solution
- Local anesthetic (lidocaine 1% without epinephrine), syringe, and needles
- Straight hemostat
- Straight scissors
- 4-0 or 5-0 Vicryl suture
- Needle holder
- Forceps
- Foley catheter

Procedure

1. Prepare and drape the dorsum of the penis in sterile fashion.
2. Using a 27-gauge needle, raise a wheal of anesthetic in the foreskin just proximal to the glans on the dorsal aspect of the penis.
3. Extend the injection along the longitudinal axis distally to the tip of the foreskin. Make sure the full thickness of the foreskin is anesthetized *(A)*.
4. After 3 or 4 minutes check to make certain anesthesia is effective.
5. Slide the closed hemostat into the space between the foreskin and the glans, and gently open it, forming a tract. Then remove the hemostat.
6. Reposition the open hemostat with one tip between the foreskin and glans and the other tip outside the foreskin, straddling the region of anesthesia. Make certain the tip of the hemostat is not in the urethral meatus *(B)*.
7. Close the hemostat over the region of anesthesia, and keep it clamped for 10 minutes *(B)*.
8. Remove the hemostat, and cut the serrated clamped tissue with the scissors *(C, D)*.
9. If the skin edges continue to ooze, a running stitch with a Vicryl suture can be placed on each side.
10. Retract the foreskin, and clean the glans.
11. Place a Foley catheter when indicated.

Complications

- Bleeding
- Infection
- Incision of the urethra
- Cosmetically poor appearance

Discussion

- Patients should be referred for urologic evaluation for possible circumcision.

Bibliography
Holman JR, Stuessi KA: Adult circumcision, *Am Fam Physician* 59(6):1514-1518, 1999.

GENITOURINARY SYSTEM

A

B

C

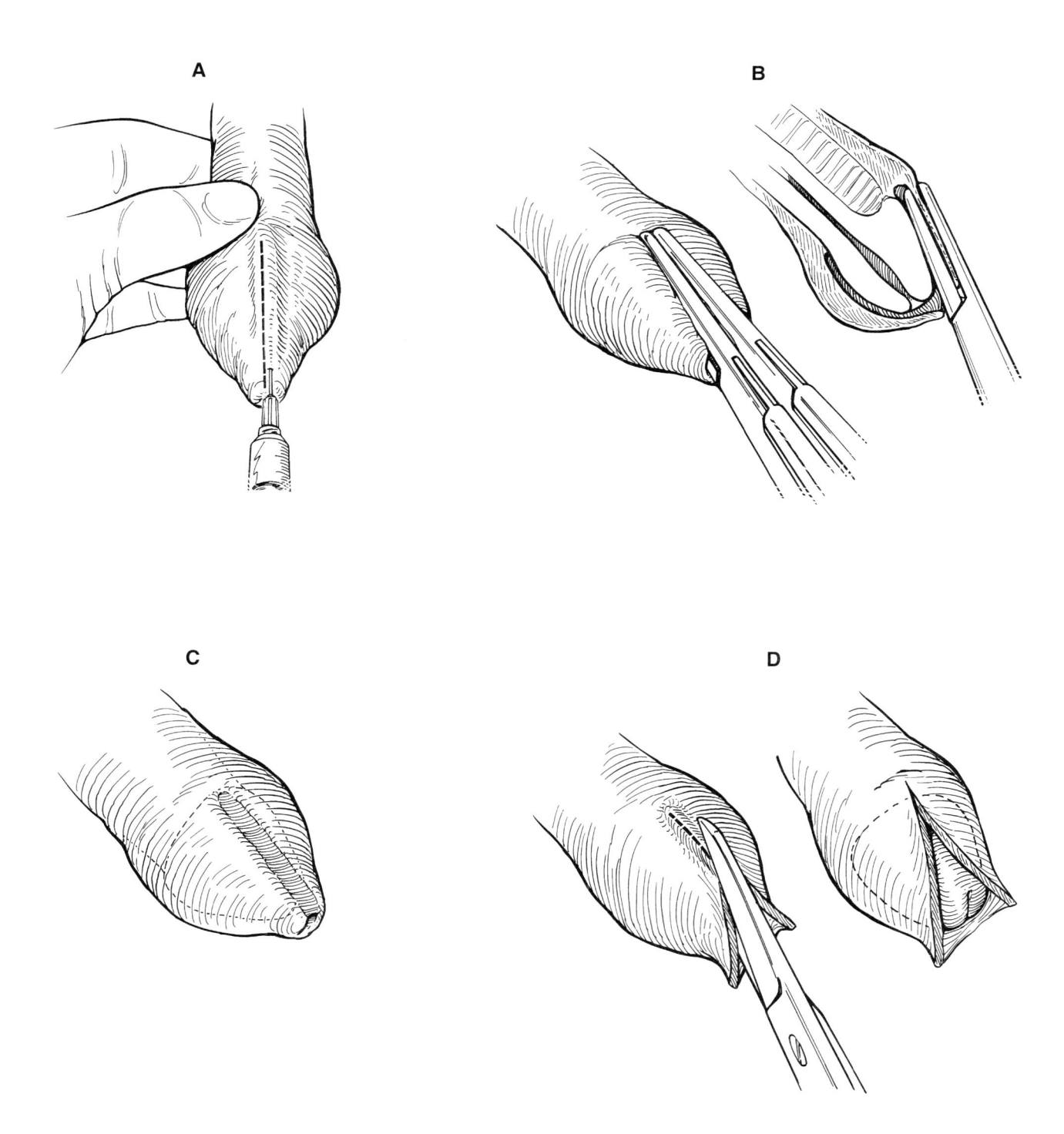

D

Manual Paraphimosis Reduction • GARY M. VILKE

Indications
- Paraphimosis *(A)*

Contraindications
- None

Equipment
- Gloves
- Lubricant jelly

Procedure

1. If a Foley catheter is in place, remove it to facilitate reduction in all but the mildest cases of paraphimosis.
2. Place a small amount of lubricant on the proximal aspect of the glans and inner surface of the foreskin.
3. Grasp the swollen foreskin with the nondominant hand, and apply slow, gentle compression for several minutes, elevating the shaft of the penis to reduce the edema *(A, B)*.
4. With the index and middle fingers of both hands, grasp the swollen foreskin and elevate upward.
5. Slowly begin pushing the glans into the foreskin with both thumbs, which are placed over the urethral meatus *(C)*. Continue until the foreskin is repositioned over the glans *(D)*.
6. Place a Foley catheter.

Complications
- Inability to reduce paraphimosis

Discussion

- Sedation and analgesia may be required if the patient is conscious and experiencing too much discomfort.
- Rather than manual compression of the swollen foreskin, a 5- to 6-cm piece of elastic bandage can be left in place for a few minutes.
- An alternative technique uses the nondominant hand to securely hold the proximal aspect of the swollen foreskin with a ring formed by the thumb and the index and middle fingers. The glans is then slowly pushed into the foreskin with the dominant thumb, which is placed over the urethral meatus.

Bibliography

Ganti SU et al: Simple method for the reduction of paraphimosis, *Urology* 25:77, 1985.

Olson C: Emergency treatment of paraphimosis, *Can Fam Physician* 44:1253-1254, 1998.

Williams JC et al: Paraphimosis in elderly men, *Am J Emerg Med* 13(3):351-353, 1995.

Genitourinary System

135

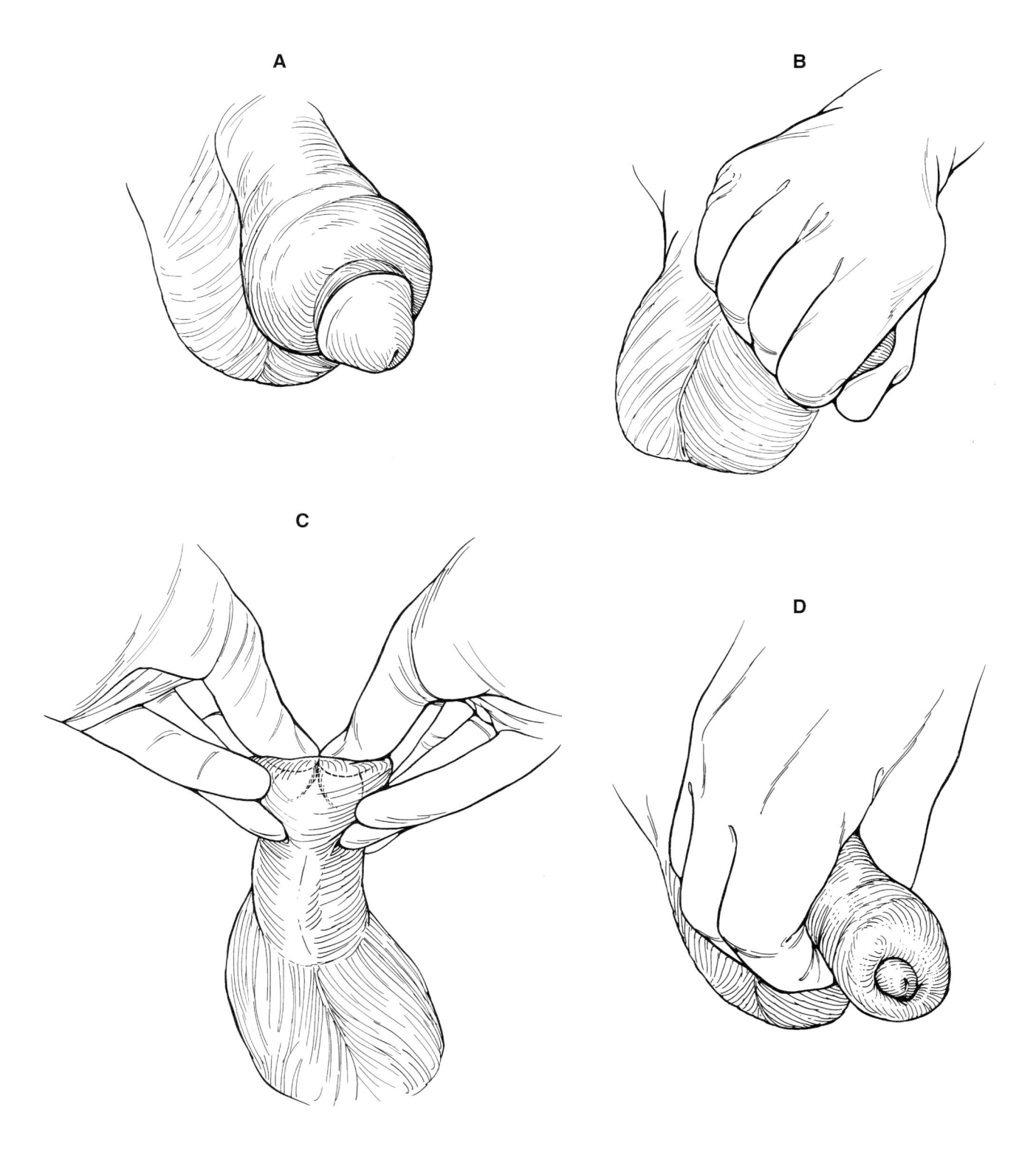

A

B

C

D

Zipper Removal ■ GARY M. VILKE

Indications
- Skin or tissue fold caught in the teeth of a zipper *(A)*

Contraindications
- None

Equipment
- Wire cutter or bone cutter
- Gloves

Procedure

1. Cut the diamond part (median bar) of the zipper in a horizontal direction *(B)*, and lift the zipper off *(C)*.
2. Locally clean injured tissue. Apply antibiotic ointment as appropriate.

Complications
- Cutting the skin or tissue with the cutter
- Infection
- Local bleeding

Discussion
- This procedure can be performed in the field.
- If the patient is too uncomfortable, 1% lidocaine can be injected locally for anesthesia.

Bibliography

Flowerdew R et al: Management of penile zipper injury, *J Urol* 115(5):671, 1977.

Strait RT: A novel method for removal of penile zipper entrapment, *Pediatr Emerg Care* 15(6):412-413, 1999.

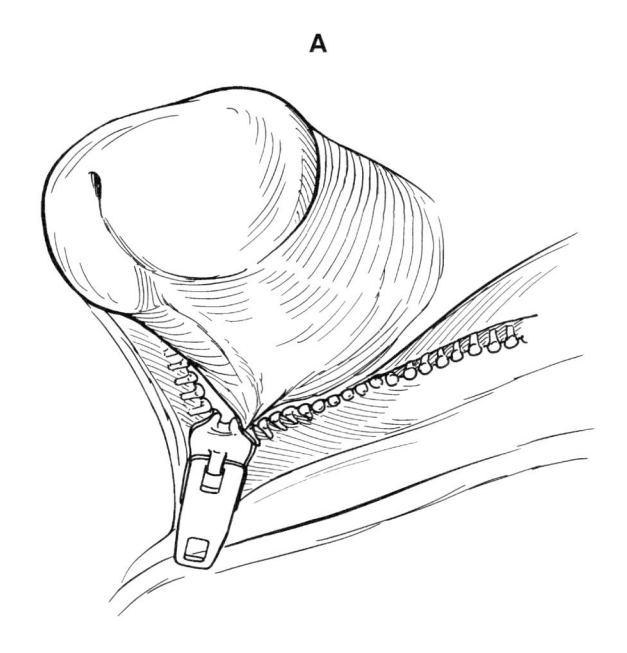

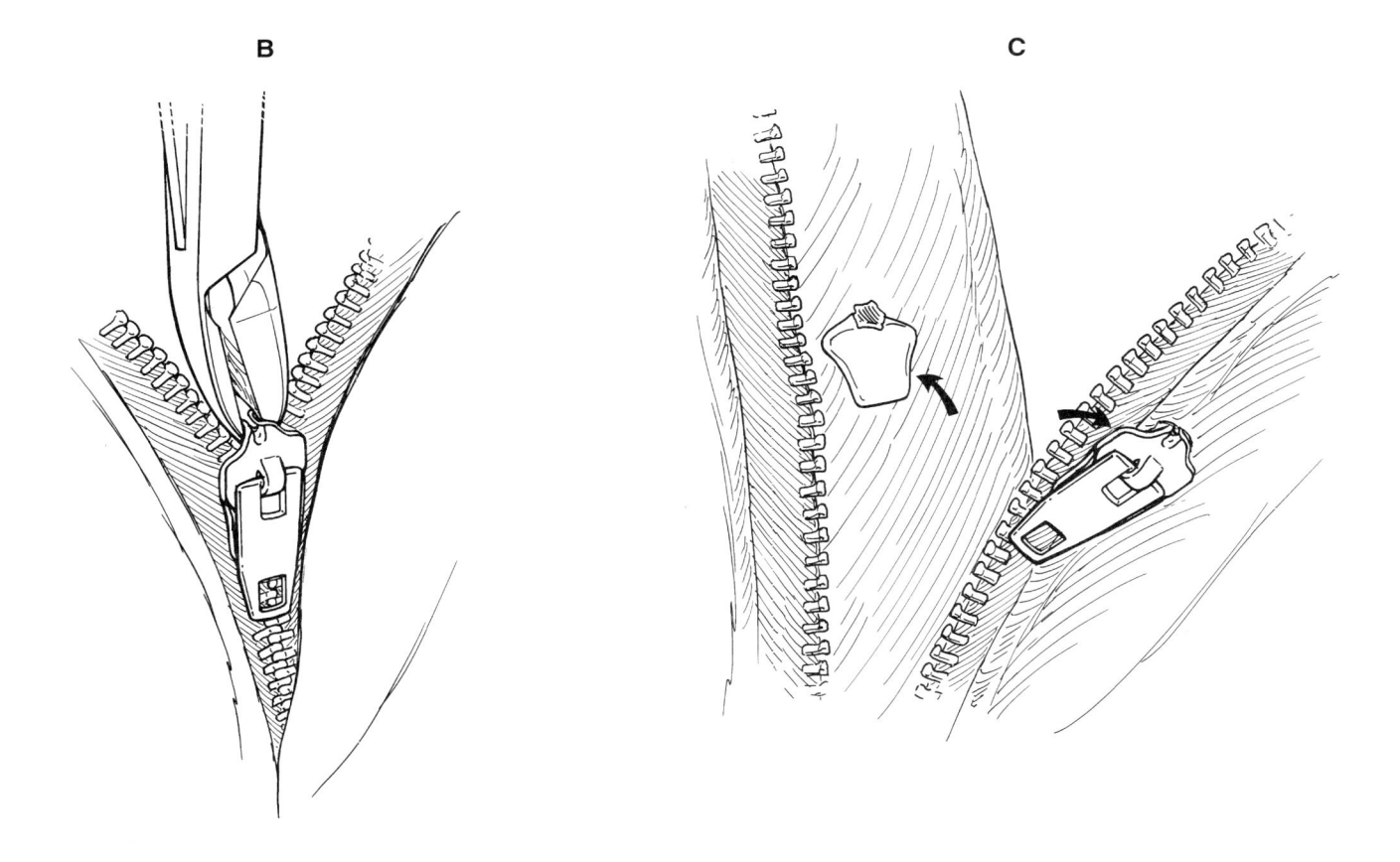

GENITOURINARY SYSTEM

A

B

C

CHAPTER 6

OBSTETRICS AND GYNECOLOGY

Culdocentesis — COLLEEN J. CAMPBELL

Indications
- Diagnosis of ectopic pregnancy, especially when the estimated gestational age is less than 6 weeks
- Diagnosis of ruptured corpus luteum cyst
- Diagnosis of pelvic inflammatory disease
- Diagnosis of intraperitoneal hemorrhage

Contraindications
- Coagulopathy
- Presence of a fixed pelvic mass
- Presence of an enlarged retroverted uterus
- Prepubertal age

Equipment
- Pelvic examination table
- Light source
- Betadine antiseptic solution
- Sterile saline
- Cotton balls
- 4 × 4 gauze pads
- Three 20-ml syringes
- Local anesthetic agent (lidocaine 1% with epinephrine), syringe, and needles
- Ring forceps
- Cervical tenaculum
- 18-gauge spinal needle or 18-gauge butterfly with ring forceps
- Vaginal speculum (preferably bivalve)
- Culture media and tubes

Procedure

1. Place the patient in dorsal lithotomy position with her head slightly elevated on the pelvic examination table (A).
2. Perform a bimanual examination to exclude large fixed pelvic masses or an enlarged retroverted uterus.
3. Place the vaginal speculum so that the cervix is easily viewed. Adjust to the maximal comfortable width and height.
4. Anesthetize the cervix by injecting local anesthetic agent into the posterior lip (B).
5. Place the cervical tenaculum on the posterior lip of the cervix, and elevate the cervix with slight longitudinal traction.
6. Prepare the posterior vaginal wall inferior to the cervix with betadine-soaked gauze sponges followed by sterile water.
7. Obtain local anesthesia by injecting 1% lidocaine (at least 2 ml in a 20-ml syringe) in the midline, 1 cm posterior to the cervix.
8. Attach a 20-ml syringe filled with 3 ml saline solution to the spinal needle.
9. Advance the spinal needle parallel to the vaginal speculum in the midline, 1 cm posterior to the vaginal-cervical junction to a depth of about 2 cm (C, D).
10. Inject the saline solution to clear the hub of the needle. Then aspirate with the syringe while withdrawing the syringe slowly.
11. If no fluid is obtained, repeat the procedure, directing the needle slightly to the left or right of midline.
12. Submit the fluid for Gram's staining, cell count, hematocrit, and culture. Observe the fluid for clotting.

Complications

- Rupture of tuboovarian abscess
- Bowel perforation
- Pelvic kidney perforation
- Uterine laceration with subsequent hemorrhage

Discussion

- A positive culdocentesis can be interpreted as more than 3 ml of nonclotting blood. The hematocrit should be above 10%. A dry tap is nondiagnostic. A negative tap is one that produces at least 3 ml of nonsanguineous fluid.
- Culdocentesis can be considered an alternative to diagnostic peritoneal lavage for female trauma victims. It has a lower complication rate and leaves no scar. It can also be used for patients with previous abdominal surgery.
- Since fluid from culdocentesis accurately reflects causative organisms, it may be useful in antibiotic selection in complicated pelvic inflammatory disease.
- Culdocentesis is most useful for a high-risk patient with a positive pregnancy test when ultrasound is indeterminate and for a patient with peritoneal signs when ultrasound is unavailable.

Bibliography
Vande Krol L, Abbott JT: The current role of culdocentesis, *Am J Emerg Med* 10:354-358, 1992.

A

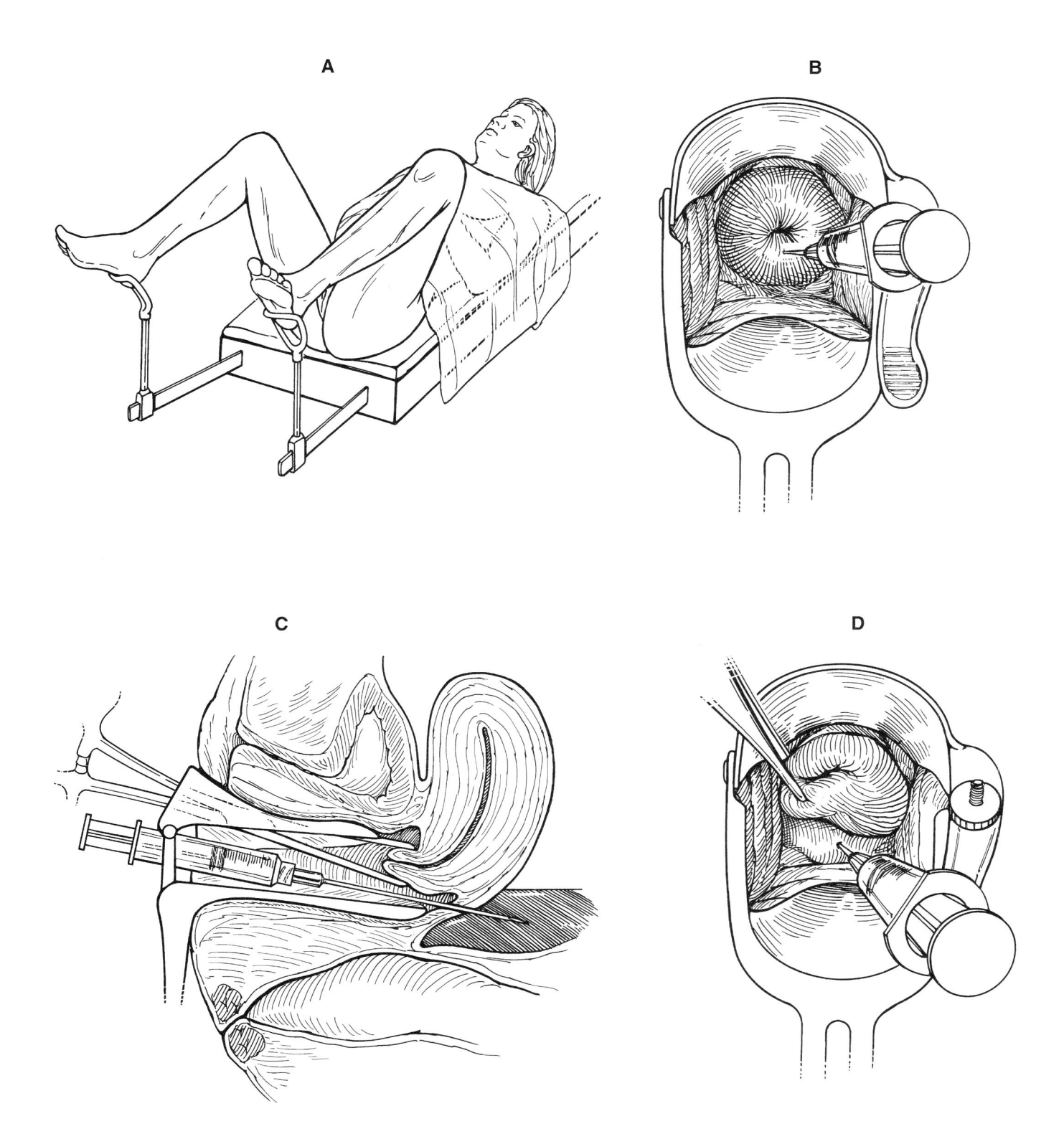

B

C

D

Vaginal Delivery · COLLEEN J. CAMPBELL

Indications
- Emergency delivery of the fetus

Contraindications
- Prolapsed cord

Equipment
- Sterile gown, shoe covers, and facemask
- Betadine antiseptic solution
- Sterile drape and towels
- Gauze
- Large basin
- Two medium Kelly clamps
- Double-grip cord clamp
- Mayo scissors
- Bulb syringe
- Baby blanket
- Oxytocin 1 ml IM injection
- Blood tubes
- Infant resuscitation tray (if available)
- Heated Isolette (if available)
- Local anesthetic (1% lidocaine), syringe, and needles

Procedure

1. Obtain a brief obstetric history: estimated gestational age, number of gestations in current pregnancy, and prenatal history.
2. Place the patient on the stretcher with her hips and knees maximally flexed and knees abducted *(A)*.
3. Using sterile gloves, perform a manual pelvic examination to assess fetal presentation.
   a. If only the cord is palpable, do not deliver the infant unless cesarean section is not an option. Otherwise, apply gentle pressure inward on the infant, tell the patient to stop pushing, and proceed to cesarean section.
   b. Examine the cervix, which should be fully dilated (10 cm).
   c. Use two fingers to ascertain the position of the anterior and posterior fontanels. The anterior fontanel is diamond shaped, and the posterior fontanel is triangular.
   d. If the fetus is presenting with the buttocks or feet, proceed to breech delivery. Otherwise, proceed to vertex delivery.

Vertex Delivery
1. Prepare and drape the vulva and introitus in sterile fashion if time permits.
2. As the infant progresses beyond crowning, place one hand over the occipital region and apply gentle inferior pressure. With the other hand, put slight upward pressure on the chin. These maneuvers will reduce vaginal tears *(B)*.
3. Once the head is delivered, wipe the baby's mouth and face and quickly suction the nose *(C)*.
4. With two fingers check the neck for coiled loops of cord. If they are found, free them over the head when possible. If you are unable to free the cord, clamp it on both ends and cut between them.
5. Exert downward gentle pressure with a hand on each side of the head to deliver the anterior shoulder.
6. Exert gentle upward pressure on the head to deliver the posterior shoulder *(D)*.
7. Hold both sides of the baby with your arms parallel to the baby's body. Cup the baby's head in your hand to maintain a secure grip as the baby is being delivered *(E)*.

Breech Delivery
1. Completion of breech delivery is imminent if the baby has spontaneously delivered to the level of the umbilicus.
2. Perform a generous episiotomy.
3. To assist with delivery of the legs in a frank breech presentation, place your fingers parallel to the femur and move the leg away from the midline.
4. Once the axillae are visible, rotate the trunk clockwise to bring the anterior shoulder to the mother's vulva and release it.
5. Rotate the body in the other direction to deliver the posterior shoulder.
6. If unable to deliver the anterior shoulder, elevate the lower body of the baby by pulling upward on the feet to deliver the posterior shoulder. Then bring the body of the baby downward in a similar manner to deliver the anterior shoulder.
7. When delivering the head, do not allow the neck to hyperextend. While supporting the baby with your bottom hand, place your index finger in the mouth to maintain the neutral position of the neck. With your other hand apply downward pressure on the shoulders while your assistant exerts suprapubic pressure.

Obstetrics and Gynecology

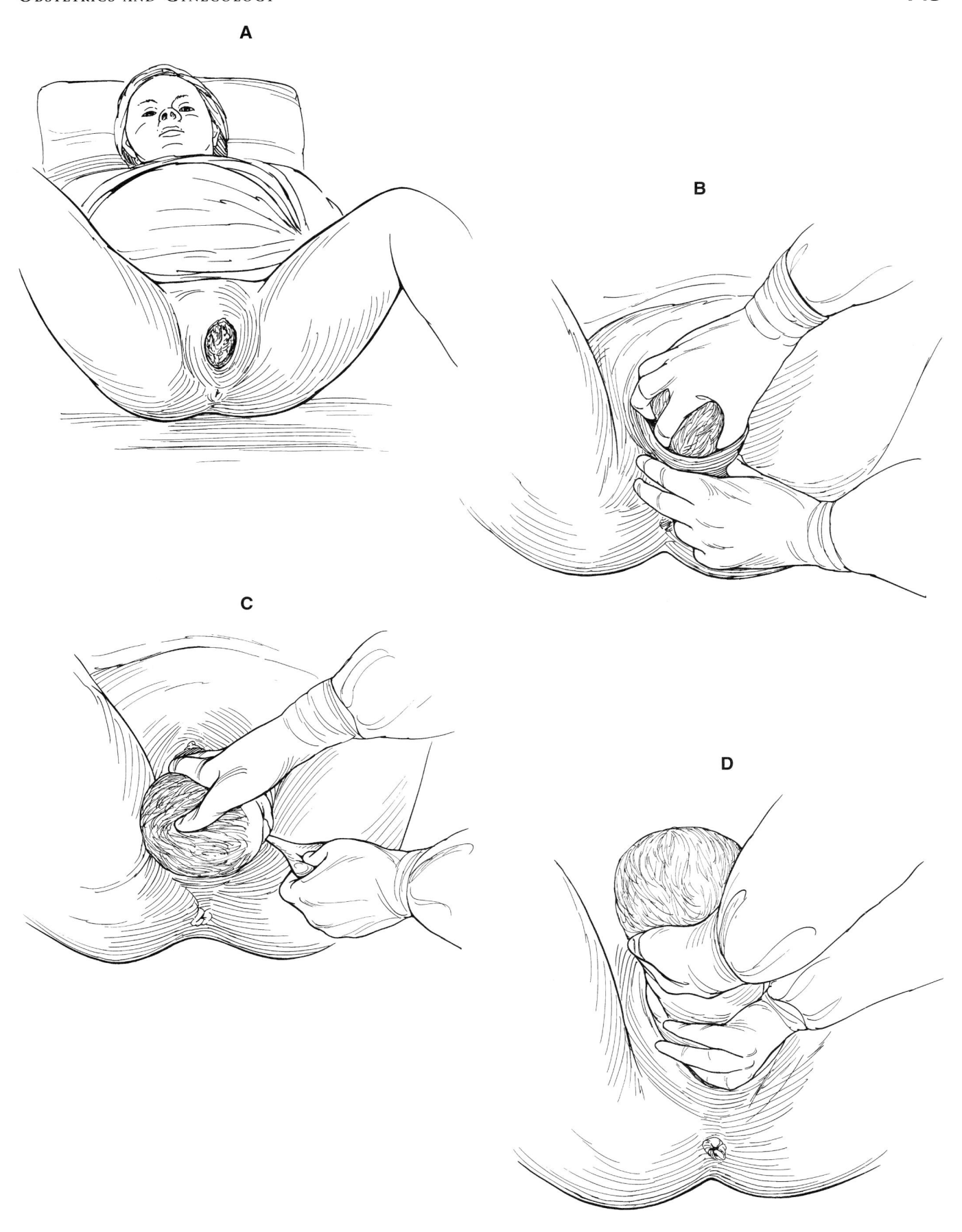

A

B

C

D

After Delivery of the Baby

1. Hold the baby slightly lower than the umbilical cord for a minute or two before clamping the cord *(E)*.
2. Place one clamp on the cord several centimeters from the baby's abdomen. Place the second clamp 2 cm distal and cut between the clamps *(F)*.
3. Obtain blood from the cord, and send it for blood typing and serologic examination.
4. Dry the baby well, and assess the Apgar scores.
5. Apply firm massage to the uterine fundus to facilitate uterine contraction and reduce bleeding.
6. Apply gentle traction to the cord. When it spontaneously loosens and blood flows out, the placenta is almost ready for delivery. Do not force its delivery.
7. As the placenta is delivered, rotate it 360° to capture loose membranes. Place the delivered specimen aside for further examination *(G)*.
8. Administer oxytocin 0.5 to 1 ml IM to help the uterus contract and reduce bleeding.
9. Inspect the vagina and cervix for tears and lacerations, applying pressure to control bleeding until definitive repair.
10. Admit the mother and child for evaluation and monitoring.

Complications

- Postpartum hemorrhage caused by uterine atony, vaginal or cervical lacerations, or uterine inversion
- Shoulder dystocia
- Rectal tears
- Urethral injuries
- Pelvic floor relaxation
- Stress incontinence
- Meconium aspiration
- Increased incidence with vaginal breech delivery:
  - Intracranial hemorrhage
  - Fractures of the clavicle, humerus, femur, and skull
  - Cervical spine injury
  - Umbilical cord prolapse
  - Brachial plexus injury
  - Sudden infant death syndrome

Discussion

- Postpartum hemorrhage caused by uterine inversion may be controlled by gently placing a fist in the mother's vagina and using the fingers to push laterally before directing the fist toward the fundus.
- If heavy meconium is noted at delivery of the head, immediate suctioning should be performed to prevent aspiration.
- In cases of shoulder dystocia the posterior shoulder should be rotated anteriorly and upward, with application of fundal pressure to deliver the anterior shoulder. If this is unsuccessful, the operator should continue rotation anteriorly to deliver the posterior shoulder. The posterior arm can be delivered by flexing the baby's elbow while looping a finger around the forearm. In cases of dystocia a generous episiotomy is recommended.
- The most common breech presentation is the frank, followed by footling and then complete breech presentations. Vaginal breech delivery should be avoided whenever possible in the emergency department. The rate of fetal complications is higher than with cesarean section, and complications are 12 times more common than with vertex deliveries. Low-birth-weight infants are especially at risk. Intracranial hemorrhage is more common because the head does not have the opportunity to mold gradually during delivery.
- Vaginal delivery can be performed safely in the prehospital setting when necessary. Keeping the baby warm and minimizing maternal hemorrhage with fundal massage are of primary importance. After delivery the mother and child should be transported to the hospital for evaluation and monitoring.

Bibliography

Eller DP, VanDorsten JP: Route of delivery for breech presentation: a conundrum, *Am J Obstet Gynecol* 173:393-398, 1995.

E

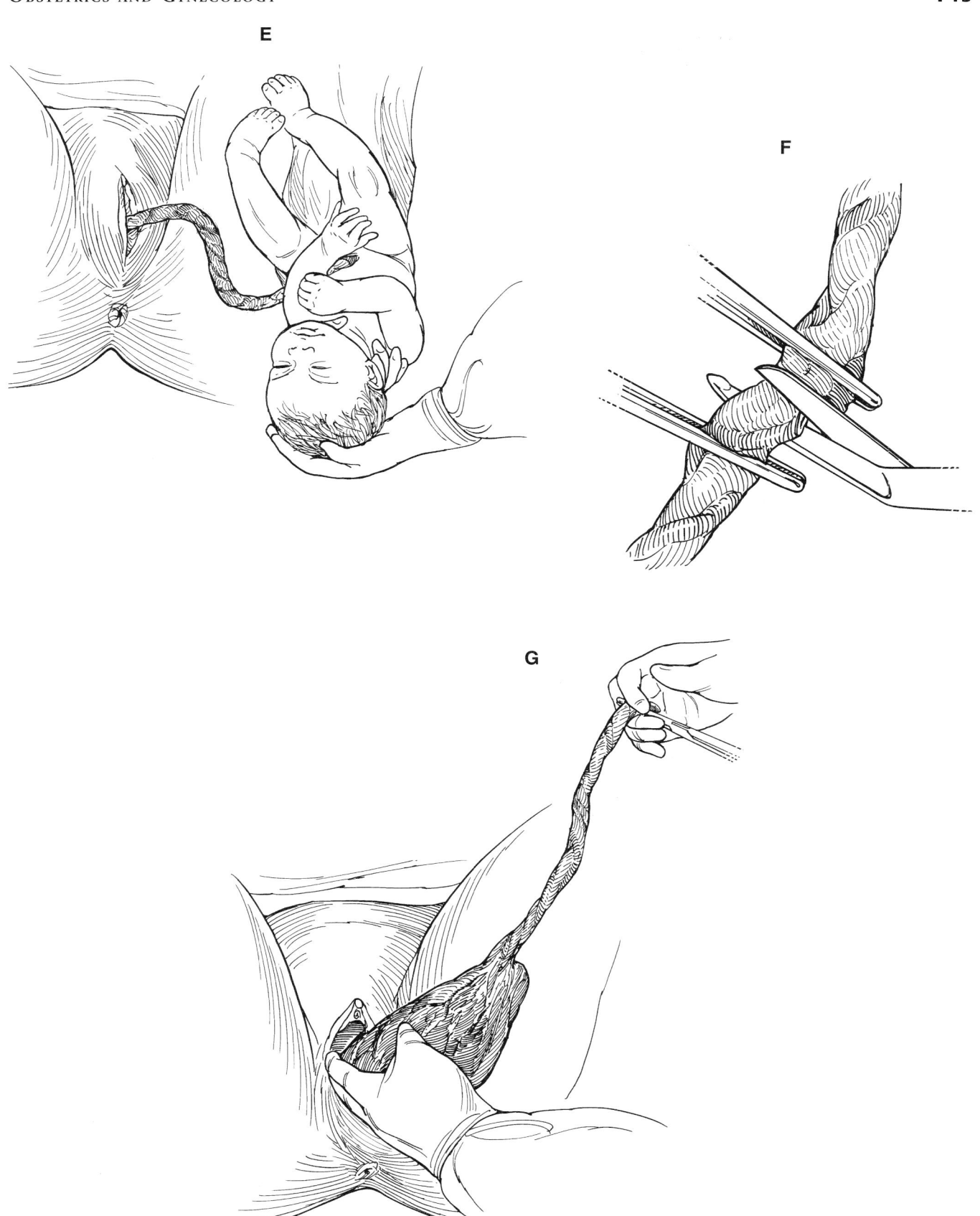

F

G

Perimortem Cesarean Section ■ COLLEEN J. CAMPBELL

Indications
- Emergency delivery of a viable fetus when maternal death is imminent or maternal vital signs have been absent for the past 15 minutes

Contraindications
- Estimated gestational age less than 28 weeks
- Prolonged maternal hypoxia (longer than 15 minutes)

Equipment
- Minimum requirements
  - Emergency department thoracotomy tray or cardiac arrest tray
  - Obstetric tray and scalpel with a No. 10 blade
  - Foley catheter
  - Sterile drapes and gloves
  - Gowns, shoe covers, facemask (at least two sets)
  - Suction (two setups)
- Ideal additional equipment
  - IV access
  - Local anesthetic (lidocaine), syringe, and needles
  - Surgical antiseptic solution
  - Foley catheter
  - Metzenbaum scissors
  - Mayo scissors
  - Suture scissors
  - Bandage scissors
  - Richardson retractors, medium and large
  - Bladder retractor
  - Hemostats, curved and straight (two of each type)
  - Two Adson forceps
  - Two smooth forceps
  - Gauze (at least four boxes)
  - Needle holders
  - Five packs of 2-0 chromic suture
  - Skin staples
  - Oxytocin
  - Bulb suction
  - Sterile towels
  - Two double cord clamps
  - Two straight clamps
  - Blood tube

Procedure
1. Place a Foley catheter to drain the bladder if time permits.
2. With the No. 10 scalpel, make a midline vertical incision to the peritoneal cavity from above the umbilicus to the margin of the pubic symphysis to the peritoneal cavity *(A-C)*.
3. Open the peritoneum by pulling up on it with two hemostats and making an incision with the Mayo scissors *(D)*. Extend the peritoneal incision superiorly to match the skin incision and inferiorly to the peritoneal bladder reflection.

OBSTETRICS AND GYNECOLOGY

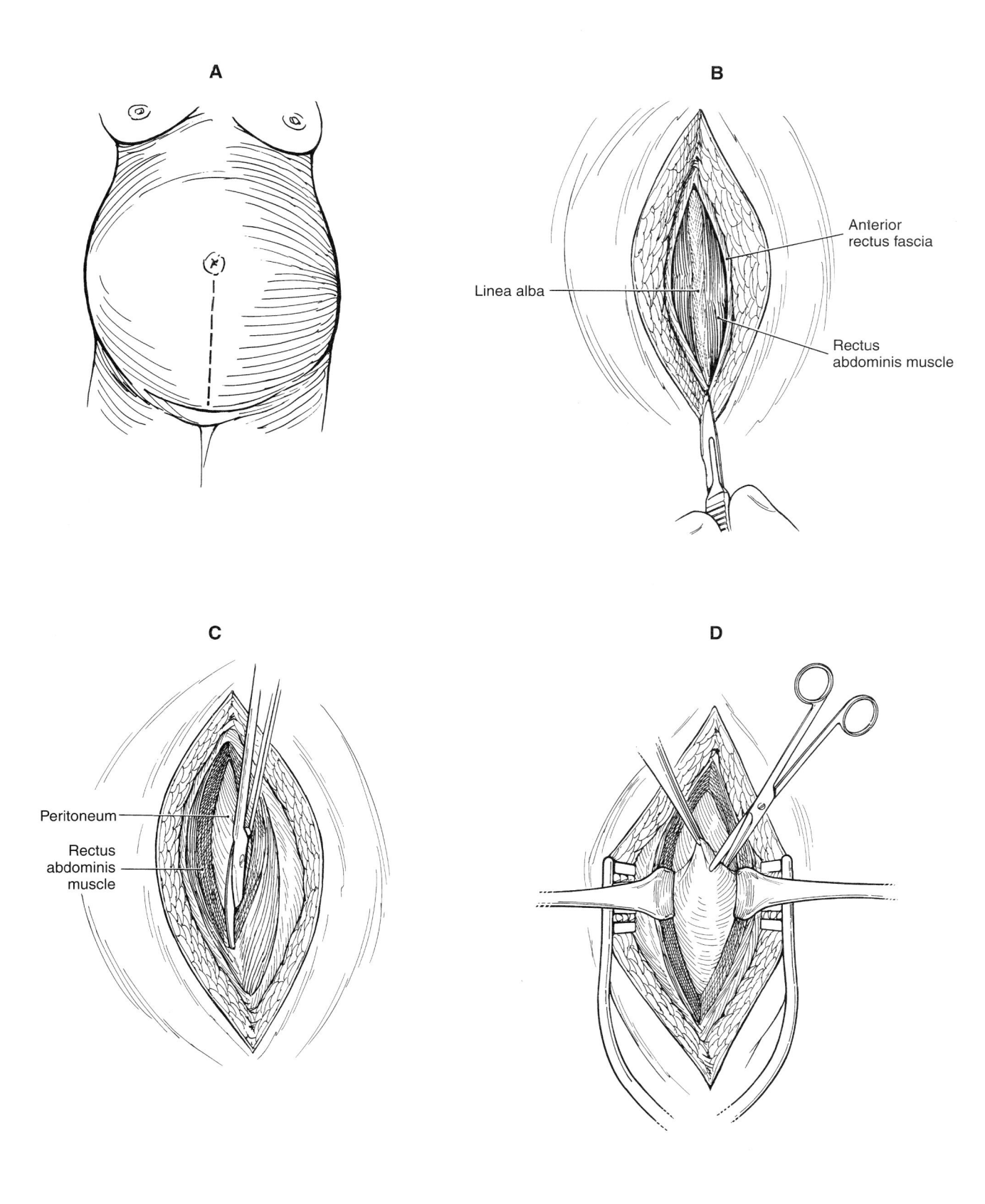

A

B

Anterior rectus fascia

Linea alba

Rectus abdominis muscle

C

Peritoneum

Rectus abdominis muscle

D

4. Use hemostats to clamp any large bleeding vessels.
5. Use retractors to open the incision laterally.
6. Identify the bladder, free it from the uterus, and retract it inferiorly.
7. Make a 5-cm vertical incision in the lower uterine segment with the scalpel.
8. Place two fingers into the uterus to clear the fetus from the incision path before extending the incision superiorly with Mayo scissors *(E)*.
9. Incise the fetal membranes as needed.
10. If the placenta is bleeding profusely, clamp and cut the cord and remove the placenta.
11. Place your hand between the symphysis pubis and the infant's head, elevate, and deliver it out of the incision *(F)*.
12. Suction the nose and mouth of the infant *(G)*.
13. Have the assistant apply fundal pressure while you are applying gentle traction on the head to deliver the shoulders *(H)*.
14. Double-clamp the cord, and cut between the clamps.
15. Begin oxytocin infusion (20 U in 1 L normal saline solution at 10 ml/hr) until the uterus contracts.
16. Place your hand between the membranes and uterus to deliver the placenta through the incision.
17. Recheck for maternal pulses, and resume maternal resuscitation if vital signs are present.
18. Close the uterus with 2-0 chromic suture in a running locking suture through the full thickness of the uterus.
19. Approximate the serosa of the bladder in its original position using 2-0 chromic suture.
20. Close the abdominal incision in three layers using 2-0 chromic suture and staples.
    a. The peritoneum is closed with running 2-0 chromic suture.
    b. The fascia is closed with interrupted 2-0 Mersiline suture.
    c. The skin is closed with skin staples or running 4-0 monofilament suture.

Complications

- Hemorrhage
- Fetal anoxic injury
- Fetal laceration and trauma

Discussion

- The physician has the legal right and responsibility to provide the unborn fetus with the maximal chance for survival in the event of maternal death.
- Cases of maternal survival after the procedure have been reported. This is thought to be due to improved venous return after uterine decompression.
- The best predictor of outcome is time from maternal loss of vital signs to delivery of the infant. In one small study 69% survived if the time was less than 5 minutes as compared with only 13% at 10 minutes.
- Outcome is also directly related to maturity of the fetus and acuity of the maternal loss of life.
- All live infants should be placed immediately in a neonatal intensive care unit.

Bibliography

Cunningham FG et al: Operative obstetrics. In *Williams obstetrics*, ed 20, Stamford, Conn, 1997, Appleton & Lange.

Doan-Wiggins L: Obstetric and gynecologic procedures. In Roberts JR, Hedges JR (eds): *Clinical procedures in emergency medicine*, ed 3, Philadelphia, 1998, WB Saunders.

Katz VL et al: Perimortem cesarean delivery, *Obstet Gynecol* 68:571, 1986.

E

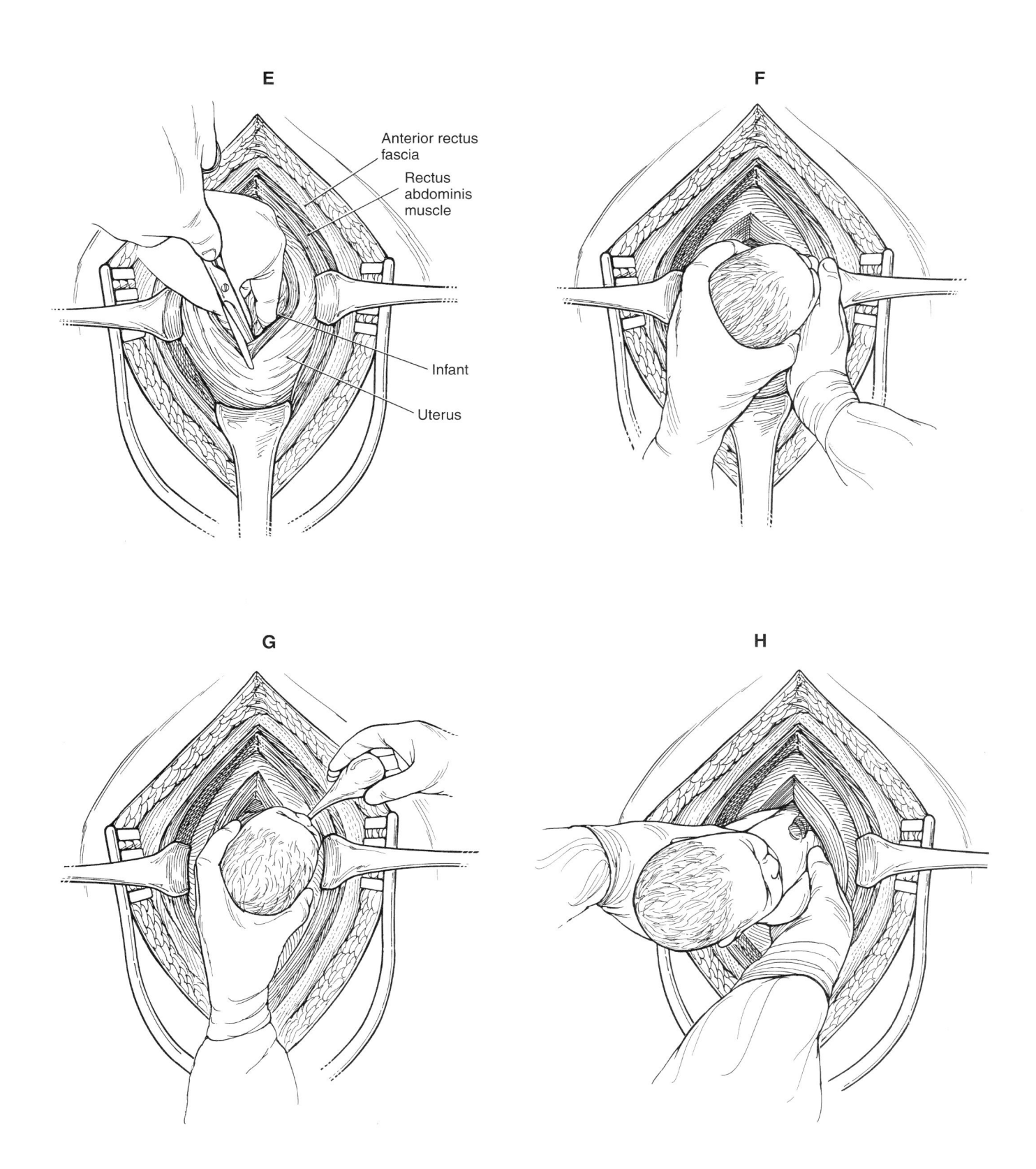

Anterior rectus fascia
Rectus abdominis muscle
Infant
Uterus

F

G

H

Episiotomy and Repair • COLLEEN J. CAMPBELL

Indications
- Enlargement of the vaginal introitus during childbirth if necessary to facilitate delivery of the fetus

Contraindications
- Early stage of labor (would cause excessive bleeding)
- Coagulopathy or bleeding disorders

Equipment
- Obstetric delivery table or vaginal examination table
- Light source
- Local anesthetic (1% lidocaine), syringe, and needles
- Sterile gauze
- Betadine antiseptic solution
- Surgical scissors
- Suture scissors
- Needle holder
- Absorbable suture (2.0 or 3.0 chromic catgut or polyglycolic acid) on a large needle

Procedure

1. As time permits, prepare the posterior vaginal introitus and posterior perineal region in sterile fashion.
2. Inject local anesthetic into the area of the posterior vaginal introitus.
3. Perform the incision when 3 to 4 cm of the fetal head is visible during contractions *(A)*.
4. To perform a midline episiotomy, incise through the median raphe of the perineum, being careful not to involve the musculature of the anal sphincter *(B, C)*.
5. To perform a mediolateral incision, direct the scissors posterior and lateral to either side of the midline sphincter.
6. After delivery of the placenta and inspection of the cervix and vaginal canal for lacerations, repair the episiotomy incision.
    a. To minimize bleeding into the surgical field, place gauze packing in the vaginal introitus.
    b. Using 2.0 or 3.0 absorbable suture, bury a knot in the deeper portion of the vaginal mucosa *(D)*.
    c. Use a continuous suture to approximate the vaginal mucosa.
    d. After approximating the hymenal ring, invert the suture and close the deep tissue, suturing in the posterior direction *(E)*.
    e. Continuing the same suture, close the subcuticular layer, burying the knot at the hymenal ring *(F)*.
    f. Alternatively, the perineal muscles may be closed with interrupted sutures.
    g. The subcuticular layer may also be closed with interrupted sutures.
    h. Repair of the mediolateral incision is performed in a similar fashion, approximating the musculature of the levator ani in the second layer.
7. The patient should have frequent sitz baths and pain relievers after the procedure. The obstetrics service should check the wound within 1 week.

Complications
- Rectal laceration or injury
- Dyspareunia
- Fecal incontinence
- Stress urinary incontinence
- Blood loss and hematoma
- Infection

Discussion
- Many obstetricians are now questioning the routine use of episiotomy because the theoretical benefits in reducing pelvic trauma, anal sphincter damage, fetal trauma, and urinary stress incontinence have not been borne out in clinical studies.
- Episiotomy has been shown to protect against anterior vaginal damage and urethral injury but is associated with a higher rate of anal sphincter damage.
- The Ipswich 2 study shows a decreased rate of dyspareunia at 3 months postpartum in women who have a two-stage repair in which the skin is left to close by secondary intention.
- The choice of midline versus mediolateral incision is stylistic. The midline approach is associated with a higher rate of anal sphincter damage but with less bleeding and less dyspareunia.

Bibliography

Gordon B et al: The Ipswich Childbirth Study: 1, 2. A randomized evaluation of two-stage postpartum perineal repair leaving the skin unsutured, *Br J Obstet Gynaecol* 105:435-445, 1998.

Robinson JN et al: Epsiotomy, operative vaginal delivery, and significant perineal trauma in nulliparous women, *Am J Obstet Gynecol* 181:1180-1184, 1999.

Sleep J et al: Care of the perineum. In Cunningham FG et al (eds): *Williams obstetrics*, ed 20, Stamford, Conn, 1997, Appleton & Lange.

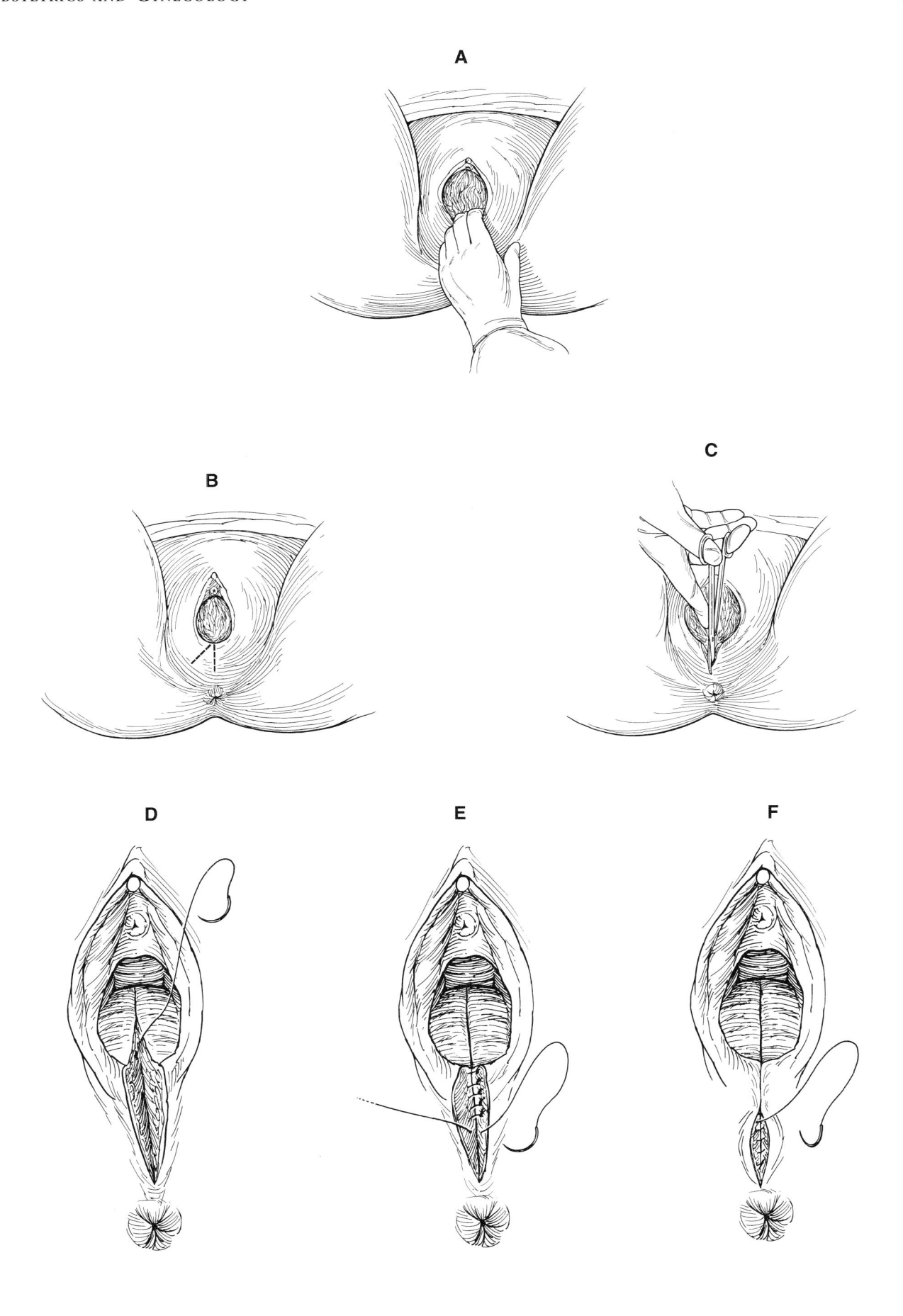

OBSTETRICS AND GYNECOLOGY

A

B

C

D

E

F

Incision and Drainage of Bartholin's Abscess
■ COLLEEN J. CAMPBELL

Indications
- Treatment of infection of Bartholin's duct and gland

Contraindications
- Painless cyst
- Coagulopathy

Equipment
- Pelvic examination table
- Betadine antiseptic solution
- Suction with catheter
- Local anesthetic agent (lidocaine 1%), syringe, and needles
- 3.0 chromic or other suture
- Word catheter (rubber catheter with inflatable tip)
- Scalpel with No. 10 or No. 11 blade
- Curved hemostat
- Toothed forceps
- 10-ml syringe
- Normal saline solution
- Culture tubes

Procedure

1. Place the patient in dorsal lithotomy position on a pelvic examination table.
2. Prepare and drape the abscessed area in sterile fashion.
3. Inject local anesthetic into the mucosal surface of the abscess and the mucocutaneous junction of the labia minora *(A)*.
4. Make a 1-cm vertical incision on the mucosal surface *(B)*.
5. Take fluid samples for culture.
6. Use a suction catheter for the remainder of the fluid.
7. Use a curved hemostat to break up loculations in the infected space.
8. Insert the Word catheter, and inflate the balloon with 5 ml normal saline. Leave in place for at least 24 hours *(C, D)*.

Complications
- Bleeding
- Recurrence
- Infection, cellulitis
- Dyspareunia

Discussion
- Most Bartholin's abscesses contain polymicrobial flora, similar to normal flora of the vagina. Antibiotics are not needed after the procedure unless surrounding cellulitis is present.
- Alternatives to the Word catheter include marsupialization of the tract with 3.0 chromic catgut suture and suturing of the everted abscess edge to the surrounding skin with simple interrupted sutures. If a Word catheter is not available, 1-inch iodoform gauze can be used to pack the abscess site after drainage. The gauze is removed in 24 hours.
- After the procedure, sitz baths should be encouraged. Oral analgesics may be prescribed.
- Necrotizing cellulitis can result from abscesses, especially in diabetic, immunocompromised, or older women.

Bibliography
Mishell DR et al: Infections of the lower genital tract. In *Comprehensive gynecology*, ed 3, St Louis, 1997, Mosby.
Ryan KJ et al: Gynecologic infections. In *Kistner's gynecology*, ed 6, St Louis, 1995, Mosby.
Sope DE: Genitourinary infections and sexually transmitted diseases. In Berek JS et al (eds): *Novak's gynecology*, ed 12, Baltimore, 1996, Williams & Wilkins.

OBSTETRICS AND GYNECOLOGY

A

B

C

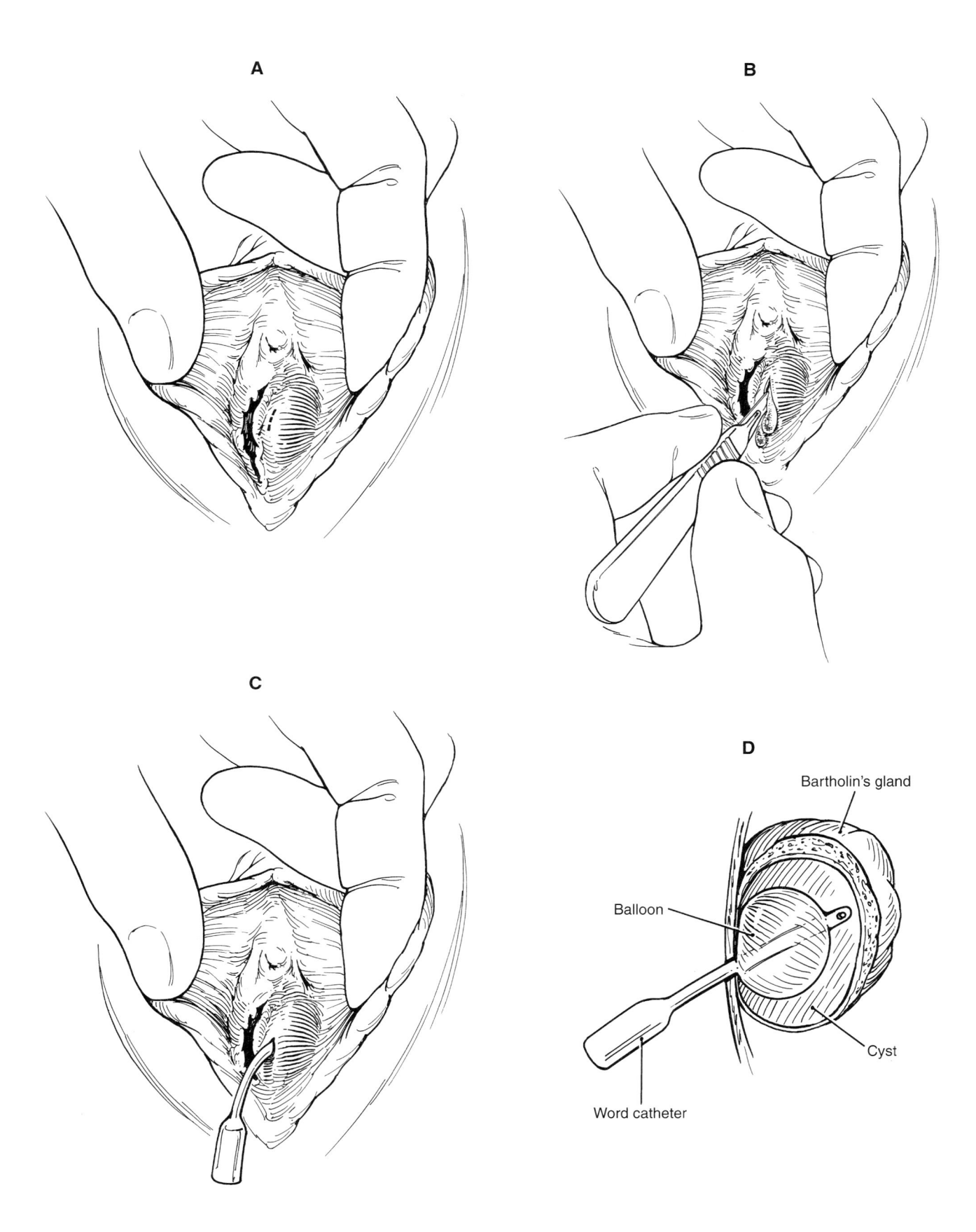

D
- Bartholin's gland
- Balloon
- Cyst
- Word catheter

CHAPTER 7

NERVOUS SYSTEM

Lumbar Puncture ■ JAMES L. LARSON, JR.

Indications
- Possible meningitis
- Possible neurosyphilis
- Possible subarachnoid hemorrhage
- Diagnosis and treatment of pseudotumor cerebri

Contraindications
- Elevation of intracranial pressure from a mass lesion
- Clinical signs of herniation
- Superficial cutaneous infection at site where procedure is to be performed
- Acquired or congenital coagulation disorders, including hemophilia, warfarin or heparin therapy, and advanced liver disease (relative contraindication)
- Thrombocytopenia (relative contraindication)

Equipment
- Prepackaged lumbar puncture kit, or the following:
  - Anesthetic (1% lidocaine without epinephrine)
  - 5-ml syringe with 25-gauge needle
  - 22-gauge 1½-inch needle
  - Betadine antiseptic solution
  - Sterile drape or towels
  - Four cerebrospinal fluid (CSF) collection tubes
  - Manometer and stopcock
  - 4 × 4 gauze pads
  - Spinal needle with stylet
  - Adhesive bandage

Procedure

1. Place the patient in the lateral decubitus or seated upright position.
2. Flex the patient to increase the intervertebral spaces.
   a. Lateral decubitus: flex knees and pelvis toward shoulders, keeping the plane of the back perpendicular to the floor *(A)*.
   b. Upright: have the patient lean over, placing arms on a table, Mayo stand, or chair *(B)*.
3. In adults the spinal cord ends at the L1-2 intervertebral space, and lumbar puncture should be performed below this level to avoid injuring the cord. To find a safe intervertebral space in which to perform the procedure, first locate the iliac crests. At the level of the crests, palpate the spinous processes and locate the intervertebral space at this level (generally, the L3-4 space) *(C)*.
4. Prepare and drape the patient in sterile fashion.
5. Inject lidocaine with the 25-gauge needle to raise a wheal over the skin surface at the intervertebral space.
6. Use the longer 22-gauge needle to inject lidocaine into the deeper tissues in order to anesthetize the intervertebral space.
7. Assemble the manometer.
8. With the spinal needle, puncture the skin at the site, aiming midline toward the umbilicus *(D)*.
9. Advance the spinal needle slowly, removing the stylet frequently to see if CSF enters the needle, which indicates that the dural space has been penetrated. If no fluid is obtained, place the stylet back into the needle and continue advancing or redirecting the needle as needed.
10. If bony resistance is encountered, withdraw the needle to the subcutaneous tissue and redirect it at a slightly different angle in the cephalocaudad direction as indicated.
11. When CSF is encountered, attach the manometer to the spinal needle to record the opening pressure (lateral decubitus position).
12. Use the four tubes to collect the CSF.
13. Replace the stylet, and remove the needle.
14. Place an adhesive bandage over the puncture site.

Complications
- Spinal subdural, epidural, or subarachnoid hematoma
- Meningitis or spinal abscess formation
- Arachnoiditis
- Post–lumbar puncture headache
- Soft tissue infection

Discussion
- Occasionally a "pop" is felt as the needle passes through the ligamentum flavum. At this point the dural space is in close proximity, and the needle should be advanced only a few millimeters before the stylet is withdrawn to determine whether the dural space has been penetrated.
- The amount of CSF to be removed depends on the clinical presentation and the information being evaluated. A minimum of 1 ml of CSF per tube is needed to evaluate for meningitis or subarachnoid hemorrhage. More CSF would be required for cytology studies.
- If difficulty is encountered in locating the dural space or obtaining cerebrospinal fluid, the patient's body position should be reassessed and the needle should be checked to confirm that is indeed midline.

Nervous System

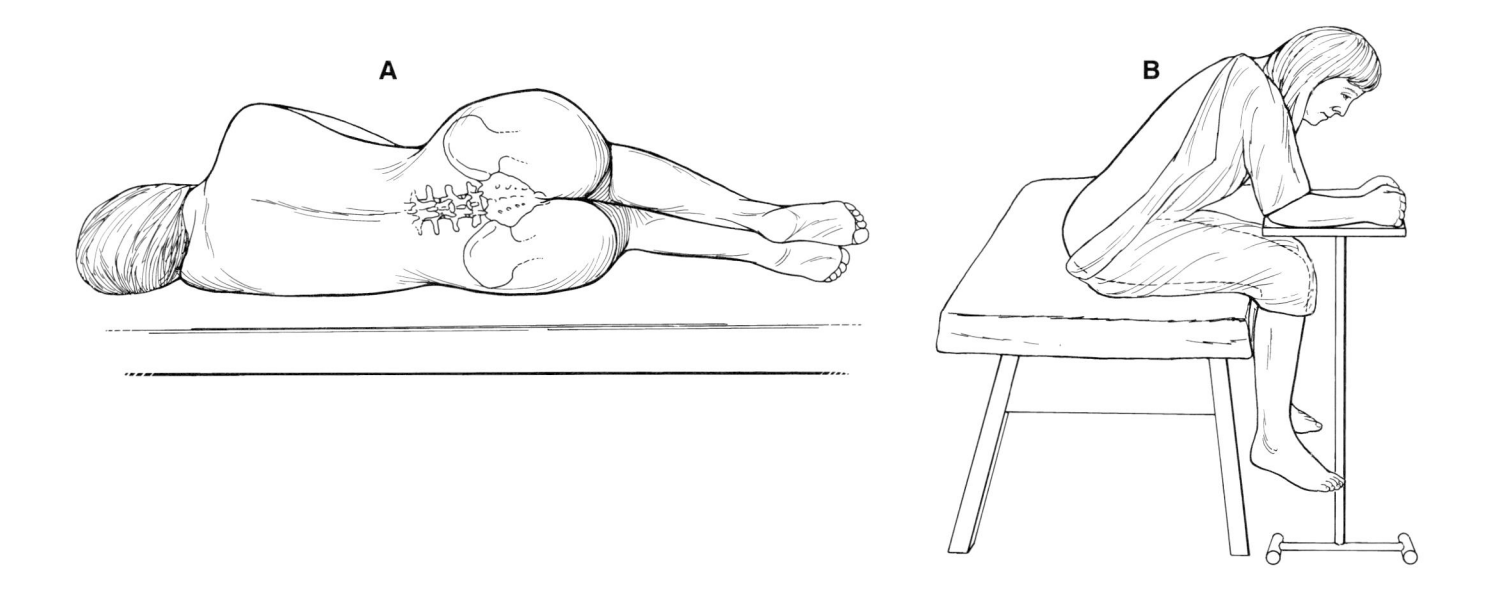

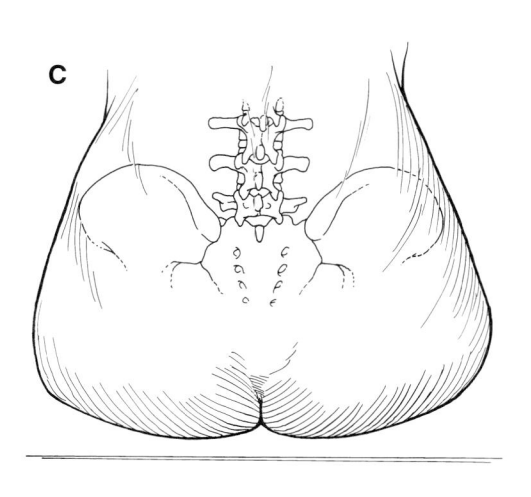

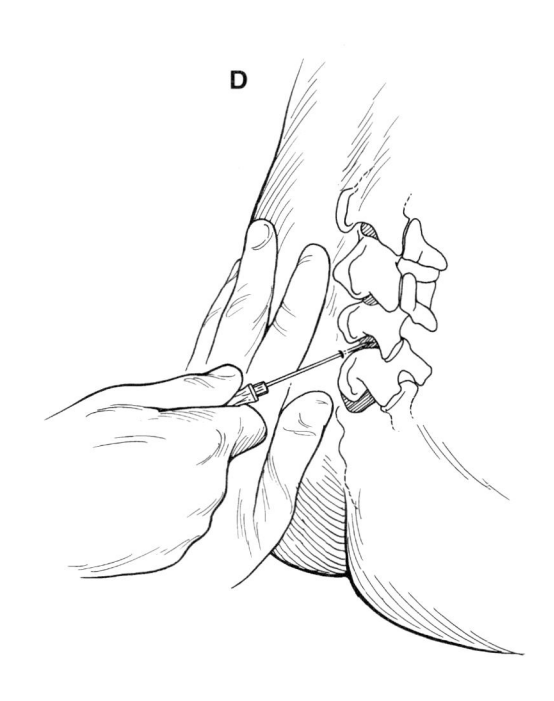

- For obese patients the upright sitting approach is often preferred because it allows easier determination of and access to the midline posteriorly. If indicated, therapeutic measures (e.g., antibiotics or coagulopathy reversal) should be instituted before or during the lumbar puncture.
- Administering IV fluids and maintaining the patient in the supine position for 30 minutes after lumbar puncture have been reported to reduce the risk of post–lumbar puncture headaches.

Bibliography

Gorelick PB, Biller J: Lumbar puncture, technique, indications and complications, *Postgrad Med* 79:257-268, 1986.

Leibold RA et al: Post dural-puncture headache: characteristics, management, and prevention, *Ann Emerg Med* 12(12):1863-1870, 1993.

Martin KM, Gean AD: The "spinal tap": a new look at an old test, *Ann Intern Med* 104:840-848, 1986.

Wee N et al: Detection of subarachnoid hemorrhage on early CT: is lumbar puncture still needed after a negative scan? *J Neurol Neurosurg Psychiatry* 58:357-359, 1995.

Facial and Oral Blocks

Supraorbital Nerve Block N. NOUNOU TALEGHANI AND GEORGE STERNBACH

Indications
- Need for anesthesia of the region of the face innervated by the supraorbital nerve

Contraindications
- Allergy to anesthetic agent
- Grossly distorted landmarks
- Infection at the site of injection

Equipment
- 27-gauge 1½-inch needle with 5-ml syringe
- 2 × 2 sterile gauze
- Betadine antiseptic solution
- 2% lidocaine with 1:100,000 epinephrine
- 0.5% bupivacaine with 1:200,000 epinephrine

Procedure
1. Palpate the superior orbital foramen or notch along the medial aspect of the supraorbital ridge *(A, B)*.
2. Prepare the site of the superior orbital foramen in sterile fashion.
3. Raise a wheal with a 50/50 mixture of lidocaine and bupivacaine above the superior orbital foramen.
4. Insert the 27-gauge needle parallel to the eyebrow, and slowly deposit 5 ml of the anesthetic agent under the skin above the entire length of the eyebrow *(C)*.

Complications
- Nerve injury
- Intravascular injection of agent
- Infection
- Allergic reactions

Discussion
- Regional blocks provide good anesthesia without distorting local landmarks for laceration repairs.

Bibliography

Kretzschmer JL, Peters JE: Nerve blocks for regional anesthesia of the face, *Am Fam Physician* 55(5):1701-1704, 1997.

A

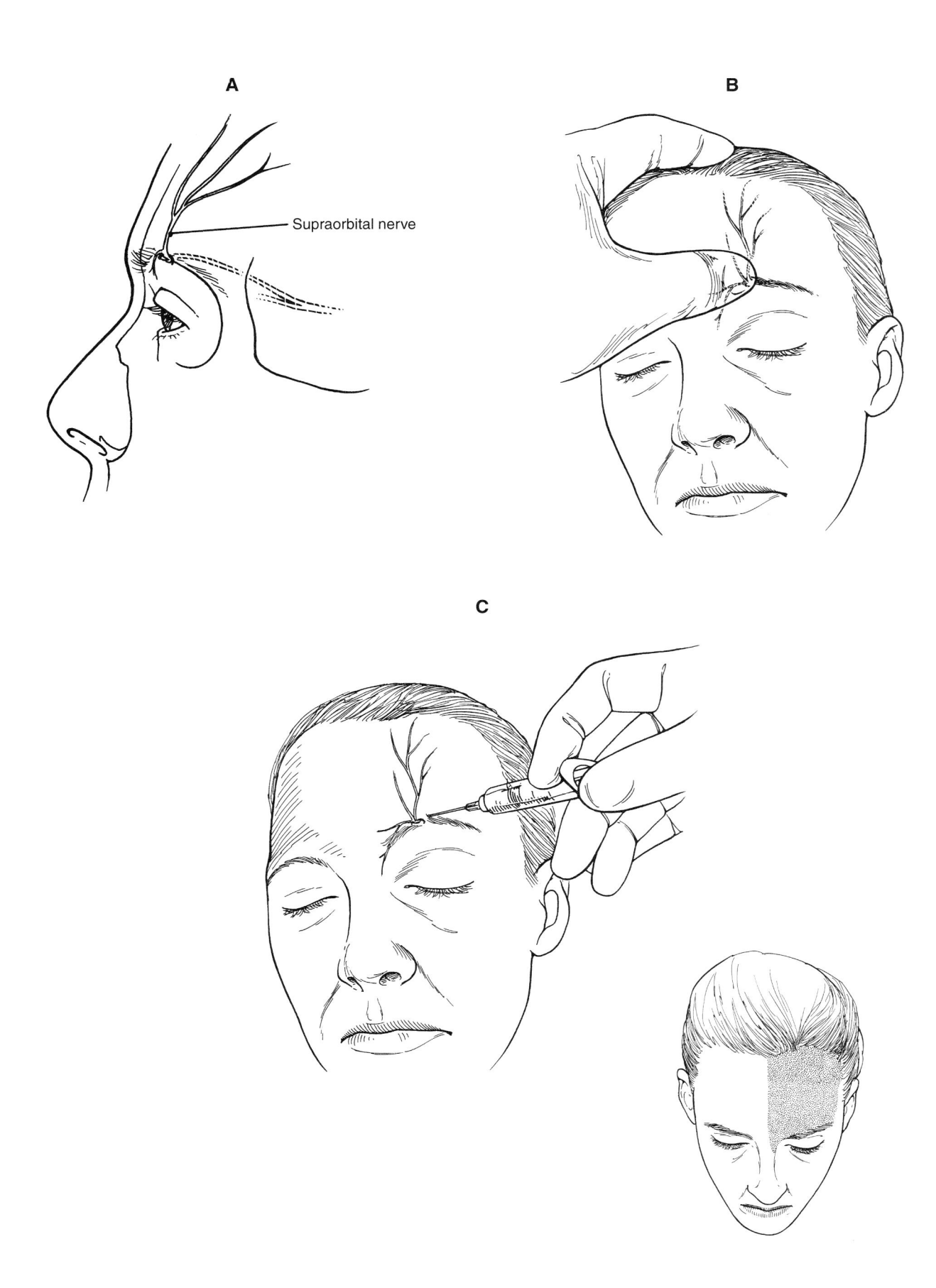

Supraorbital nerve

B

C

INFRAORBITAL NERVE BLOCK   N. NOUNOU TALEGHANI AND GEORGE STERNBACH

Indications
- Need for anesthesia of the region of the face innervated by the infraorbital nerve (A, B)

Contraindications
- Allergy to anesthetic agent

Equipment
- Dental aspirating syringe or standard 27-gauge 1½-inch needle with 3-ml syringe
- 2 × 2 sterile gauze
- Cotton-tipped applicator
- Suction
- 2% lidocaine with 1:100,000 epinephrine
- 0.5% bupivacaine with 1:200,000 epinephrine

Procedure
1. Locate the landmark of the infraorbital foramen (A, B).
2. Swab the labial mucosa just anterior to the apex of the first premolar tooth of the maxilla with topical 2% lidocaine on a cotton-tipped applicator.
3. Once the anesthetic has taken effect, retract the maxillary lip with the nondominant thumb and index finger.
4. Position and insert the needle into the mucolabial fold, just anterior to the apex of the first premolar tooth.
5. Place a finger over the infraorbital foramen, and advance the needle tip along the axis of the tooth toward the foramen. Total depth should be 5 to 10 mm (C).
6. Slowly inject 1 to 2 ml of anesthetic (50/50 mix of lidocaine and bupivacaine).

Complications
- Nerve injury
- Intravascular injection of agent
- Infection
- Allergic reactions

Discussion
- Regional blocks provide good anesthesia without distorting local landmarks for laceration repairs.
- If the patient complains of paresthesia after the needle is in place but before injection of the anesthetic, the needle is probably in the infraorbital nerve and should be withdrawn 1 or 2 mm before injection.
- Divert the patient's attention from the injection by retracting the lip back and forth during the delivery of the anesthetic.
- Anesthesia is confirmed by a subjective feeling of numbness or tingling in the lip or the patient's stating that the lip feels "fat."

Bibliography
Kretzschmer JL, Peters JE: Nerve blocks for regional anesthesia of the face, *Am Fam Physician* 55(5):1701-1704, 1997.

A

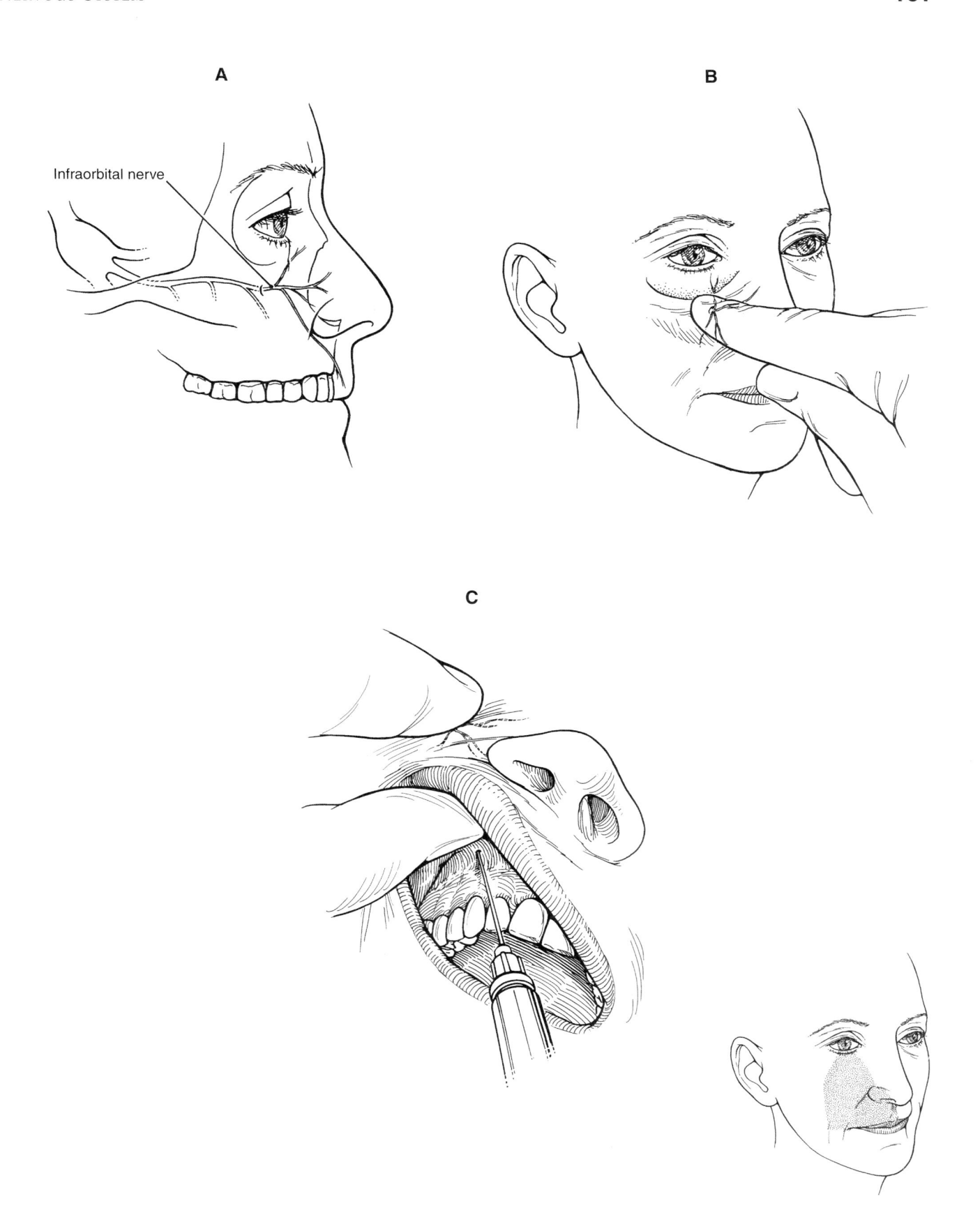

Infraorbital nerve

B

C

Internal Maxillary–Superior Alveolar Nerve Block   JAMES T. AMSTERDAM

Indications
- To achieve anesthesia of the maxillary (upper) teeth and surrounding soft tissue
- Relief of dental pain from caries or trauma to the upper teeth
- Incision and drainage of dental infection involving the upper teeth
- Anesthesia for facial soft tissue repair involving the upper lip or surrounding region

Contraindications
- Necessity for passing injection through infected tissue
- Inability to perform aspiration
- Uncooperative patient
- Patient with bleeding disorder or receiving anticoagulants (relative contraindication)

Equipment
- Ear, nose, and throat (ENT)/dental chair
- Adequate lighting or headlamp
- Gauze
- Topical anesthetic spray (benzocaine)
- Dental aspirating syringe (monojet) or standard plastic syringe that allows aspiration
- Local anesthetic agent or carpules of dental local anesthetic agent (lidocaine with epinephrine 1:100,000, 3% mepivacaine, 0.5% bupivacaine)
- Standard aspiration syringe
- 25- to 27-gauge hypodermic needles

Procedure

Seat the patient in the ENT/dental chair in semi-Fowler's position.

Identify the region of injection based on area of anesthesia needed (generally along the mucobuccal fold of the upper gum just above the teeth; see below) *(A)*.

Apply topical anesthetic over this area.

Prepare the dental aspiration syringe.

Draw 2 to 5 ml anesthetic agent into the syringe, and attach needle.

If using a dental carpule, slide the carpule into the barrel of the syringe and slip the needle into the carpule. Tap the handle with force so that the barb engages the rubber stopper in the carpule.

Have the patient open the mouth slightly. Grasp the lip with thumb and forefinger.

Expose the mucobuccal fold and injection site.

7. Identify the specific region for the block, and proceed as follows:
   a. Supraperiosteal injection (anesthesia of maxillary anterior teeth—canine to canine teeth, anterior to premolars)
      i. Insert the needle directly above the apex of the specific tooth.
      ii. Inject 2 ml of anesthetic with the needle bevel facing bone.
   b. Anterosuperior alveolar injection and canine space block (anesthesia of maxillary canine and half of upper lip and surrounding soft tissues) *(B)*
      i. Insert the needle above the apex of the canine tooth into the canine fossa.
      ii. Inject 2 ml of anesthetic with the needle bevel facing bone.
   c. Middle superior alveolar injection and block (anesthesia of the maxillary premolar teeth and mesiobuccal root of the maxillary first molar) *(C)*
      i. Insert needle above the apex of the second premolar tooth.
      ii. Inject 2 ml of anesthetic with the needle bevel facing bone.
   d. Posterosuperior alveolar injection (anesthesia of maxillary molar teeth and surrounding soft tissue) *(D)*
      i. Stand on the ipsilateral side of the patient.
      ii. Have the patient close the jaw gently and swing the jaw toward you.
      iii. Insert the needle into the mucosa above the maxillary second molar, holding the syringe at a 30° angle to the sagittal plane.
      iv. Direct the needle posteriorly and superiorly around the tuberosity (at the third molar or directly behind the area of the third molar) to a depth of approximately 2 cm.
      v. Aspirate (to avoid the pterygoid plexus of vessel), and inject 2 ml of anesthetic with the needle bevel facing bone.

Complications

- Bleeding, hematoma
- Intravascular injection
- Infection
- Needle breakage
- Facial nerve anesthesia (iatrogenic Bell's palsy)
- Vasovagal syncope

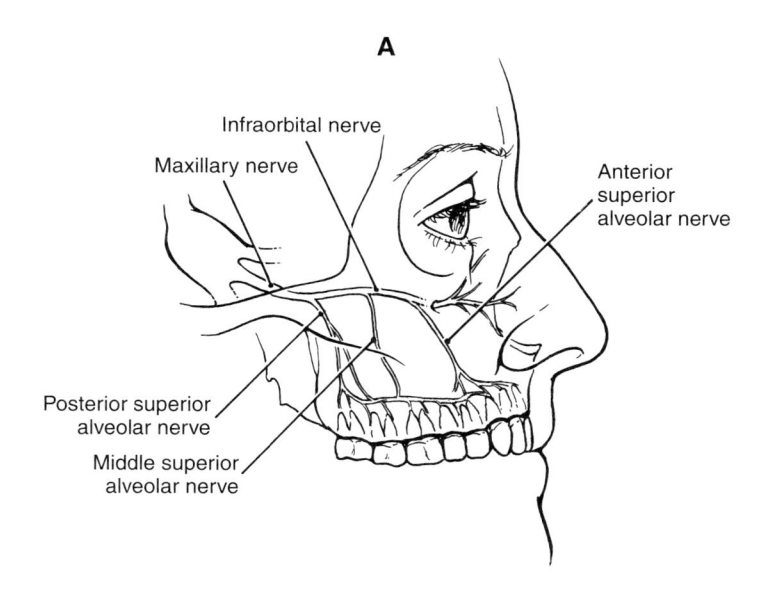

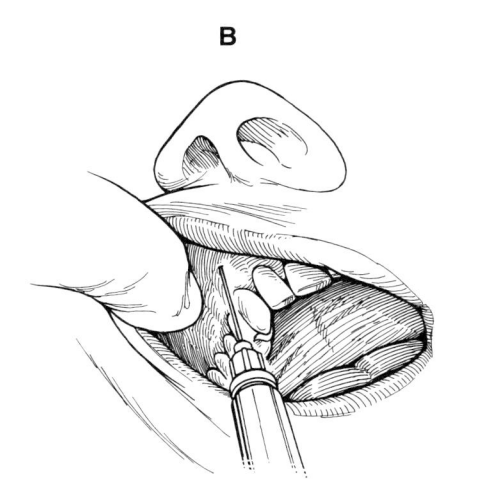

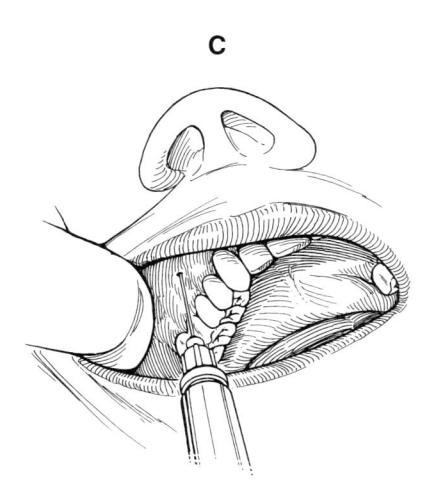

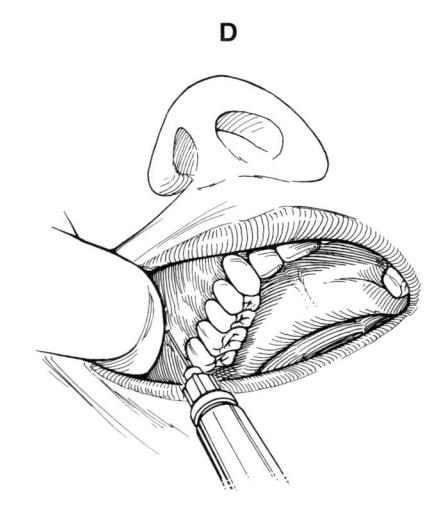

A

Infraorbital nerve
Maxillary nerve
Anterior superior alveolar nerve
Posterior superior alveolar nerve
Middle superior alveolar nerve

B **C** **D**

Discussion

- Aspiration is important before any injection to prevent intravascular injection of the anesthetic agent. Dental aspirating syringes are ideal for aspiration and injection. A standard syringe can also be used, particularly one with a ring on the handle to make aspiration easier.
- The anterosuperior alveolar block is useful for repair of upper lip lacerations. However, when this block is used for a midline lip laceration, additional anesthesia (local or similar nerve block) may be necessary for the contralateral side. Only one side should be blocked to prevent bite damage to the lips that might occur if the lips were totally anesthetized.
- The posterosuperior alveolar block is technically more difficult than the other blocks. In addition to the posterior block, a middle superior alveolar block may be necessary to supplement anesthesia of the molar region.
- Patients should be given oral analgesics if the anesthesia is expected to wear off before dental follow-up.

Bibliography

Amsterdam JT: Regional anesthesia of the head and neck. In Roberts JR, Hedges JR (eds): *Clinical procedures in emergency medicine*, ed 3, Philadelphia, 1998, WB Saunders.

Bennett CR: *Manheim's local anesthesia and pain control in dental practice*, St Louis, 1978, Mosby.

Lynch MT et al: Comparison of intraoral and percutaneous approaches for intraorbital nerve block, *Acad Emerg Med* 1:514, 1994.

Mandibular and Inferior Alveolar Nerve Block   James T. Amsterdam

Indications
- Anesthesia of the mandibular teeth to one side of the midline, buccal gingiva and mucosa, and lower lip (inferior alveolar nerve); anterior two thirds of the tongue (lingual nerve); and gingival and buccal mucosa opposite the second and third molars (buccal nerve) *(A)*
- Relief of dental pain from caries, infection, or trauma to the mandibular teeth
- Incision and drainage of dental infection involving the mandibular teeth
- Relief of pain associated with mandible fracture

Contraindications
- Necessity for injection to pass through infected tissue
- Inability to perform aspiration
- Uncooperative patient
- Patient with bleeding disorder or receiving anticoagulant (relative contraindication)

Equipment
- ENT/dental chair
- Adequate lighting or headlamp
- Gauze
- Topical anesthetic spray (benzocaine)
- Dental aspirating syringe (monojet) or standard plastic syringe that allows aspiration
- Local anesthetic agent or carpules of dental local anesthetic agent (lidocaine with epinephrine 1:100,000, 3% mepivacaine, 0.5% bupivacaine)
- 25- to 27-gauge hypodermic needles
- Standard aspiration syringe

Procedure

1. Seat the patient in the ENT/dental chair in the semi-Fowler's position.
2. Spray topical anesthetic over the area.
3. Prepare the dental aspiration syringe.
   a. Load 2 to 5 ml anesthetic agent into the syringe, and attach the needle.
   b. If using a dental carpule, slide the carpule into the barrel of the syringe and slip the needle into the end. Tap the handle with force so that the barb engages the rubber stopper in the carpule.
4. Stand facing the patient.
5. Palpate the coronoid process of the mandible with your thumb, and retract the cheek laterally *(B)*.
6. Use gauze to dry the mucosal area.
7. Visualize the mucosa posterior to the molars, where a small triangle of tissue (formed by the ptyergomandibular raphe of tissues) is generally seen.
8. Slide the thumb farther laterally once this area is identified.
9. Insert the needle into the center of the triangle with the syringe held parallel to the occlusal surface of the teeth and over the contralateral first and second premolars *(C)*.
10. Direct the needle posteriorly until encountering bone.
11. Withdraw the needle slightly, and aspirate (to avoid the inverior alveolar artery).
12. Inject 2 ml of anesthetic into the region.
13. Obtain additional blocks, if needed, at this time.
    a. Lingual nerve: continue to withdraw the needle slowly, and right before the needle exits the mucosa, inject 0.5 ml of anesthetic to anesthetize the lingual nerve.
    b. Long buccal nerve: after the needle is withdrawn, deposit 0.5 ml of anesthetic in the buccal mucosa opposite the second molar to anesthetize the long buccal nerve.

Complications

- Bleeding, hematoma
- Intravascular injection
- Infection
- Needle breakage
- Facial nerve anesthesia (iatrogenic Bell's palsy)
- Vasovagal syncope

Discussion

- Aspiration is important before any injection to prevent intravascular injection of the anesthetic agent. Dental aspirating syringes are ideal for aspiration and injection. A standard syringe can also be used, particularly one with a ring on the handle to make aspiration easier.
- If the patient experiences an electric shock sensation, the needle has entered the nerve. The operator should withdraw the needle slightly and aspirate. Nothing should be injected directly into the nerve, since this can cause permanent paresthesia.
- If the patient's lips do not become numb, the block was incomplete or unsuccessful. An alternative approach

A

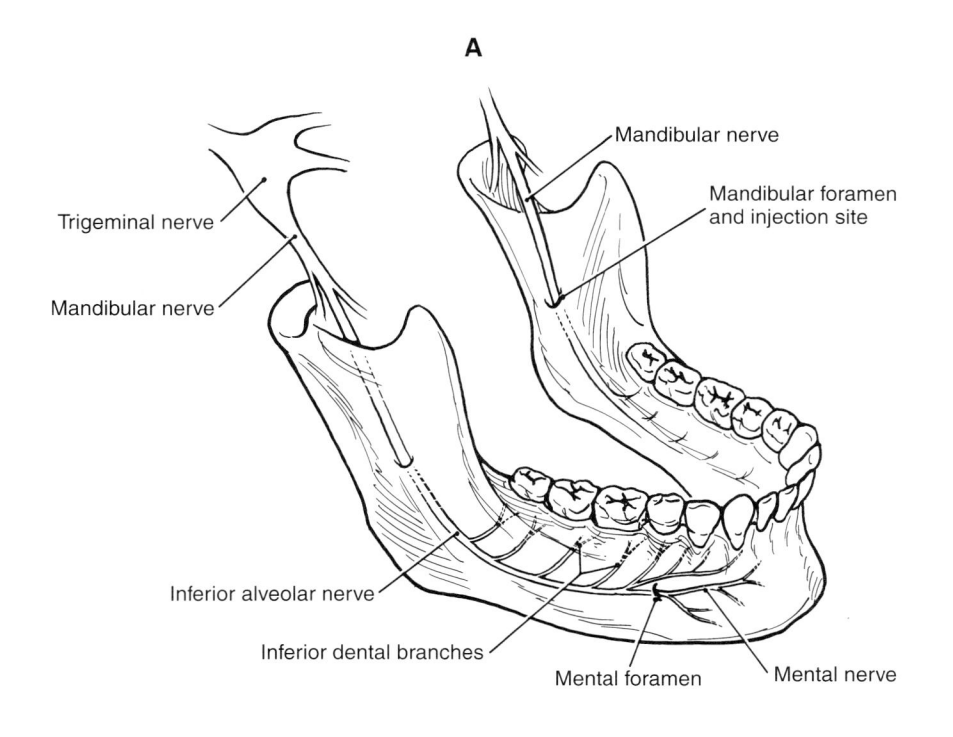

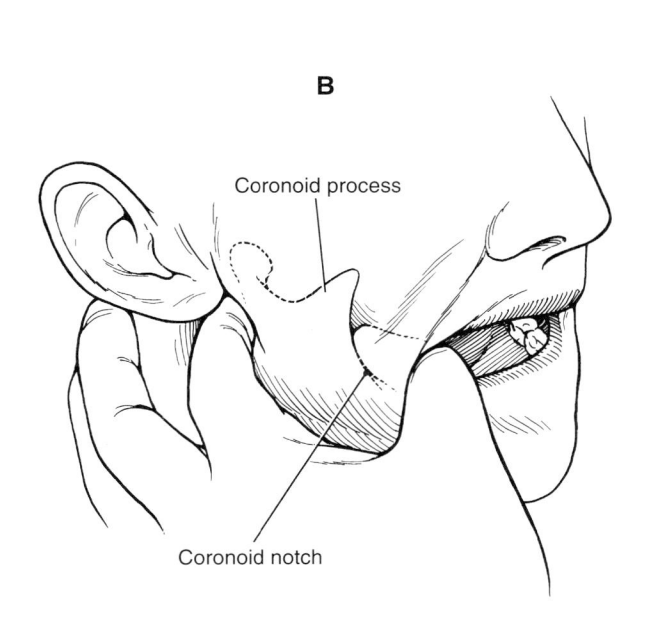

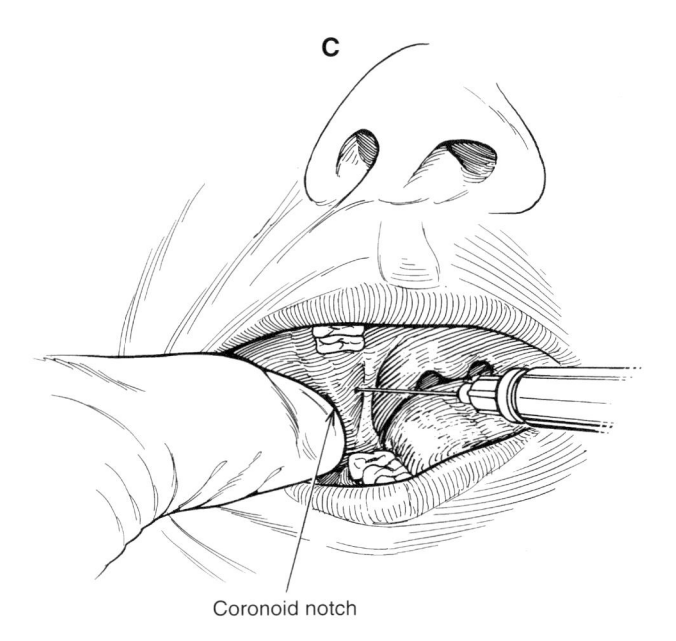

- Trigeminal nerve
- Mandibular nerve
- Mandibular nerve
- Mandibular foramen and injection site
- Inferior alveolar nerve
- Inferior dental branches
- Mental foramen
- Mental nerve

B

- Coronoid process
- Coronoid notch

C

- Coronoid notch

can be used. After the needle is inserted to the bone, the syringe can be swung toward the midline (from its position overlying the contralateral second and third molars). With the syringe in this position the needle is inserted another 0.5 cm posteriorly. The syringe is swung back to its original position. The needle is inserted again until contact is made with bone and anesthetic agent is injected as above. This technique allows passage around the lingula, a prominence of bone that protects the inferior alveolar foramen.

- Patients should be given oral analgesics if the anesthesia is expected to wear off before dental follow-up.

Bibliography

Amsterdam JT: Regional anesthesia of the head and neck. In Roberts JR, Hedges JR (eds): *Clinical procedures in emergency medicine,* ed 3, Philadelphia, 1998, WB Saunders.

Bennett CR: *Manheim's local anesthesia and pain control in dental practice,* St Louis, 1978, Mosby.

Lynch MT et al: Comparison of intraoral and percutaneous approaches for infraorbital nerve block, *Acad Emerg Med* 1:514, 1994.

Mental Nerve Block JAMES T. AMSTERDAM

Indications
- Anesthesia of the lower lip and associated soft tissues almost to the level of the chin
- Anesthesia for facial soft tissue repair involving the lower lip or surrounding region

Contraindications
- Necessity for injection to pass through infected tissue
- Inability to perform aspiration
- Uncooperative patient
- Patient with bleeding disorders or receiving anticoagulants (relative contraindication)

Equipment
- ENT/dental chair
- Adequate lighting or headlamp
- Gauze
- Topical anesthetic spray (benzocaine)
- Dental aspirating syringe (monojet) or standard plastic syringe that allows aspiration
- Local anesthetic agent or carpules of dental local anesthetic agent (lidocaine with epinephrine 1:100,000, 3% mepivacaine, 0.5% bupivacaine)
- 25- to 27-gauge hypodermic needles
- Standard aspiration syringe

Procedure
1. Seat the patient in an ENT/dental chair in semi-Fowler's position.
2. Spray topical anesthetic over the area.
3. Prepare the dental aspiration syringe.
   a. Load 2 to 5 ml anesthetic agent into the syringe, and attach the needle.
   b. If using a dental carpule, slide the carpule into the barrel of the syringe and slip the needle into the end. Tap the handle with force so that the barb engages the rubber stopper in the carpule.
4. Palpate the mental foramen between the two lower premolar teeth in adults and between the first and second primary molars in children *(A)*.
5. Retract the cheek laterally.
6. Insert the needle into the mucobuccal fold between the two premolar teeth near the foramen *(B)*.
7. Administer 2 to 3 ml of anesthetic into this area.

Complications
- Bleeding, hematoma
- Intravascular injection
- Infection
- Needle breakage
- Facial nerve anesthesia (iatrogenic Bell's palsy)
- Vasovagal syncope

Discussion
- Aspiration is important before any injection to prevent intravascular injection of the anesthetic agent. Dental aspirating syringes are ideal for aspiration and injection. A standard syringe can also be used, particularly one with a ring on the handle to make aspiration easier.
- If the lower lip laceration involves the midline, anesthetic should be deposited in the supraperiosteal soft tissue or a mental nerve block should be performed on the contralateral side. Lacerations involving the corner of the lip may require both a mental nerve block and an anterosuperior alveolar nerve block (see section on maxillary block) for adequate anesthesia.
- If the mental foramen cannot be identified, the anesthetic should simply be deposited somewhere near where the mental nerve exits the foramen (i.e., in the mucobuccal fold between the premolars). Direct infiltration into the foramen can damage the neurovascular bundle, causing a permanent paresthesia.
- The mental nerve block is used for anesthesia for soft tissue repair and not for anesthetizing the teeth.
- Patients should be given oral analgesics if the anesthesia is expected to wear off before dental follow-up.

Bibliography
Amsterdam JT: Regional anesthesia of the head and neck. In Roberts JR, Hedges JR (eds): *Clinical procedures in emergency medicine*, ed 3, Philadelphia, 1998, WB Saunders.

Bennett CR: *Manheim's local anesthesia and pain control in dental practice*, St Louis, 1978, Mosby.

Lynch MT et al: Comparison of intraoral and percutaneous approaches for infraorbital nerve block, *Acad Emerg Med* 1:514, 1994.

Syverud SA et al: A comparative study of percutaneous versus intraoral technique for mental nerve block, *Acad Emerg Med* 1:509, 1994.

NERVOUS SYSTEM

A

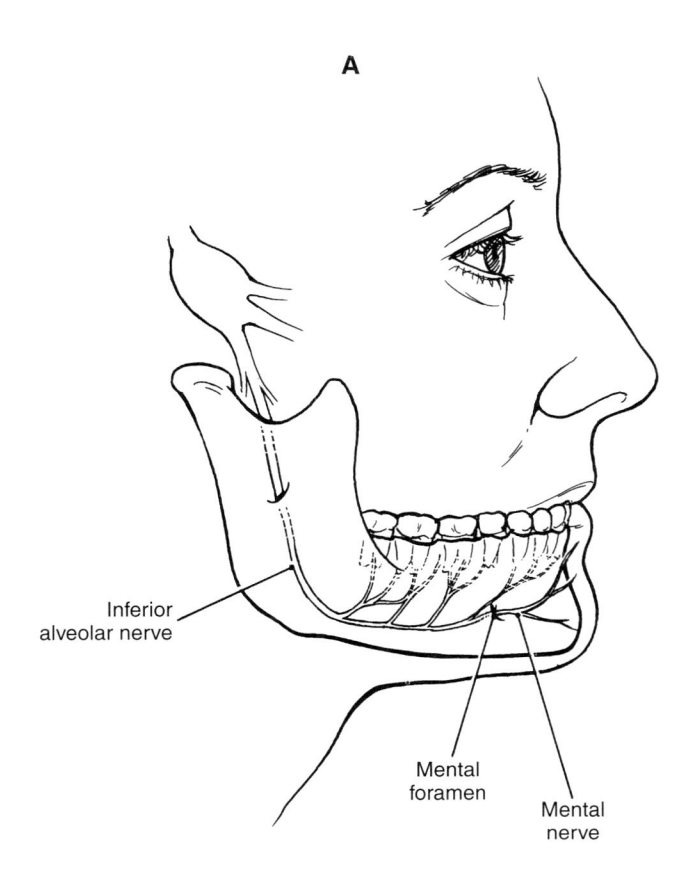

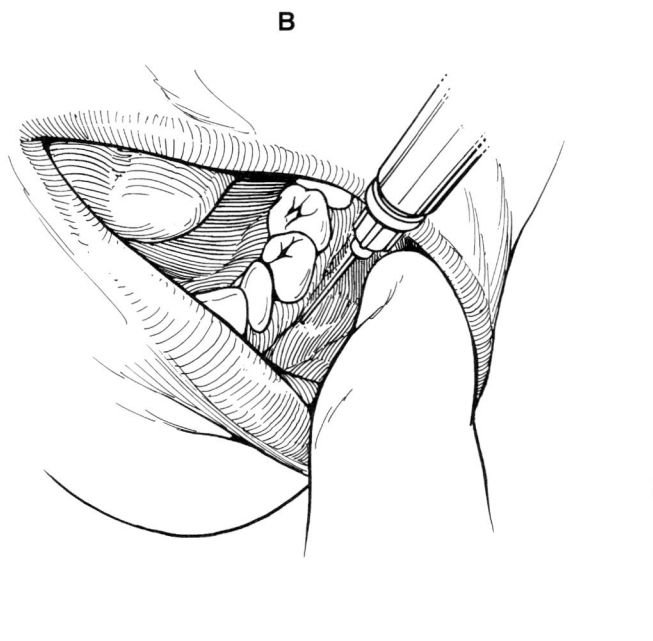

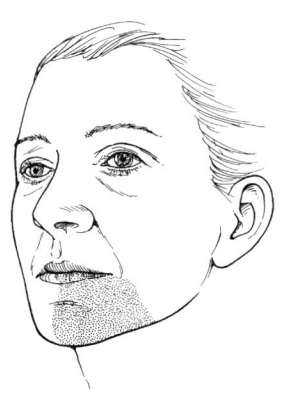

Inferior alveolar nerve

Mental foramen

Mental nerve

B

Extremity Blocks

BIER BLOCK   JAMES DUCHARME

Indications
- Anesthesia of upper or lower extremity for complex laceration repairs, fracture reduction, or extensive debridement

Contraindications
- Extensive soft tissue injury or swelling in the proximal extremity
- Severe peripheral vascular disease
- Infection or phlebitis in the region of intended anesthesia
- Allergy to anesthetic agent

Equipment
- Double-cuffed tourniquet, allowing separate inflation and deflation
- Pressure source
- IV catheter (22 or 25 gauge)
- Saline lock
- Lidocaine without epinephrine
- Esmarch or elastic bandage

Procedure

1. Place an IV catheter with a saline lock into the dorsum of the injured hand (or foot), located as distally as possible *(A)*.
2. Place the double-cuffed tourniquet on the proximal portion of the extremity.
3. Either elevate the extremity for 3 to 4 minutes, or gently but firmly wrap the elastic bandage over the extremity, starting distally and working proximally *(B)*.
4. Before removing the wrap, inflate the proximal cuff to at least 50 mm Hg above the systolic blood pressure *(C)*.
5. After the cuff is inflated, the extremity may be lowered or the bandage removed *(D)*.
6. Inject lidocaine through the IV cannula. The dose should be 50 ml of 0.5% lidocaine for the upper extremity and 80 to 100 ml for the lower extremity *(D)*.
7. Anesthesia should start taking effect in about 5 minutes.
8. Once the extremity is anesthetized, inflate the distal cuff to the same pressure as the proximal cuff, then deflate the proximal cuff (this leaves the cuff pressure over the insensate region, decreasing discomfort) *(D)*.
9. Remove the IV catheter before starting the intended procedure.
10. Leave the cuff inflated for at least 25 minutes.

Complications
- Systemic lidocaine toxicity
- Hematoma or bleeding from the IV site
- Infection
- Local tissue injury if the cuff pressure is greater than 300 mm Hg

Discussion
- If the 25-minute minimum time interval for inflation of the cuff after lidocaine injection is not observed, the patient may receive a systemic bolus, which could cause paresthesias, hypotension, agitation, or seizure.
- This type of anesthesia is ideal for elderly patients or those at higher risk with general anesthesia.

Bibliography

Bolte RG et al: Mini-dose Bier block intravenous regional anesthesia in the emergency department treatment of pediatric upper-extremity injuries, *J Pediatr Orthop* 14:534-537, 1994.

Graham CA et al: Anesthesia for the management of distal radius fractures in adults in Scottish hospitals, *Eur J Emerg Med* 4:210-212, 1997.

Kendall JM et al: Hematoma block or Bier's block for Colles' fracture reduction in the accident and emergency department—which is best? *J Accid Emerg Med* 14:352-356, 1997.

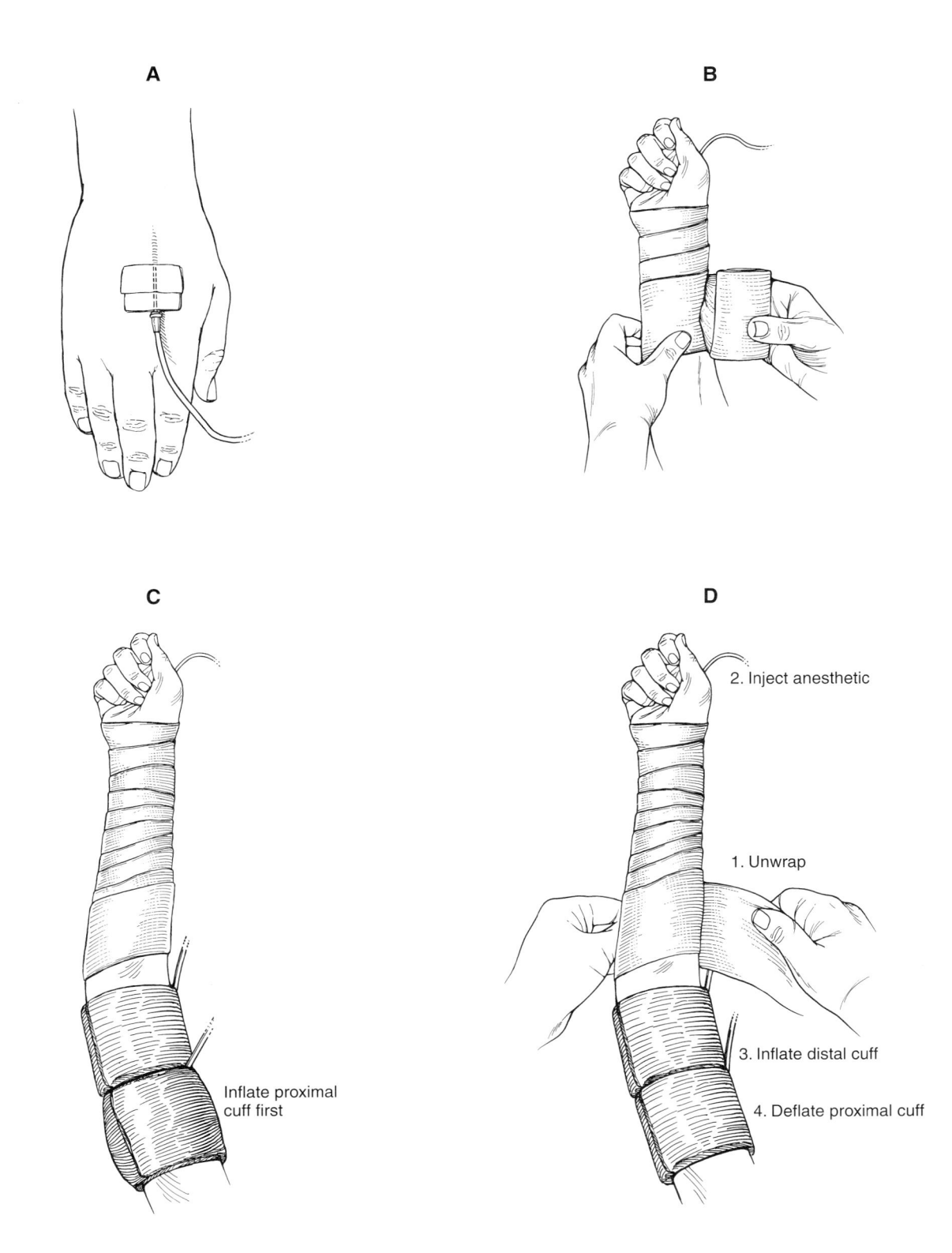

Nervous System

A

B

C

Inflate proximal cuff first

D

2. Inject anesthetic

1. Unwrap

3. Inflate distal cuff

4. Deflate proximal cuff

WRIST BLOCKS   JAMES DUCHARME

Indications
- Anesthesia for procedures involving the hand or more than one finger

Contraindications
- Allergy to anesthetic agent

Equipment
- 27-gauge ½-inch needle
- 10-ml syringe
- Betadine antiseptic solution
- 2% lidocaine without epinephrine
- 2% mepivacaine without epinephrine

Procedure

Radial Nerve Block
1. Identify the radial artery, the radial styloid, and the anatomic snuffbox *(A)*.
2. Prepare the site in sterile fashion.
3. Starting just lateral to the artery, at the level of the styloid, inject about 3 ml of a 50/50 mixture of lidocaine and mepivacaine *(B)*.
4. Raise a subcutaneous wheal from this point proceeding dorsally, crossing both the radial styloid and the snuffbox *(C)*.
5. The total volume to be injected is about 5 ml.

NERVOUS SYSTEM   171

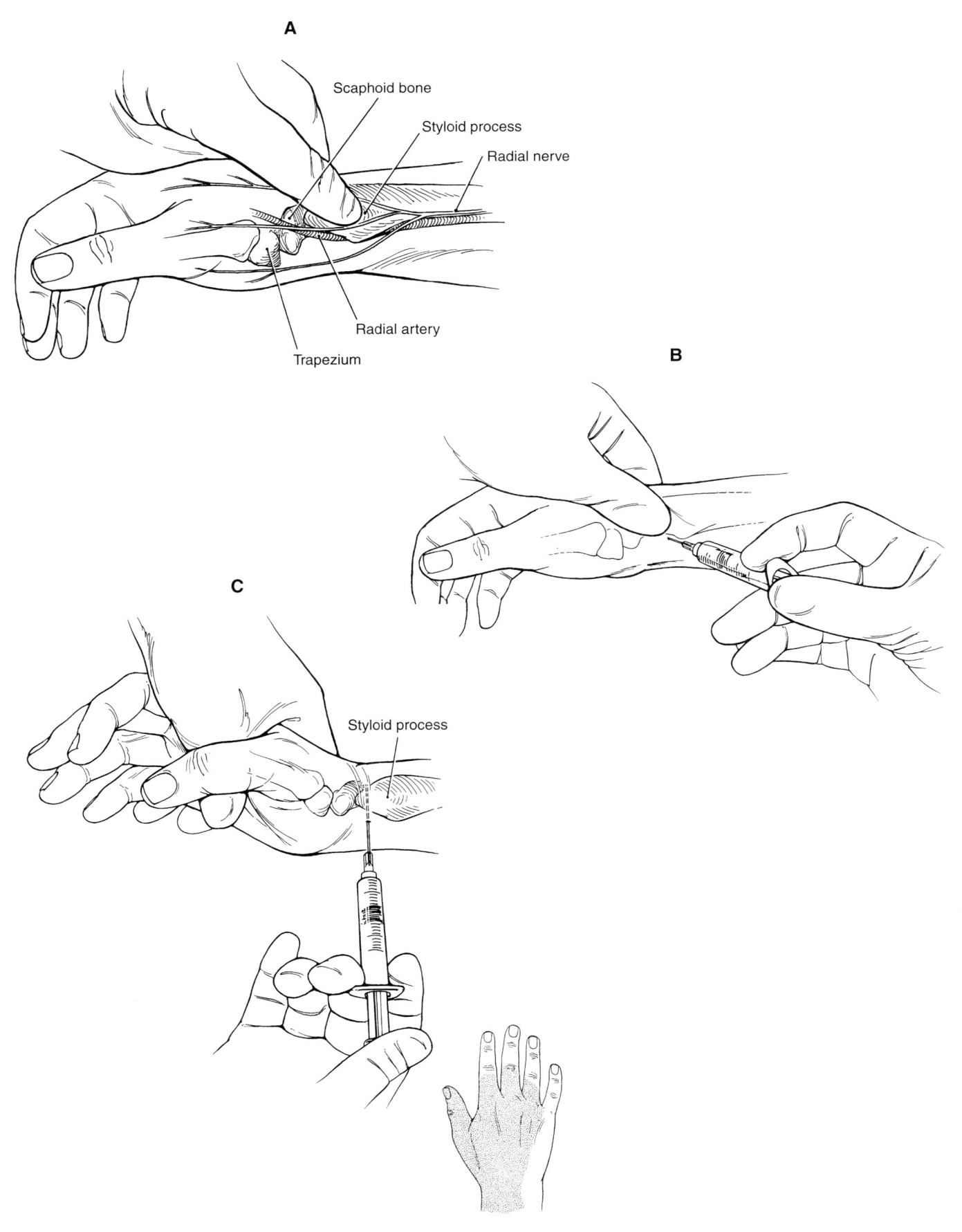

A

- Scaphoid bone
- Styloid process
- Radial nerve
- Radial artery
- Trapezium

B

C

- Styloid process

Ulnar Nerve Block

1. Identify the ulnar artery and the flexor carpi ulnaris tendon. The ulnar nerve is between these structures at the level of the ulnar styloid *(D)*.
2. Prepare the site in sterile fashion.
3. Insert the needle vertically between the artery and the tendon to the depth of the ulnar styloid from either the volar *(E)* or the dorsal *(F)* aspect.
4. Inject a total of about 5 to 7 ml of a 50/50 mixture of lidocaine and mepivacaine.

Median Nerve Block

1. Identify the flexor carpi radialis tendon and the palmaris longus tendon (found in about 85% of patients). The median nerve is located between these tendons at the level of the proximal volar crease *(G)*.
2. Prepare the site in sterile fashion.
3. Enter the skin with the needle perpendicular to the volar surface, being sure to penetrate through the deep fascia (if a cutaneous wheal develops, the needle is not through the fascia) *(H)*.
4. Inject a total of about 5 to 7 ml of a 50/50 mixture of lidocaine and mepivacaine.

Complications

- Nerve injury
- Hematoma formation
- Infection
- Allergic reactions

Discussion

- Regional blocks will give good anesthesia without distorting local landmarks for laceration repairs.
- Many patients find regional blocks more comfortable than local wound injection.
- Many operators prefer the volar approach over the dorsal approach to the ulnar nerve block.

Bibliography

Ferrera PC, Chandler R: Anesthesia in the emergency setting. 1. Hand and foot injuries, *Am Fam Physician* 50:569-573, 1994.

Leversee JH, Bergman JJ: Wrist and digital nerve blocks, *J Fam Pract* 13:415-421, 1981.

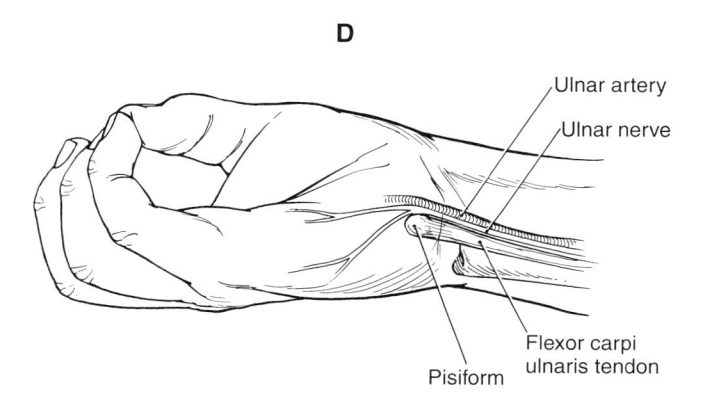

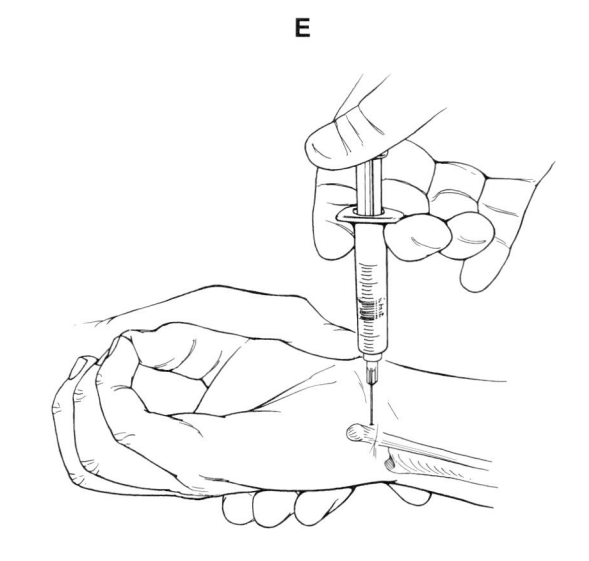

D

E

NERVOUS SYSTEM

F

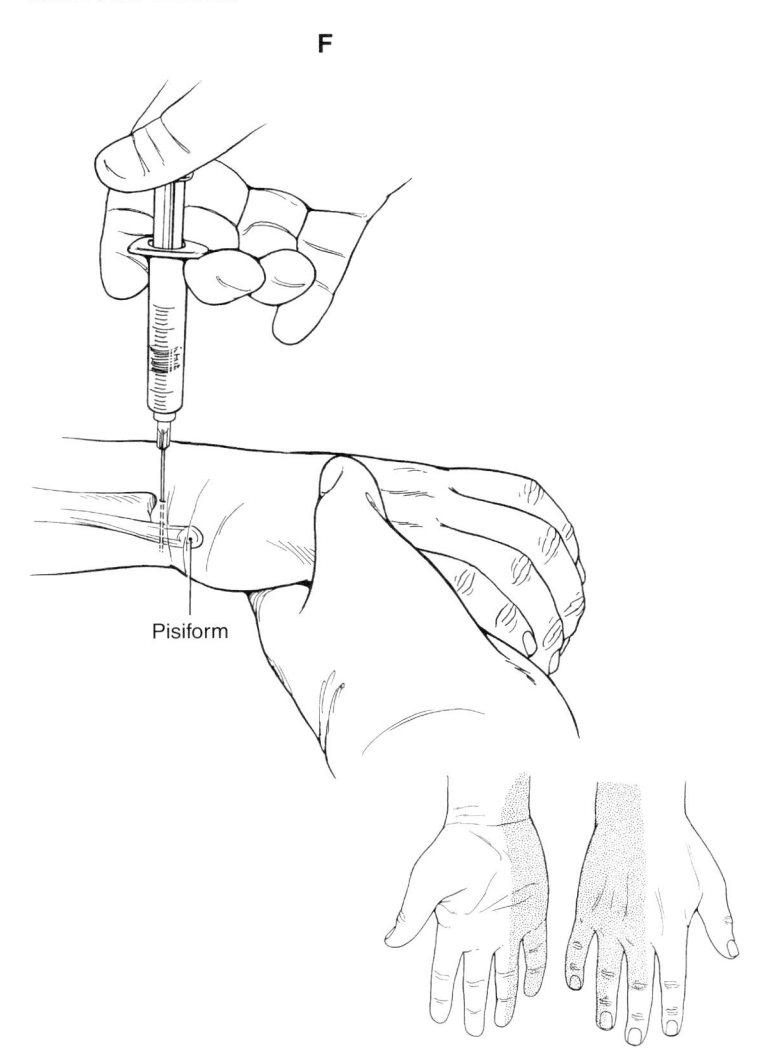

G

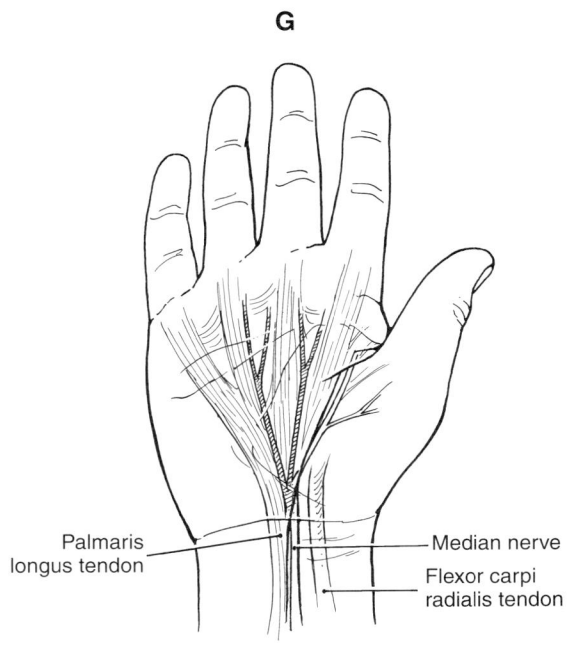

Palmaris longus tendon
Median nerve
Flexor carpi radialis tendon

Pisiform

H

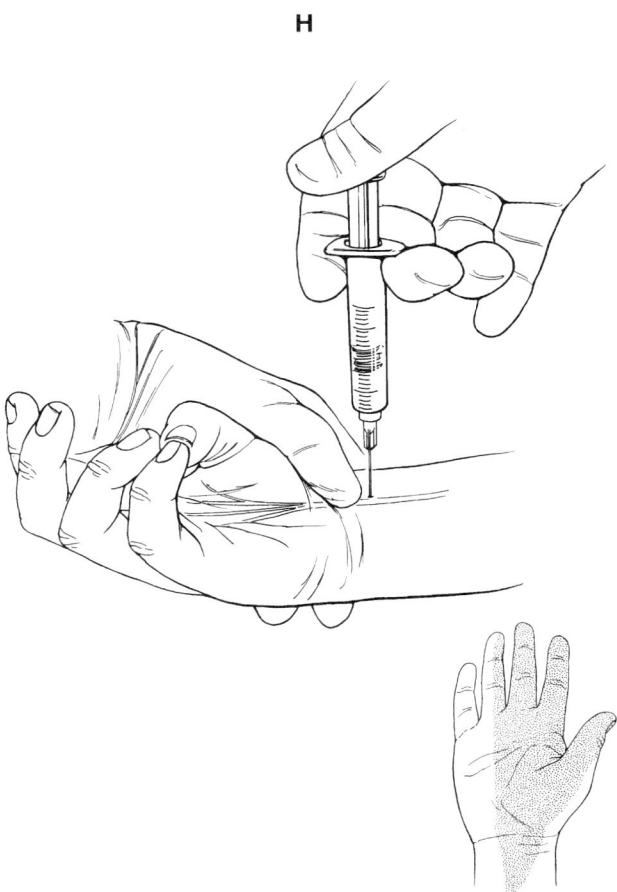

Digital Nerve Block N. NOUNOU TALEGHANI AND GEORGE STERNBACH

Indications
- Anesthesia of a single finger

Contraindications
- Allergy to anesthetic agent
- Grossly distorted landmarks
- Infection at the site of injection

Equipment
- 27-gauge 1½-inch needle with 5-ml syringe
- 2 × 2 sterile gauze pads
- Betadine antiseptic solution
- 2% lidocaine without epinephrine
- 0.25% bupivacaine without epinephrine

Procedure
1. Prepare in sterile fashion the injection site in the metacarpophalangeal joint region of the finger *(A)*.
2. Inject a 50/50 mixture of lidocaine and bupivacaine to raise a wheal between the metacarpal bones on the dorsum of the hand *(B)*.
3. Enter the wheal with the needle. After aspiration confirms that the needle is not in an intravascular position, slowly inject 2 to 3 ml of anesthetic.
4. Repeat steps 2 and 3 on the other side of the metacarpal region on the finger being anesthetized *(C, D)*.

Complications
- Nerve injury
- Intravascular injection of agent
- Vascular injury
- Infection
- Allergic reactions

Discussion
- Use of excessive amount of solution can create a fluid tourniquet and result in vascular compromise.
- Regional blocks provide good anesthesia without distorting local landmarks for laceration repairs.
- Allow 5 to 10 minutes for the anesthetic to take effect. Never use vasoconstrictive agents (e.g., epinephrine) on the digits.

Bibliography
Mulroy MF, Thompson GE: Blockade of digital nerves. In Hahn MB et al (eds): *Regional anesthesia: atlas of anatomy and technique*, St Louis, 1997, Mosby, pp 121-124.

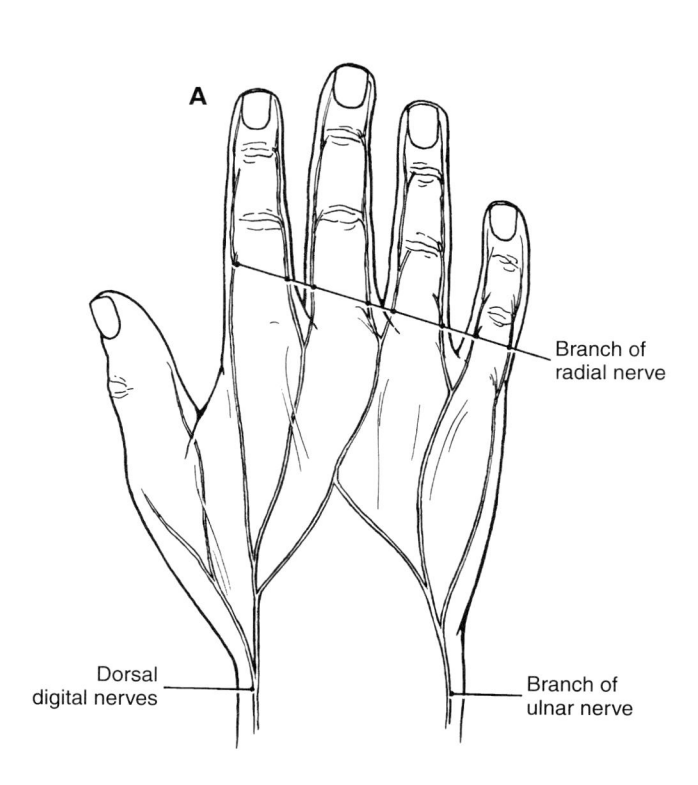

NERVOUS SYSTEM   **175**

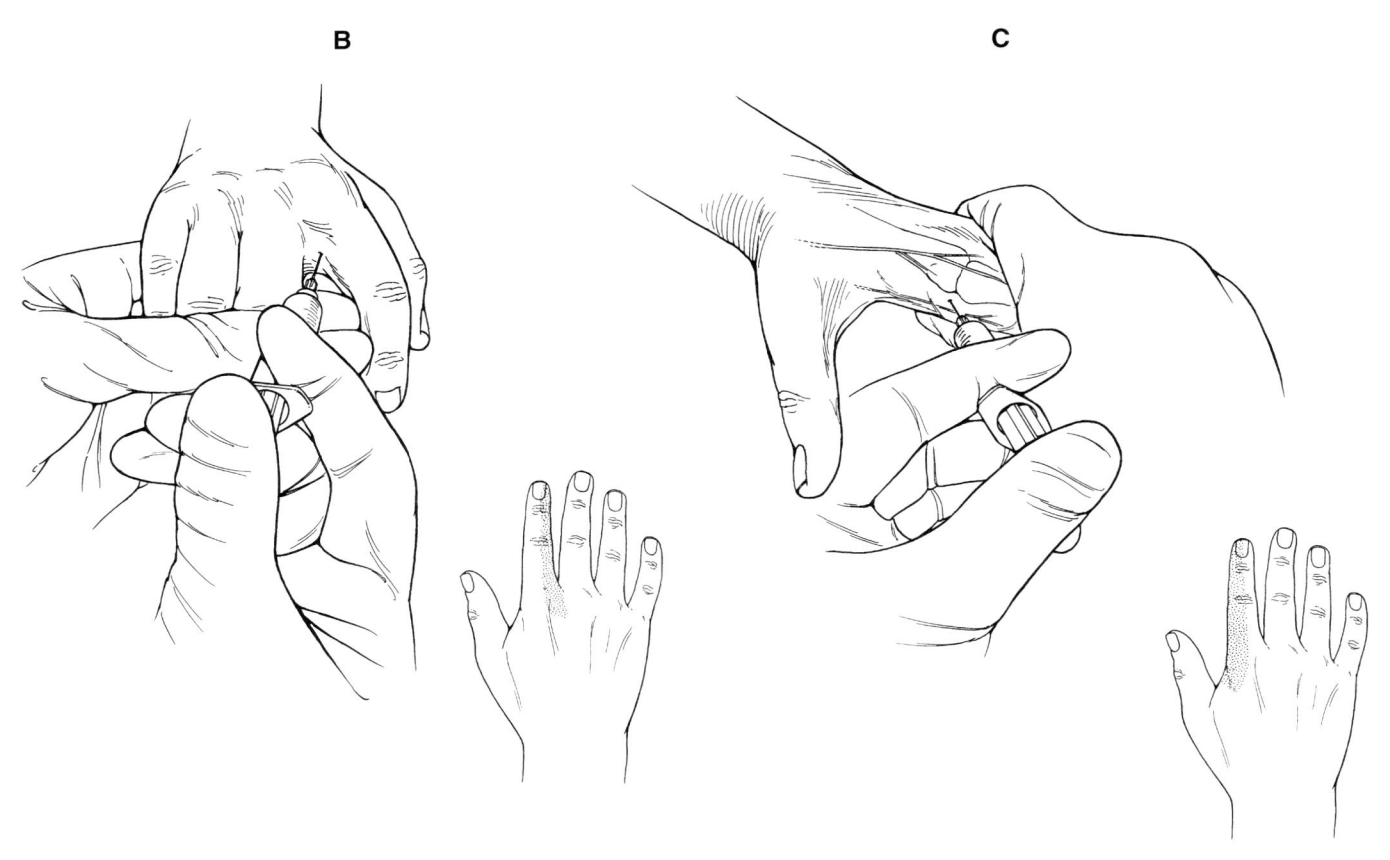

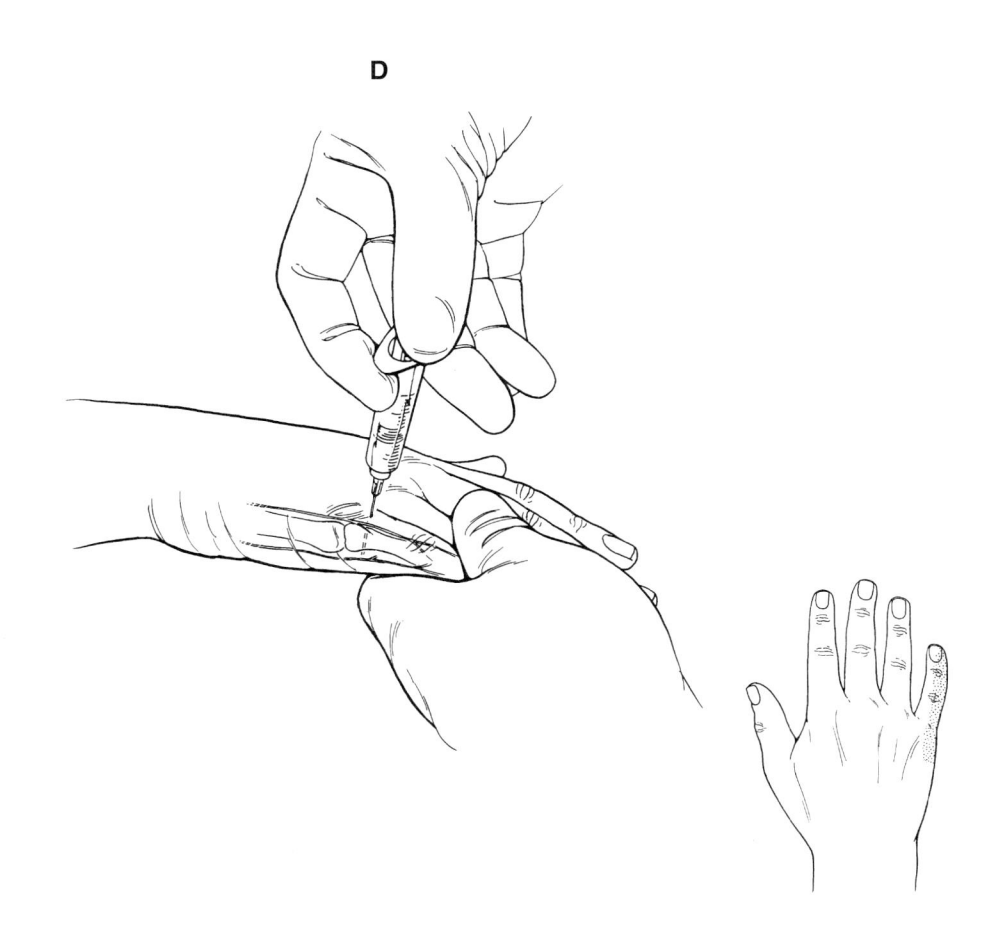

B

C

D

Foot Blocks N. NOUNOU TALEGHANI AND GEORGE STERNBACH

Indications
- Need for anesthesia of specific regions of the foot

Contraindications
- Allergy to anesthetic agent
- Grossly distorted landmarks
- Infection at the site of injection
- Lower extremity ischemia or diabetic foot disorders

Equipment
- 27-gauge 1½-inch needle with 10-ml syringe
- 2 × 2 sterile gauze
- Betadine antiseptic solution
- 2% lidocaine without epinephrine
- 0.25% bupivacaine without epinephrine

Procedure

Posterior Tibial Nerve Block
1. Position the patient prone with the foot extended beyond the end of the stretcher and held in light dorsiflexion.
2. Prepare in sterile fashion the skin over the medial malleolus, extending posteriorly to the Achilles' tendon.
3. Palpate the posterior tibial artery just posterior to the medial malleolus. Hold the position of the artery with fingers of the nondominant hand.
4. Insert the needle just posterior to the artery, perpendicular to the skin at the level of the top of the medial malleolus. If a pulse is not palpable, insert the needle to the medial side of the Achilles' tendon where it levels with the lower border of the medial malleolus *(A)*.
5. Slowly deposit 3 to 4 ml of anesthetic agent (usually a 50/50 mixture of lidocaine and bupivacaine). Then, while slowly withdrawing the needle, inject another 5 ml of anesthetic.

Sural Nerve Block
1. Position the patient prone with the foot extended beyond the end of the stretcher and held in light dorsiflexion.
2. Use betadine for sterile preparation of the skin over the lateral malleolus, extending posteriorly to the Achilles' tendon.
3. Insert the needle lateral to the Achilles' tendon, approximately 1 cm superior to the lateral malleolus *(B)*.
4. Block the branches of the sural nerve by creating a subcutaneous band of anesthesia. This is done by infiltrating 3 to 5 ml of anesthetic from the posterior aspect of the lateral malleolus to the anterior margin of the Achilles' tendon.

Superficial Peroneal Nerve Block
1. Place the patient in a supine position.
2. Use betadine for sterile preparation of the skin over the lateral malleolus.
3. Insert the needle subcutaneously immediately above and lateral to the lateral malleolus *(C)*.
4. Make a wheal with 0.5 to 1 ml of anesthetic midway between the anterior tibial surface and the lateral malleolus.

Deep Peroneal Nerve Block
1. Place the patient in a supine position.
2. Use betadine for sterile preparation of the skin over the lateral malleolus and slightly proximal.
3. Identify the extensor hallucis longus (EHL) tendon by dorsiflexing the great toe.
4. Raise a wheal just medial to the EHL tendon *(D)*.
5. Direct the needle 30° laterally beneath the EHL tendon, and advance it 0.5 to 1 cm until it strikes the tibia.
6. Deposit 3 to 5 ml of anesthetic.

Complications
- Nerve injury
- Intravascular injection of agent
- Vascular injury
- Infection
- Allergic reactions

Discussion
- If paresthesia is produced before the anesthetic is injected, the needle should be withdrawn 1 to 2 mm to prevent inadvertent intraneuronal injection.
- Use of an excessive amount of solution can create a fluid tourniquet and result in vascular compromise.
- Regional blocks provide good anesthesia without distorting local landmarks for laceration repairs.

Bibliography
Hess J: A review of regional blocks for the foot, *AANA J* 66(1):82-91, 1998.

NERVOUS SYSTEM

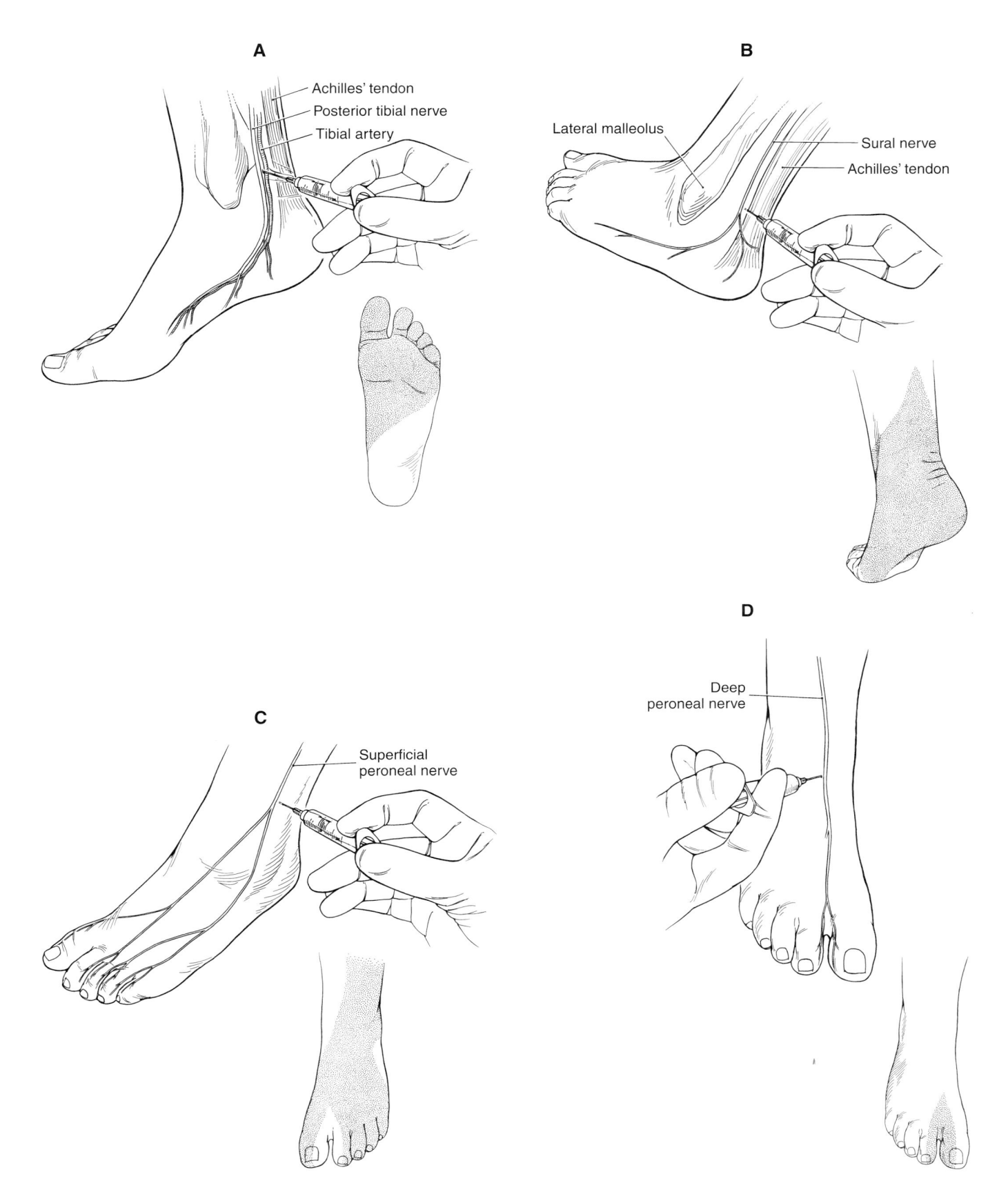

A
- Achilles' tendon
- Posterior tibial nerve
- Tibial artery

B
- Lateral malleolus
- Sural nerve
- Achilles' tendon

C
- Superficial peroneal nerve

D
- Deep peroneal nerve

CHAPTER 8

EYE

Corneal Foreign Body Removal ■ PASCAL S.C. JUANG

Indications
- Foreign body in the eye

Contraindications
- Ruptured globe
- Foreign body penetrating globe
- Patient noncompliance

Equipment
- Slit lamp
- Proparacaine or tetracaine eyedrops
- 22-gauge needle

Procedure

1. Place the patient in a slit lamp, and instill anesthetic drops into the affected eye *(A)*. Make sure the patient's chin and forehead are firmly resting forward in the slit lamp *(B)*.
2. Instruct the patient to fixate the noninjured eye on the examiner's ear or a distant object and not to speak or open the mouth during the procedure.
3. Rest the hand holding the needle on the patient's zygomatic arch, not the slit lamp.
4. While viewing the cornea through the slit lamp, approach the eye with the needle in a plane tangential to the curve of the cornea.
5. Position the needle with the bevel facing away from the cornea, and use the tip to pick up the foreign body from the corneal surface *(C)*.
6. Reexamine the eye after removal.

Complications
- Ruptured globe
- Infection
- Retained foreign body

Discussion

- Make sure the patient's head is stabilized and the eyes are fixated to minimize risk of eye injury with the needle.
- Rather than a needle, a plastic IV catheter tip can be used. It should be cut short so that it will not bend as the foreign body is retrieved. A burr instrument may also be used to remove foreign bodies *(D)*.
- For some looser foreign bodies a cotton-tipped swab can be used for blunt removal.

Bibliography
Cullom R, Chang B: *The Wills eye manual: office and emergency room diagnosis and treatment of eye disease,* ed 2, Philadelphia, 1994, JB Lippincott.

Juang P, Rosen P: Ocular examination techniques for the emergency department, *J Emerg Med* 15(6):793-810, 1997.

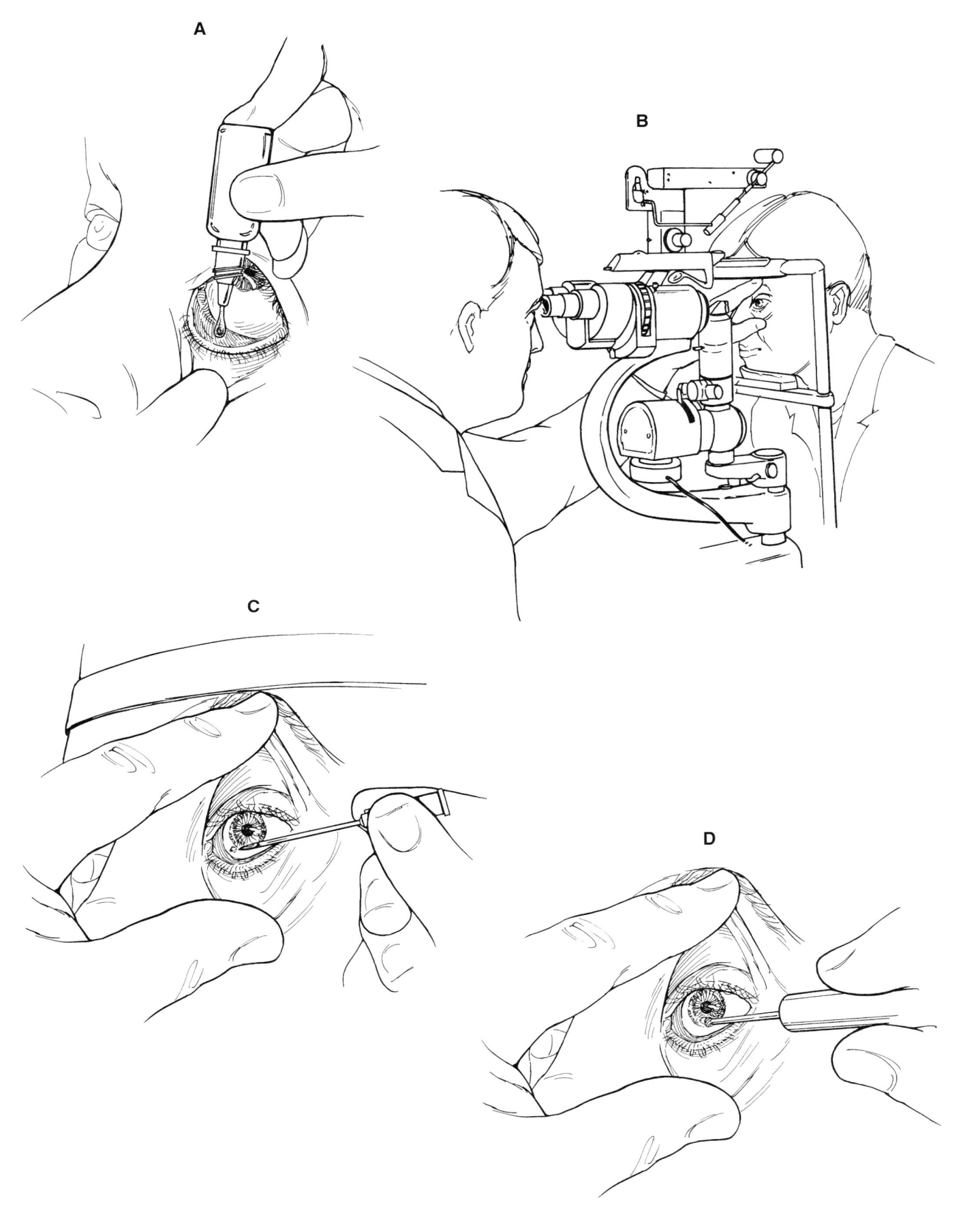

EYE

Eversion of Upper Eyelid ▪ PASCAL S.C. JUANG

Indications
- Assessment for foreign body

Contraindications
- Ruptured globe

Equipment
- Cotton-tipped swab

Procedure

1. Place a cotton-tipped swab 8 to 10 mm above the margin of the upper eyelid *(A)*.
2. Hold the eyelashes with the fingers of the other hand.
3. In one motion, pull the eyelash toward the eyebrow while moving the tip of the cotton-tipped swab down *(B)*.
4. After the eyelid is everted, the swab tip may be placed on the underside of the eyelid to hold the eyelid in eversion.

Complications

- Ruptured globe

Bibliography

Juang P, Rosen P: Ocular examination techniques for the emergency department, *J Emerg Med* 15(6):793-810, 1997.

A

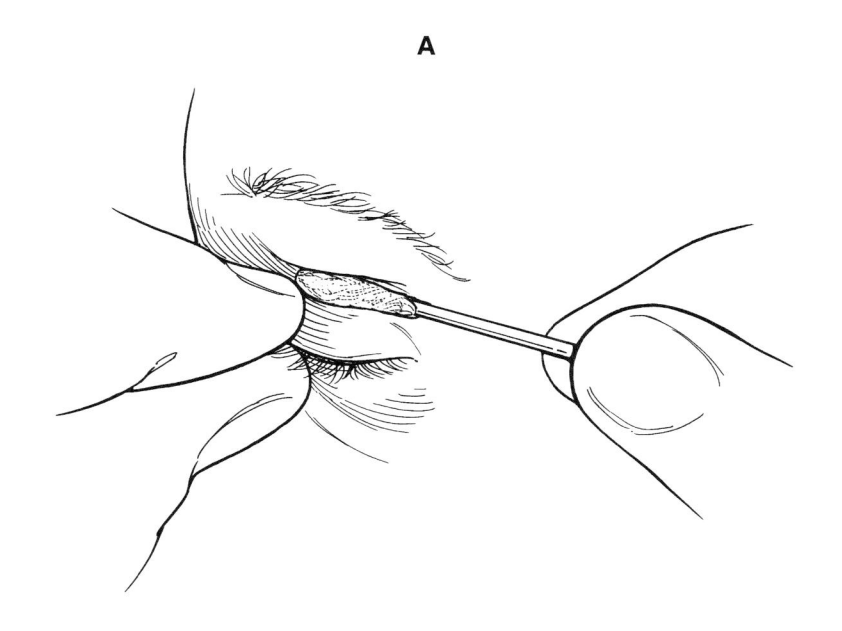

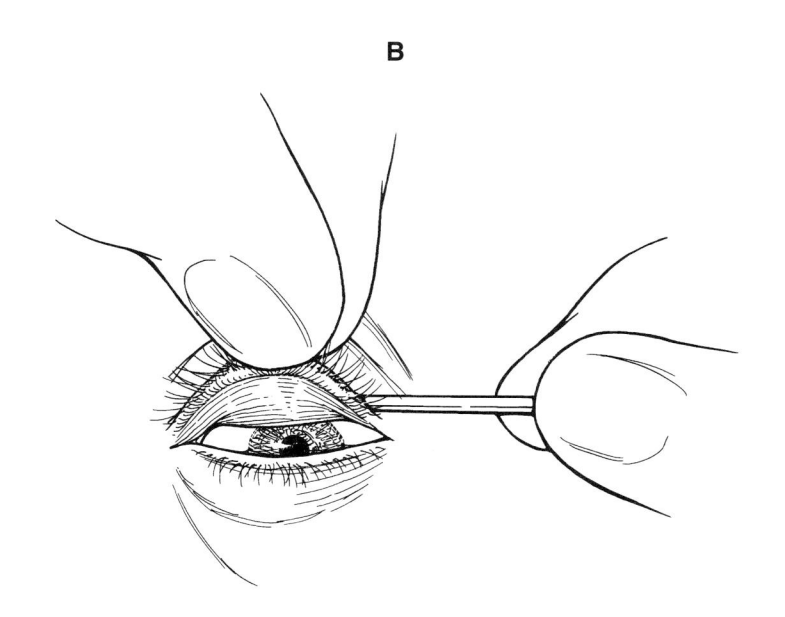

B

Contact Lens Removal ▪ PASCAL S.C. JUANG

Indications
- Inability of the patient to remove the contact lens

Contraindications
- Ruptured globe

Equipment
- Artificial tears
- Lens suction cup

Procedure

Hard Lens
1. Lubricate the eye with artificial tears.
2. Place the suction cup onto the contact lens *(A)*. Do not pull on the contact lens until it has been moved off the cornea and onto the sclera *(B)*.
3. Once on the sclera, the lens may be pulled off.

Soft Lens
1. Lubricate the eye with artificial tears.
2. Gently place a moistened cotton-tipped swab on the lens surface.
3. Use the swab to move the lens onto the sclera *(C)*.
4. The contact lens will fold as it moves off the cornea.
5. When the lens folds, use the swab or fingers to remove the lens *(C, D)*.

Complications
- Infection
- Corneal abrasion

Discussion

- Pulling the lens away from the eye while it is still on the cornea may cause corneal damage.
- Hard contact lenses are 8 to 10 mm in diameter and do not extend past the limbus of the eye, whereas soft lenses are 12 to 14 mm and usually extend past the limbus.
- If a suction cup is not available for hard lens removal, the lens can be removed using the patient's eyelid. Place the thumb and index finger of each hand on the patient's eyelids, medially and laterally. Make sure the eyelid margins are outside the circumference of the contact lens. While closing the eyelids, place medial and lateral traction on them so that the margins become taut *(E)*. This will make the eyelid margins catch the superior and inferior edges of the lens, causing the lens to bend and pop out of the eye *(F)*.

Bibliography
Juang P, Rosen P: Ocular examination techniques for the emergency department, *J Emerg Med* 15(6):793-810, 1997.

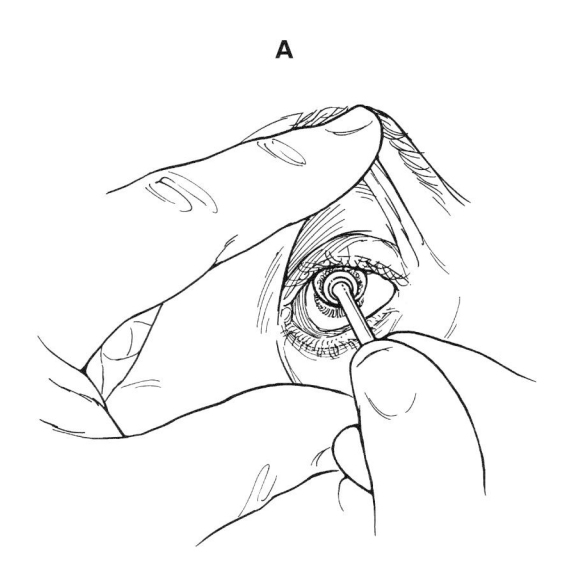

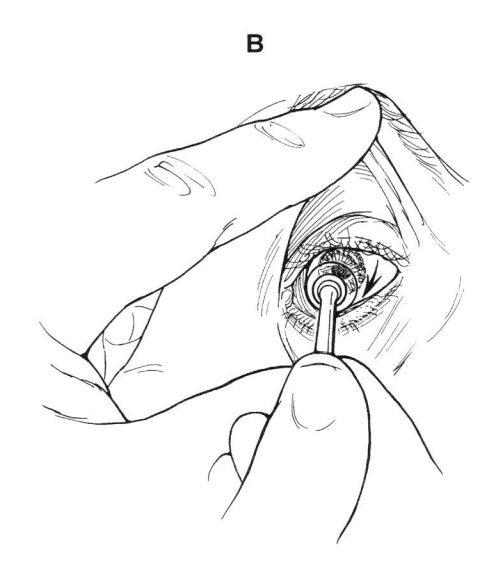

A

B

EYE **185**

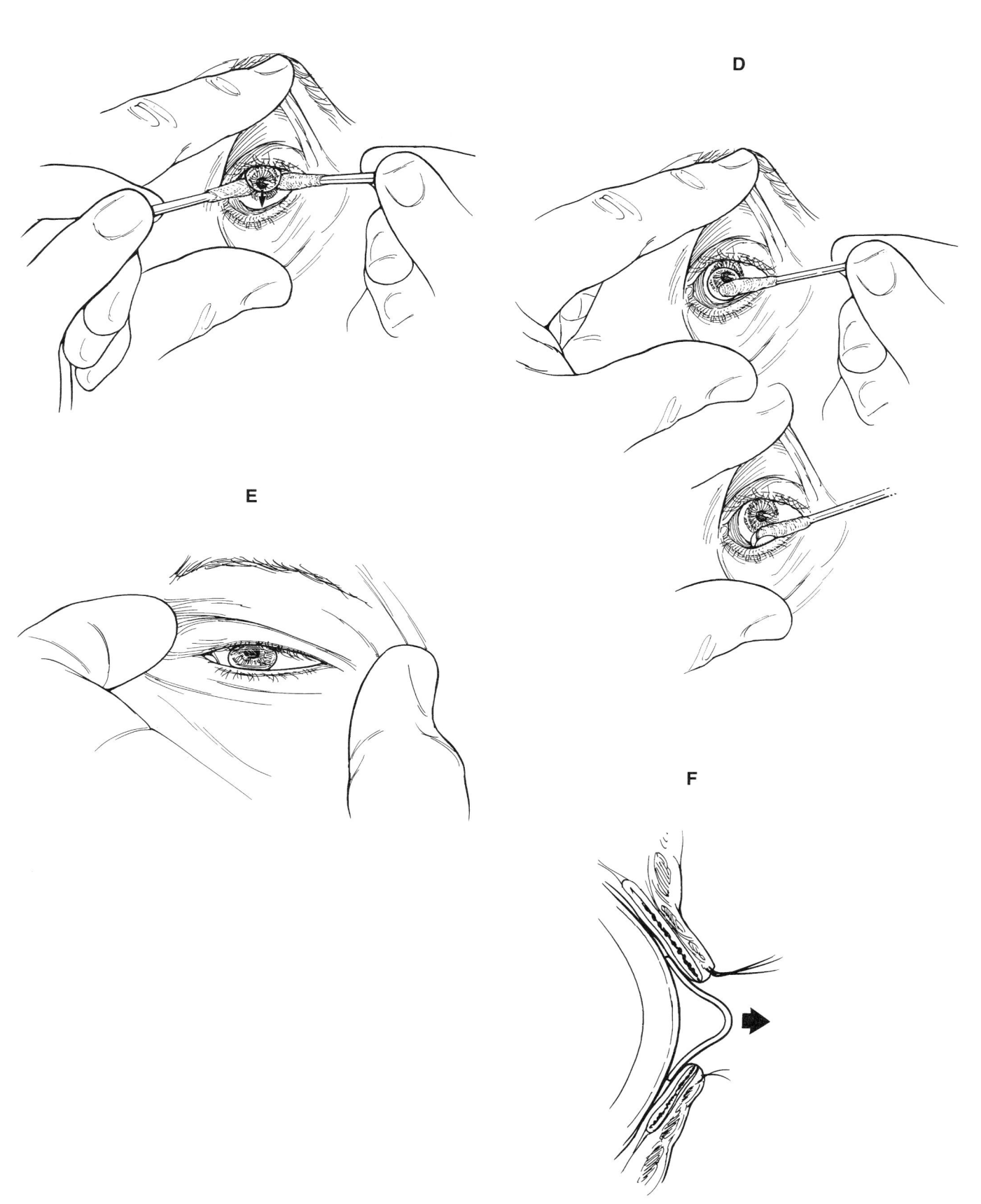

C

D

E

F

Measurement of Intraocular Pressure–Schiøtz Tonometry
■ PASCAL S.C. JUANG

Indications
- Need to measure intraocular pressure

Contraindications
- Ruptured globe

Equipment
- Schiøtz tonometer
- Proparacaine or tetracaine eyedrops

Procedure

1. Make sure the tonometer is sterilized per manufacturer's recommendations.
2. Instill anesthetic eyedrops into the eye.
3. Position the head so that the plane of the face is parallel to the ceiling.
4. Hold the patient's eye open by using the thumb and index finger of the nondominant hand, making sure the fingers are pressed against the bones of the orbital rim.
5. Place the tonometer onto the surface of the eye, and record the measurement *(A)*.
6. Correlate this measurement with the conversion chart provided with the Schiøtz tonometer to determine the intraocular pressure.

Complications
- Infection
- Corneal abrasion

Discussion
- Make sure the fingers holding the eye open are pushing on the orbital rim rather than the eye, which could falsely elevate intraocular pressure.
- An electronic hand-held tonometer is now available and can be used to measure intraocular pressure.

Bibliography

Juang P, Rosen P: Ocular examination techniques for the emergency department, *J Emerg Med* 15(6):793-810, 1997.

A

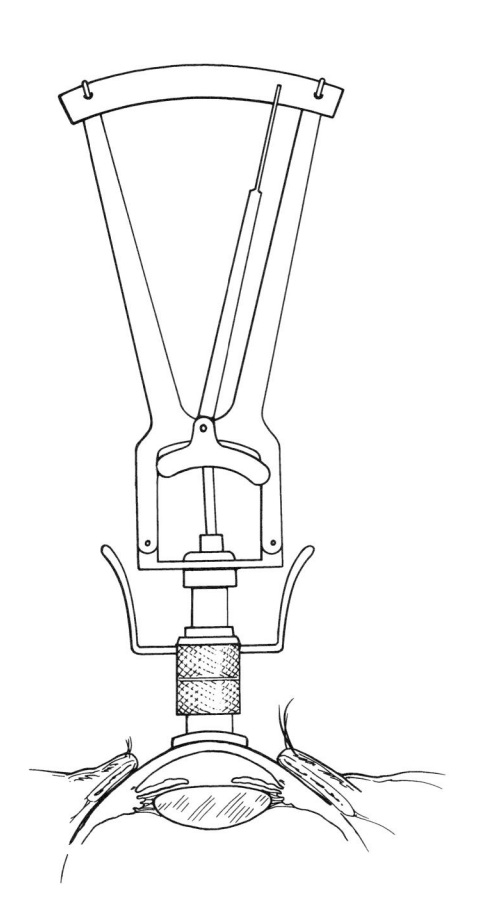

CHAPTER 9

EAR, NOSE, AND THROAT

Anterior Packing ■ THEODORE C. CHAN

Indications
- Persistent epistaxis from anterior source
- High risk of rebleeding after bleeding from anterior source has resolved
- Posterior epistaxis (performed in combination with posterior packing)

Contraindications
- Suspected cribriform plate fracture
- Evidence of cerebrospinal fluid rhinorrhea

Equipment
- For epistaxis:
  - Ear, nose, and throat (ENT) light source
  - Nasal speculum
  - Gowns (for patient and physician) and goggles
  - Frazier tip suction
  - Cotton balls and pledgets
  - Topical vasoconstrictor and anesthetics (2% to 4% cocaine; 2% to 4% lidocaine with epinephrine; 0.05% oxymetazoline or 1% phenylephrine plus 2% tetracaine)
  - Local hemostatic agents (silver nitrate, electrocautery, cellulose sponge)
- For anterior packing:
  - Commercially available anterior packing device, or the following:
    - Bayonet forceps
    - ¼- to ½-inch ribbon petroleum gauze
    - Antibiotic ointment

Procedure

1. Take resuscitative measures (airway, breathing, circulation) as needed. Reassure and calm the patient.
2. Have the patient sit up (to decrease swallowing of blood) and blow the nose to remove residual clots.
3. Have the patient hold external pressure by nose pinch or other device (to compress the alae just below the nasal cartilage) for 5 to 10 minutes.
4. Prepare equipment.
5. Insert the nasal speculum horizontally, and open in superoinferior access to view the nasal cavity *(A)*. Suction blood and secretions as needed.
6. If an anterior source is identified, cauterize the site. (Avoid cauterizing large areas on both sides of the septum.)
7. If no source is identified or bleeding is too brisk, insert cotton pledgets soaked in a vasoconstrictor-anesthetic agent for 10 to 15 minutes. Remove the pledgets, and reassess for bleeding and source.
8. Place anterior packing if there is continued bleeding from a suspected anterior site or a high risk for rebleeding after epistaxis is resolved.
9. To perform anterior packing:
    a. Grasp the ribbon gauze 2 to 3 cm from the end with bayonet forceps.
    b. Insert the gauze along the floor of the nasal cavity parallel to the palate as far as the patient tolerates (the nasal cavity in an adult is approximately 6 to 8 cm) *(B)*.
    c. Remove the forceps, and grasp the ribbon gauze again (approximately 6 to 8 cm from the nares) to form a loop. Reinsert into the nasal cavity above the first layer.
    d. Repeat layering multiple times to form an "accordion" mattress pack. Forceps may be used to compress previously placed layers against the floor of the nasal cavity.
    e. Each layer should lie anterior and superior to the previous layer to prevent the gauze from falling into the posterior nasopharynx *(C)*.
    f. Up to 6 feet of ribbon gauze may be necessary to complete the packing.
10. Antibiotic ointment should be placed around the nares to prevent desiccation and crusting.
11. Systemic treatment with a prophylactic antistaphylococcal antibiotic is prudent for patients with unilateral packing and mandatory for patients with bilateral anterior packing.
12. A follow-up check and packing removal should occur at 48 to 72 hours.

Complications

- Nasal injury
- Local infection
- Airway obstruction
- Sinusitis
- Toxic shock syndrome

Ear, Nose, and Throat

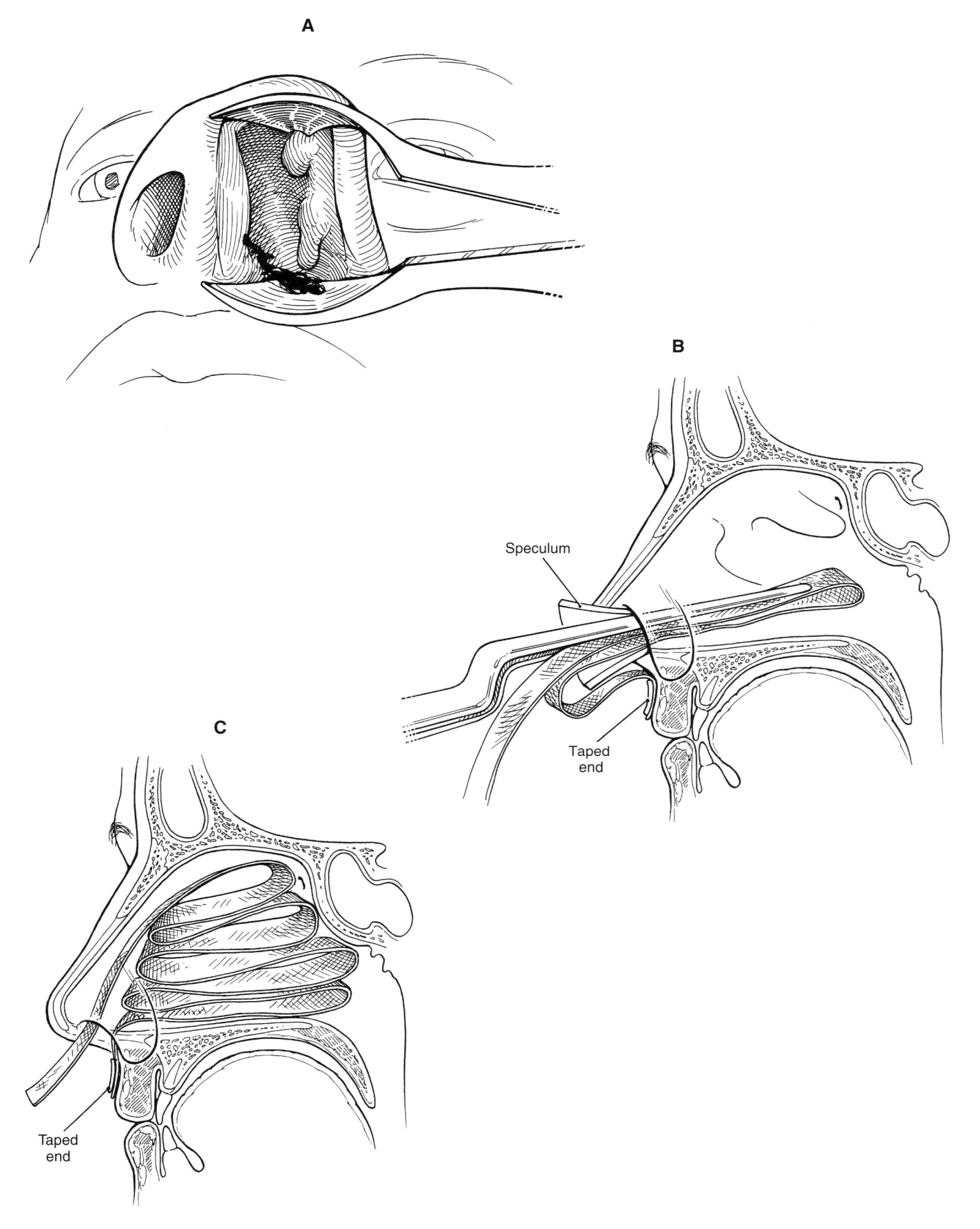

A

B

Speculum

Taped end

C

Taped end

Discussion

- A number of commercial anterior nasal packs are available. The packing material is generally a self-expanding sponge that absorbs fluid and expands on insertion into the nasal cavity. The sponge should be inserted along the nasal cavity floor, lying parallel to the palate *(D-F)*.
- Bilateral anterior packing should be considered in cases of severe anterior epistaxis or an unstable nasal septum.
- Patients should be advised to apply Vasoline or antibiotic ointment to the nares and to use humidified air to prevent desiccation. Patients should also be advised to avoid forceful nose blowing or sneezing through the nose. Mild sedatives may be required if the patient has difficulty tolerating the nasal packing.

Bibliography

Alvi A, Joyner-Triplett N: Acute epistaxis: how to spot the source and stop the flow, *Postgrad Med* 99(5):83-90, 1996.

Perretta LJ et al: Emergency evaluation and management of epistaxis, *Emerg Med Clin North Am* 5(2):265-277, 1987.

Pollice PA, Yoder MG: Epistaxis: a retrospective review of hospitalized patients, *Otolaryngol Head Neck Surg* 117(1):49-53, 1997.

Sugarman PM, Alderson DJ: Training model for nasal packing, *J Accid Emerg Med* 12(4):276-278, 1995.

Votey S, Dudley JP: Emergency ear, nose and throat procedures, *Emerg Med Clin North Am* 7(1):117-154, 1989.

D

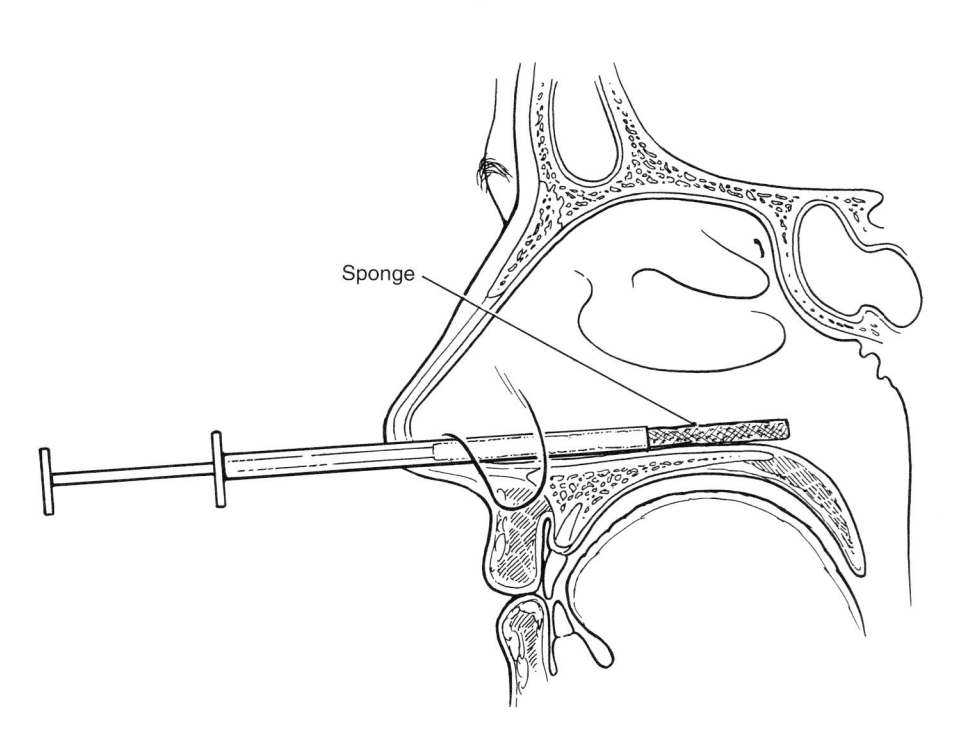

Sponge

E

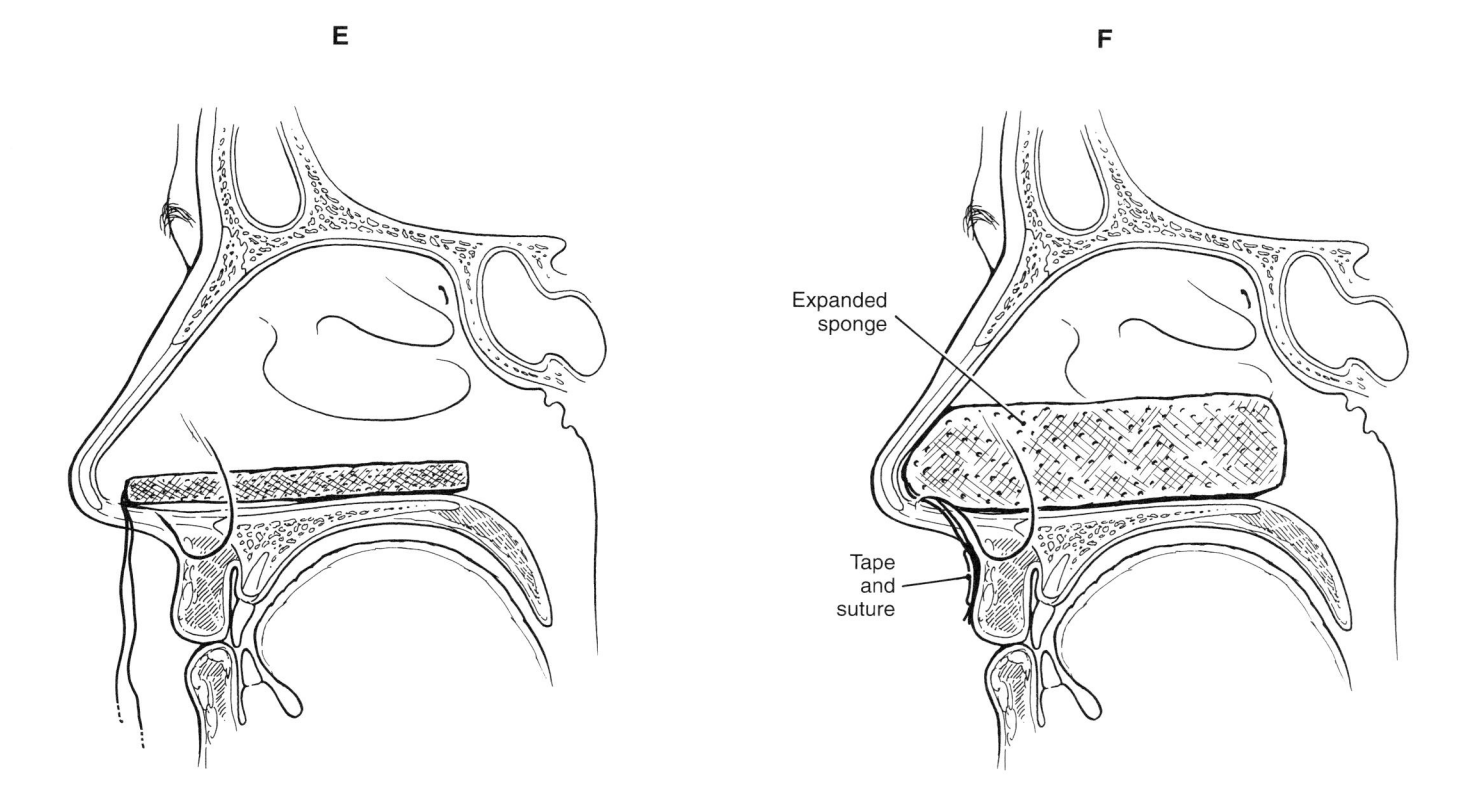

F

Expanded sponge

Tape and suture

Posterior Packing ▪ THEODORE C. CHAN

Indications
- Posterior epistaxis (profuse, recurrent, cyclical, uncontrolled epistaxis for which no anterior source is found)

Contraindications
- Suspected cribriform plate fracture
- Evidence of cerebrospinal fluid rhinorrhea
- High risk for airway obstruction

Equipment
- For epistaxis:
  - Ear, nose, and throat (ENT) light source
  - Nasal speculum
  - Gowns (for patient and physician) and goggles
  - Frazier tip suction
  - Cotton balls and pledgets
  - Topical vasoconstrictor and anesthetics (2% to 4% cocaine; 2% to 4% lidocaine with epinephrine; 0.05% oxymetazoline or 1% phenylephrine plus 2% tetracaine)
  - Local hemostatic agents (silver nitrate, electrocautery, cellulose sponge)
- For packing:
  - 20% topical benzocaine spray
  - 4 × 4 gauze roll
  - 3-0 silk ties or umbilical tape
  - Two red rubber catheters (8 to 10 Fr)
  - Hemostats
  - Or, as an alternative to the above:
    - Foley catheter (14 Fr)
    - Commercially available posterior pack kit
  - Anterior packing materials

Procedure

1. Follow the approach to the patient with epistaxis outlined in the section on anterior packing.
2. If posterior epistaxis is present, prepare the equipment for posterior packing.
3. To perform posterior packing:
   a. Anesthesize the posterior pharynx with 20% benzocaine spray to decrease the gag reflex.
   b. Tie the ends of 3-0 silk or umbilical tape ties around gauze to form a cylinder roll.
   c. Insert a red rubber catheter through the naris into the oropharynx.
   d. Through the oral cavity, use a hemostat to grab the end of the red rubber catheter and pull it out of the mouth. The catheter should form a loop, entering the naris and exiting the mouth.
   e. Attach the silk or umbilical tape tie (at the ends opposite the gauze roll) to the catheter tip exiting the mouth *(A)*.
   f. Pull the catheter out of the naris, inserting the gauze roll into the mouth.
   g. Guide the gauze roll into the posterior nasopharynx behind the soft palate and uvula, occluding the posterior choanae *(B)*.
   h. Once the roll is in place, remove the red rubber catheter, leaving the tie in place exiting the naris *(B)*.

EAR, NOSE, AND THROAT 195

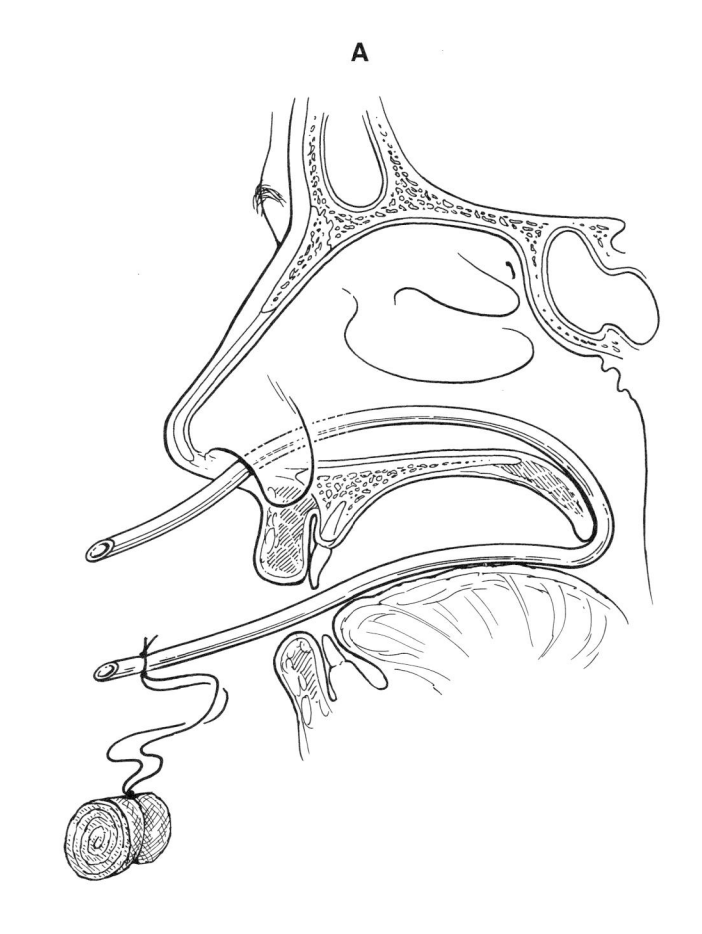

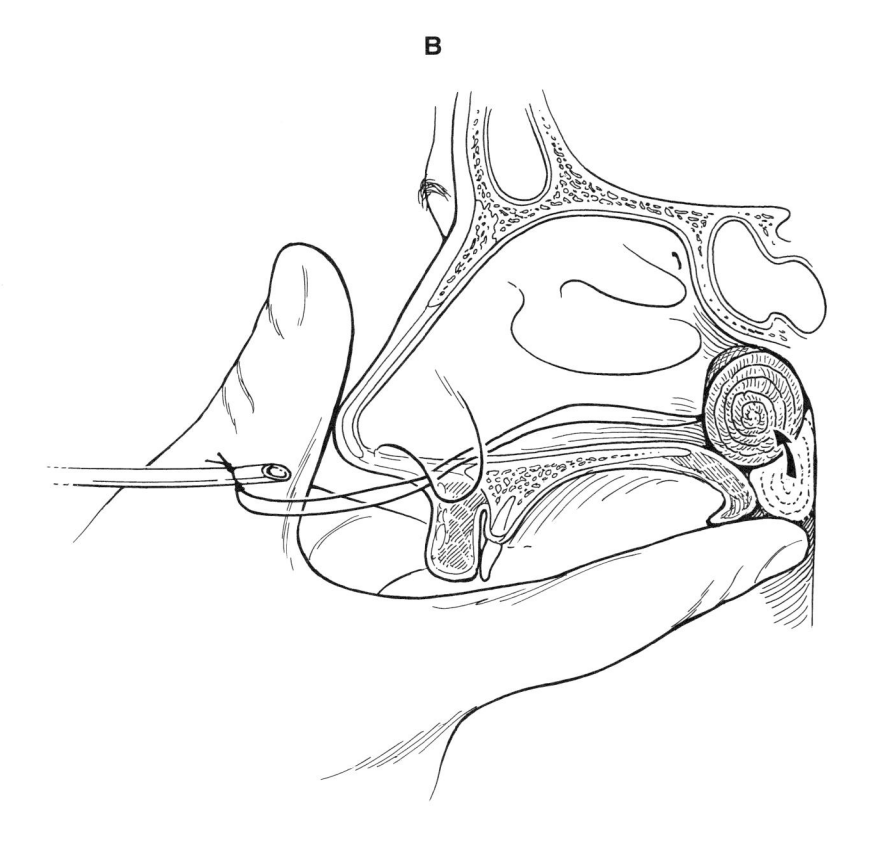

A

B

4. To use the alternative Foley posterior pack:
   a. Cut the tip off the Foley catheter.
   b. Insert the Foley catheter through the nares into the oropharynx.
   c. Once the catheter is seen in the oropharynx, inflate the Foley catheter balloon with 10 to 20 ml of normal saline solution.
   d. Pull the catheter back out of the nares until the balloon enters into the posterior nasopharynx and applies adequate pressure to the region *(C)*.
5. After posterior packing is complete, perform anterior packing as described in the section on anterior packing.
6. Ensure that the patient receives humidified oxygen, antibiotics, adequate sedation, and close monitoring. All patients with posterior packing should be admitted for observation and further care.

Complications

- Nasal and pharyngeal injuries
- Local infection
- Airway obstruction
- Sinusitis
- Toxic shock syndrome
- Hemoptysis
- Hematemesis

Discussion

- A number of commercial posterior nasal packs are available. These packs generally include two balloons or sponges to provide tamponade pressure, one in the posterior nasopharynx and the other in the nasal cavity. The device should be inserted along the nasal cavity floor into the oropharynx, where the posterior balloon may be inflated and pulled back into the posterior nasopharyx. Once this is done, the anterior balloon may be inflated to provide packing in the nasal cavity *(D, E)*.
- In cases of a deviated septum, posterior packing may be placed through the single patent naris.

Bibliography

Alvi A, Joyner-Triplett N: Acute epistaxis: how to spot the source and stop the flow, *Postgrad Med* 99(5):83-90, 1996.

Perretta LJ et al: Emergency evaluation and management of epistaxis, *Emerg Med Clin North Am* 5(2):265-277, 1987.

Pollice PA, Yoder MG: Epistaxis: a retrospective review of hospitalized patients, *Otolaryngol Head Neck Surg* 117(1):49-53, 1997.

Votey S, Dudley JP: Emergency ear, nose and throat procedures, *Emerg Med Clin North Am* 7(1):117-154, 1989.

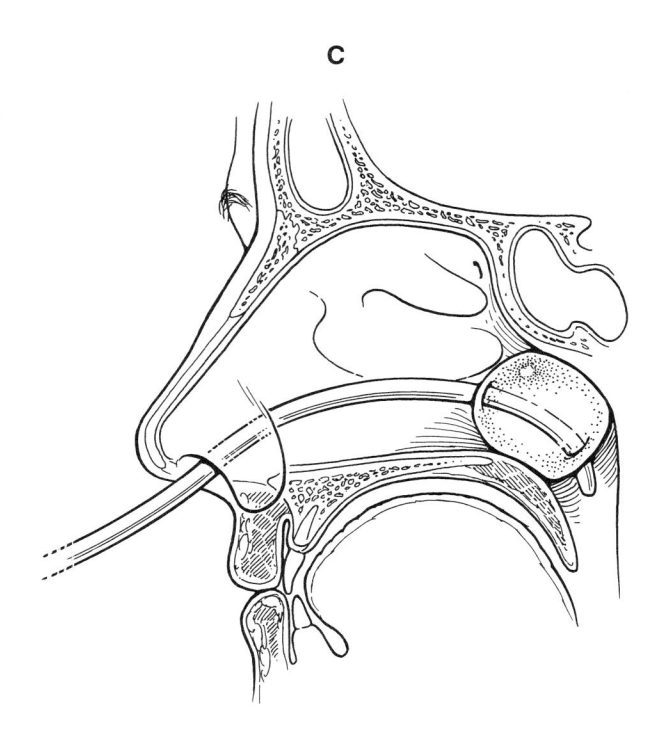

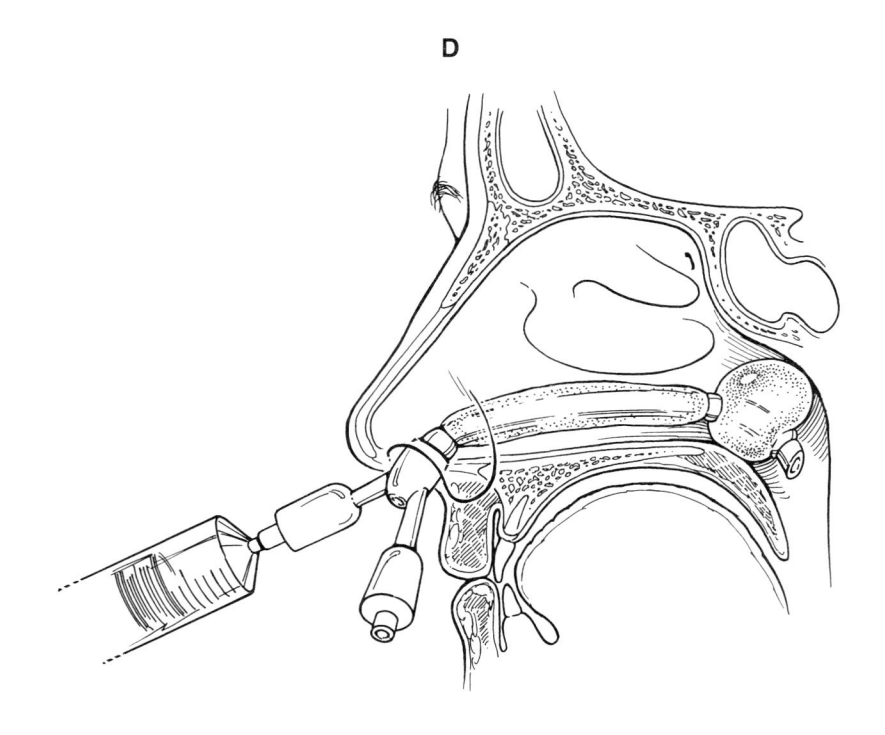

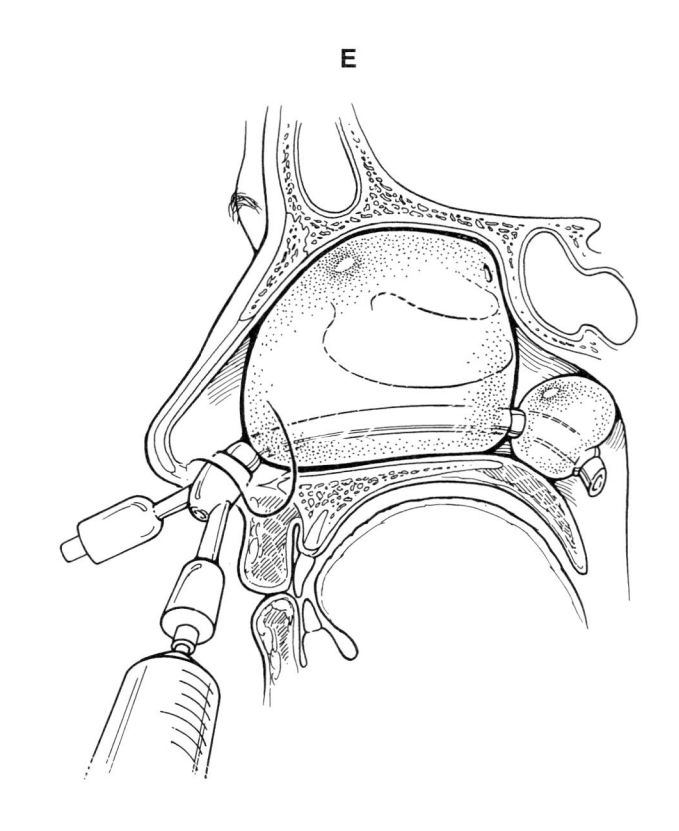

D

E

Septal Hematoma Drainage ■ THEODORE C. CHAN

Indications

- Subperichondral hematoma located at septum (usually associated with trauma); drainage is necessary to restore blood supply from the perichondrium to cartilage and thus prevent abscess formation, cartilage necrosis, and deformity

Contraindications

- Suspected cribriform plate fracture
- Evidence of cerebrospinal fluid rhinorrhea

Equipment

- Topical anesthetic (cocaine, tetracaine, benzocaine, lidocaine)
- Scalpel with No. 11 blade
- Small cup forceps or scissors
- Frazier tip suction if needed
- Anterior packing equipment
- Sterile rubber drain (optional)

Procedure

1. Identify the location of the septal hematoma (soft, bluish swelling below the mucosa of the septum) *(A)*.
2. Remove debris from the area (use suction if necessary).
3. Apply topical anesthetic.
4. Using the scalpel with a No. 11 blade, make a small L-shaped incision inferiorly in the most dependent part of the hematoma *(B)*.
5. Use forceps or scissors to open and drain the hematoma and to prevent reaccumulation.
6. Place anterior nasal packing (see the section on nasal packing).
7. Arrange a follow-up check in 48 hours.

Complications

- Mucosal or septal injury
- Local infection
- Abscess formation
- Bleeding
- Hematoma reaccumulation
- Aseptic necrosis of septal cartilage
- Deformity

Discussion

- Needle aspiration of the hematoma followed by nasal packing may be considered. The likelihood of hematoma reaccumulation is high. Daily checks are prudent.
- A small rubber drain may be placed in the incision site before anterior packing to prevent reaccumulation of the hematoma.
- Prophylactic antibiotics are recommended because of the risk of infection and the presence of anterior packing.

Bibliography

Altreuter RW: Nasal trauma, *Emerg Med Clin North Am* 5(2):293-300, 1987.
Ginsburg CM: Nasal septal hematoma, *Pediatr Rev* 19(4):142-143, 1998.
Votey S, Dudley JP: Emergency ear, nose and throat procedures, *Emerg Med Clin North Am* 7(1):117-154, 1989.

A

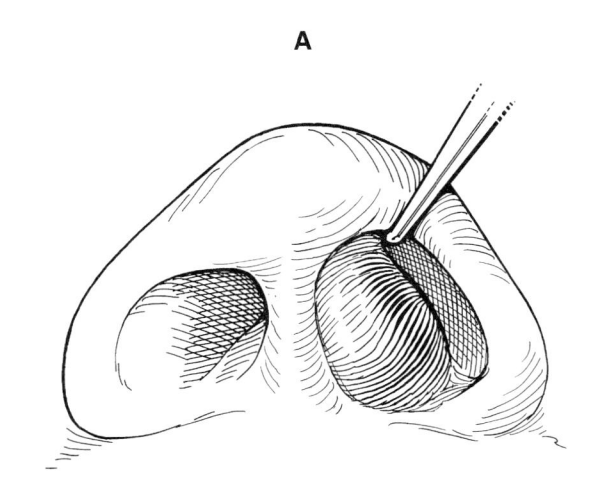

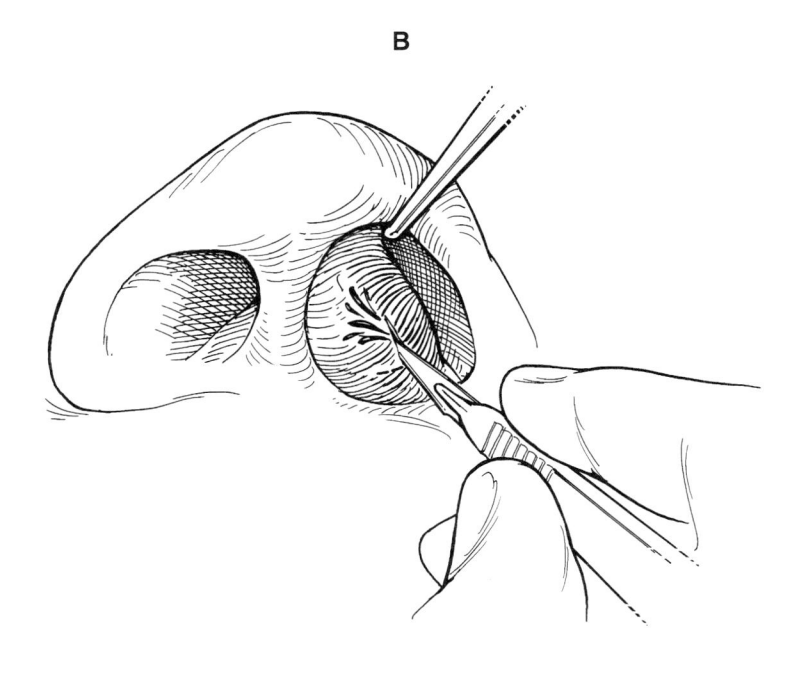

B

Auricular Hematoma Drainage · THEODORE C. CHAN

Indications
- Subperichondral hematoma around the auricle of the ear (usually associated with blunt trauma); drainage is necessary to restore blood supply from the perichondrium to cartilage and thus prevent abscess formation, cartilage necrosis, and deformity

Contraindications
- Severe trauma requiring operative debridement and repair of the ear

Equipment
- Local anesthetic (lidocaine without epinephrine), syringe, and needles
- Scalpel with No. 11 blade
- Frazier tip suction if needed
- Compression (mastoid) dressing materials: bulk cotton, gauze pads, xeroform gauze, gauze wrap, and normal saline solution or mineral oil
- Sterile rubber drain (optional)

Procedure

1. Identify the location of the auricular hematoma *(A)*.
2. Cleanse and prepare the area in sterile fashion.
3. Apply the anesthetic agent.
   a. Locally infiltrate the region around the incision site.
   b. Infiltrate around the posterior base of the ear and tragus for complete ear block.
4. Using the scalpel with a No. 11 blade, make an incision in the most dependent part of the hematoma *(B)*.
5. Once the hematoma is fully drained, prepare a compression dressing to prevent it from reforming.
6. Apply the compression (mastoid) dressing.
   a. Place bulk cotton dressing behind the auricle (posterior ear).
   b. Apply cotton or gauze pads moistened with normal saline solution or mineral oil in a xeroform dressing wrap.
   c. Press the wrap into the auricle, forming a "cast" in the concha (bowl) of the auricle.
   d. Apply bulk cotton dressing over the ear.
   e. Place a circumferential gauze wrap around the dressing and head to maintain compression of the dressing.
7. Arrange a wound check and dressing changes in 24 to 48 hours to assess for hematoma reaccumulation. Patients may require the compression dressing up to 7 days for proper healing.

Complications
- Auricular soft tissue or cartilage injury
- Local infection
- Abscess formation
- Bleeding
- Hematoma reaccumulation
- Aseptic necrosis of auricular cartilage
- Deformity (cauliflower ear)

Discussion
- Needle aspiration of the auricular hematoma may be considered but is not recommended because the risk of hematoma reaccumulation is high.
- Daily rechecks are strongly suggested for patients at high risk of hematoma reaccumulation.
- A small rubber drain may be placed in the incision site before application of the compression dressing to prevent reformation of the hematoma.
- Prophylactic systemic antibiotics should be administered.

Bibliography
Quine SM et al: Treatment of acute auricular haematoma, *J Laryngol Otol* 110(9):862-863, 1996.
Turbiak TW: Ear trauma, *Emerg Med Clin North Am* 5(2):243-251, 1987.

A

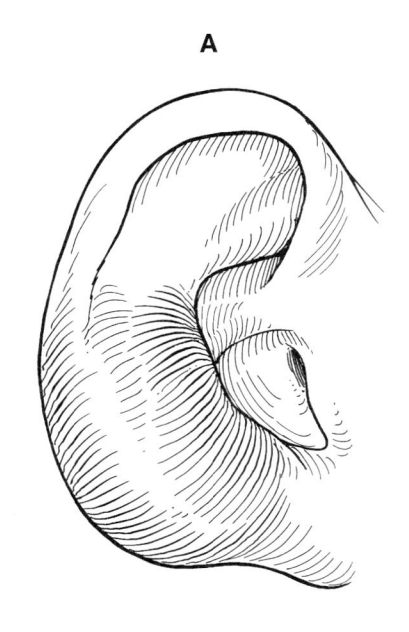

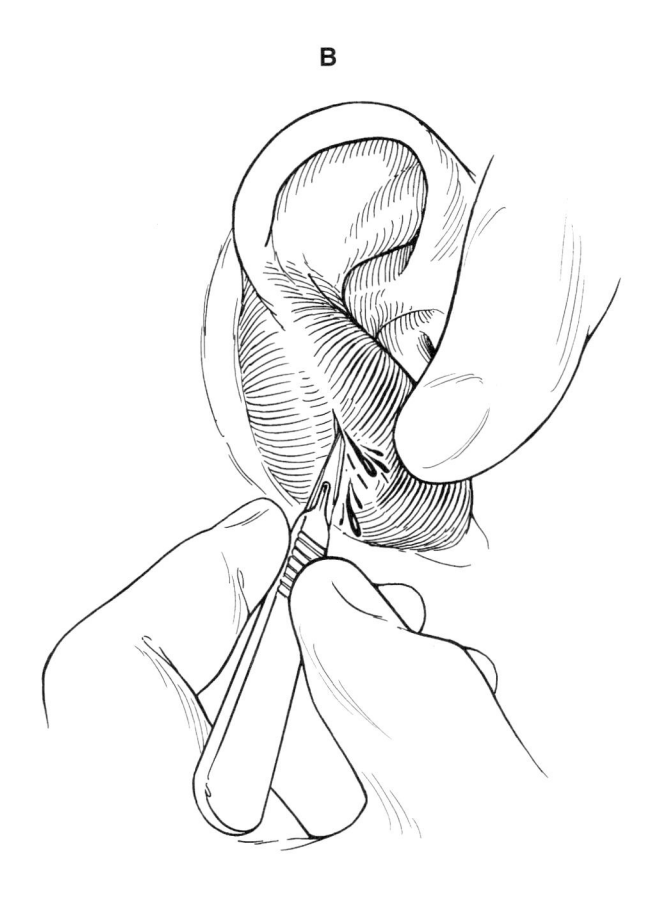

B

Peritonsillar Abscess Drainage ▪ JAMES T. AMSTERDAM

Indications
- Fluctuant peritonsillar abscess
- Peritonsillar pus collection as identified by intraoral ultrasound or computed tomography

Contraindications
- Trismus
- Uncooperative patient
- Toxic-appearing patient who requires hospital admission or drainage in the operating room

Equipment
- Ear, nose, and throat (ENT)/dental chair
- Adequate lighting or headlamp
- Tongue blade
- Topical anesthetic spray (benzocaine)
- Local anesthetic with vasoconstrictor agent (lidocaine with epinephrine 1:10,000), syringe, and needles
- 18-gauge needle with syringe (retain plastic needle cap with distal 1 cm cut off to act as a stop)
- No. 11 scalpel blade
- Hemostat (mosquito)
- Yankauer suction
- Gauze

Procedure

1. Seat the patient in the ENT/dental chair with the head slightly extended and supported by the headrest.
2. Identify the peritonsillar abscess, and locate the point of maximum fluctuance.
3. Spray topical anesthetic over the area.
4. Depress the tongue with a blade, and inject a small amount (1 to 2 ml) of local anesthetic agent superficially over the area (if a vasoconstrictor agent is used, the mucosa should be injected until blanching occurs).
5. Perform needle aspiration.
   a. Prepare an 18-gauge needle and syringe by retaining the plastic needle cap with the distal 1 cm cut off and removed; the modified cap remains on the needle (so that only the distal 1 cm of the needle is exposed) and prevents insertion of the needle into the deeper tissues *(A)*.
   b. Depress the tongue with the blade, and penetrate the point of maximal fluctuance with the needle and syringe. Do not penetrate farther than 1 cm into the tissues *(B)*.
   c. Aspirate purulent material.
   d. If no pus is aspirated, the needle and syringe may be removed and repositioned to be inserted slightly more inferiorly, or subsequently laterally if inferior aspiration is unsuccessful.
6. Perform incision and drainage.
   a. Consider preparing the scalpel with No. 11 blade by wrapping tape around the proximal end of the blade so that only the distal 1 cm of the blade is exposed.
   b. Prepare to suction with the Yankauer suction tip.
   c. Make a small stab incision at the point of maximal fluctuance, and suction as needed *(C)*.
   d. Use the hemostat to gently spread the incision and break up any loculations. Avoid deep dissection because of the proximity of the internal carotid artery.
7. Have the patient rinse and spit after the procedure.
8. Use gauze packs for oozing at the procedure site.
9. Discharged patients should be directed to continue intraoral rinses several times a day with warm saline solution to promote continued drainage.
10. Patients who appear toxic or markedly dehydrated should be admitted for IV fluid administration, ENT consultation, and possible drainage in the operating room.

Complications

- Bleeding
- Perforation of internal carotid artery
- Dry tap

Discussion

- Although needle aspiration is easy to perform, the risk of abscess recurrence is greater with this technique. The incision and drainage procedure is technically more complicated and may be reserved for the ENT consultant.
- Failure to obtain pus is not uncommon. The physician must then decide whether to treat the patient with antibiotics with or without steroids, obtain ENT consultation and admit the patient, or pursue further studies, including ultrasound and computed tomography.

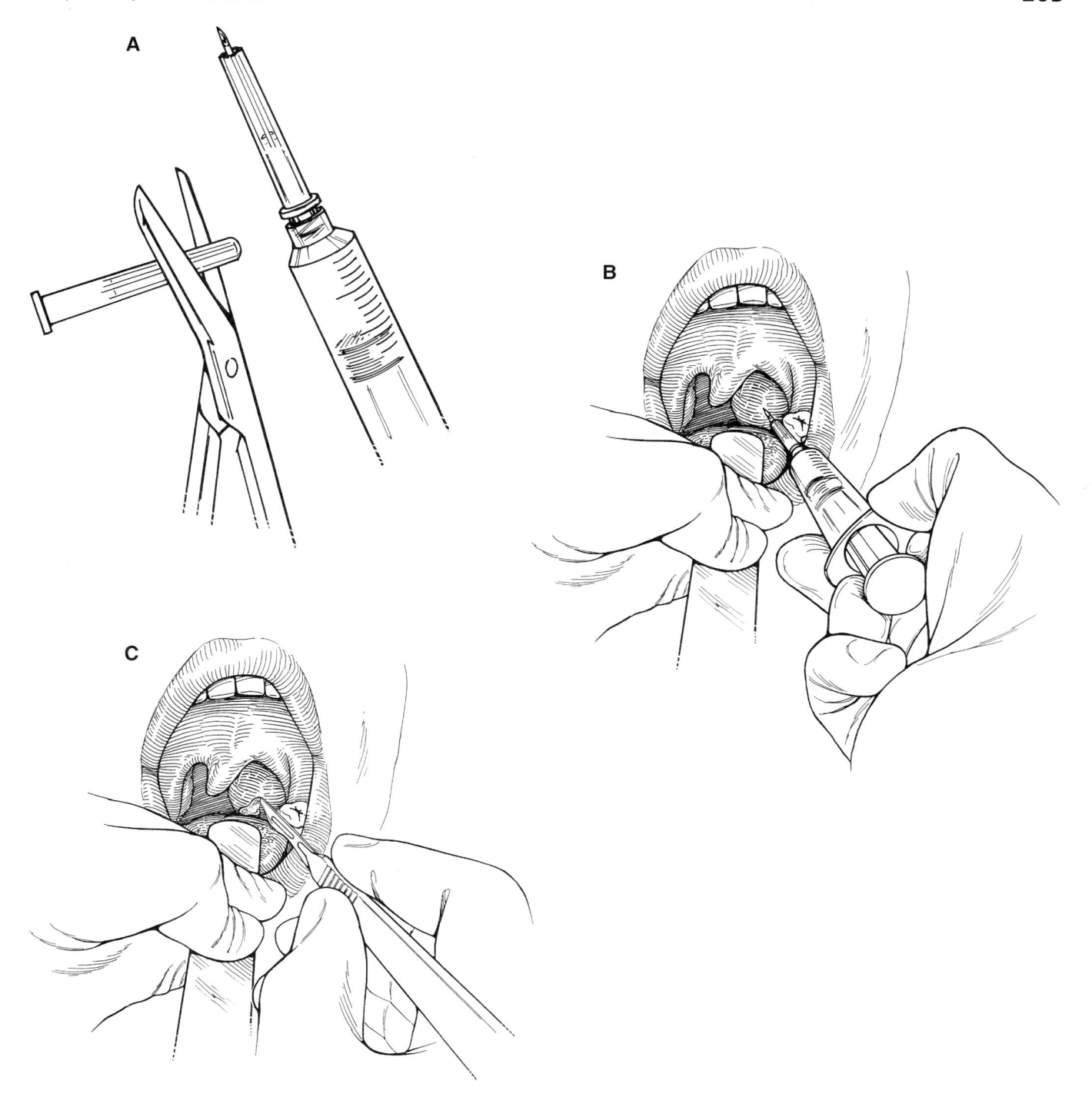

- Patients with a pathologic heart murmur, valvular disease, mitral valve prolapse, or prosthetic valve will require prophylaxis against subacute bacterial endocarditis before aspiration or incision of a peritonsillar abscess.

Bibliography

Friedman NR et al: Peritonsillar abscess in early childhood: presentation and management, *Arch Otolaryngol Head Neck Surg* 123(6):630-632, 1997.

Prior A et al: The microbiology and antibiotic treatment of peritonsillar abscess, *Clin Otolaryngol* 20(3):219-223, 1995.

Wolf M, Even-Chen I, Kronenberg J: Peritonsillar abscess: repeated needle aspiration versus incision and drainage, *Ann Otol Rhinol Laryngol* 103(7):554-557, 1994.

Mandibular Reduction • JAMES T. AMSTERDAM

Indications
- Mandibular dislocation, most commonly resulting in dislocation of the condyles anterior to the eminence with resulting masseter muscle spasm *(A)*

Contraindications
- Mandible fracture
- Recurrent dislocations that required general anesthesia in the past
- Contraindication to conscious sedation

Equipment
- Ear, nose, and throat (ENT)/dental chair
- Conscious sedation agents per protocol
- Gloves
- Gauze
- Bite block

Procedure

1. This procedure should be performed with the aid of an assistant.
2. Reassure and calm the anxious patient.
3. In cases of trauma, obtain mandible radiographs to assess for fracture.
4. Provide IV access, oxygen, and monitoring per institutional policies for conscious sedation.
5. Sedate the patient with selected conscious sedation agents.
6. Seat the patient in an ENT/dental chair.
7. Wear gloves, and insert a bite block *(B)*.
8. Place your thumbs over the patient's lower molars.
9. Exert steady, constant pressure in the downward (inferior) direction onto the mandible.
10. As the masseter muscles relax, the mandible should move downward, backward (posteriorly) *(C)*, and then upward *(D)* as the condyles are forced below the eminences and slip posteriorly back into the fossae.
11. Muscle spasm can cause the mandible to snap shut suddenly once reduction is obtained. The bite block is intended to protect the operator's thumbs from being bitten.
12. Once the dislocation is reduced, assess the patient for normal articulation; the patient should have no malocclusion.
13. Discharge the patient with instructions to maintain a soft diet, support the jaw while yawning and laughing, and apply cold packs to the temporomandibular joint (TMJ) for the next 48 hours. The patient should also be instructed to open and close the jaw several times a day and advised to follow up with a dentist or oral and maxillofacial surgeon.

Complications

- Failure to reduce the mandible
- Spontaneous dislocation after reduction in a patient with chronic dislocation
- Thumb injury to the operator from being bitten by the patient

Discussion

- The operator's thumbs may be placed on the mandibular ridge rather than the molars. This reduces the operator's risk of being bitten during the reduction. Pressure is directed medially as well as downward from this position.
- If conscious sedation does not result in adequate muscle relaxation to allow relocation, local anesthetic can be injected into the TMJ before further attempts.
- Patients with chronic dislocation problems may require a Barton bandage (wrapping around the head and jaw) to prevent maximal jaw opening and recurrent dislocation.

Bibliography

Amsterdam JT: Emergency dental procedures. In Roberts JR, Hedges JR (eds): *Clinical procedures in emergency medicine*, ed 3, Philadelphia, 1998, WB Saunders.

Avrahami E et al: Unilateral medial dislocation of the temporomandibular joint, *Neuroradiology* 39(8):602-604, 1997.

Undt G et al: Treatment of recurrent mandibular dislocations (parts I & II), *Int J Oral Maxillofac Surg* 26(2):92-102, 1997.

EAR, NOSE, AND THROAT 205

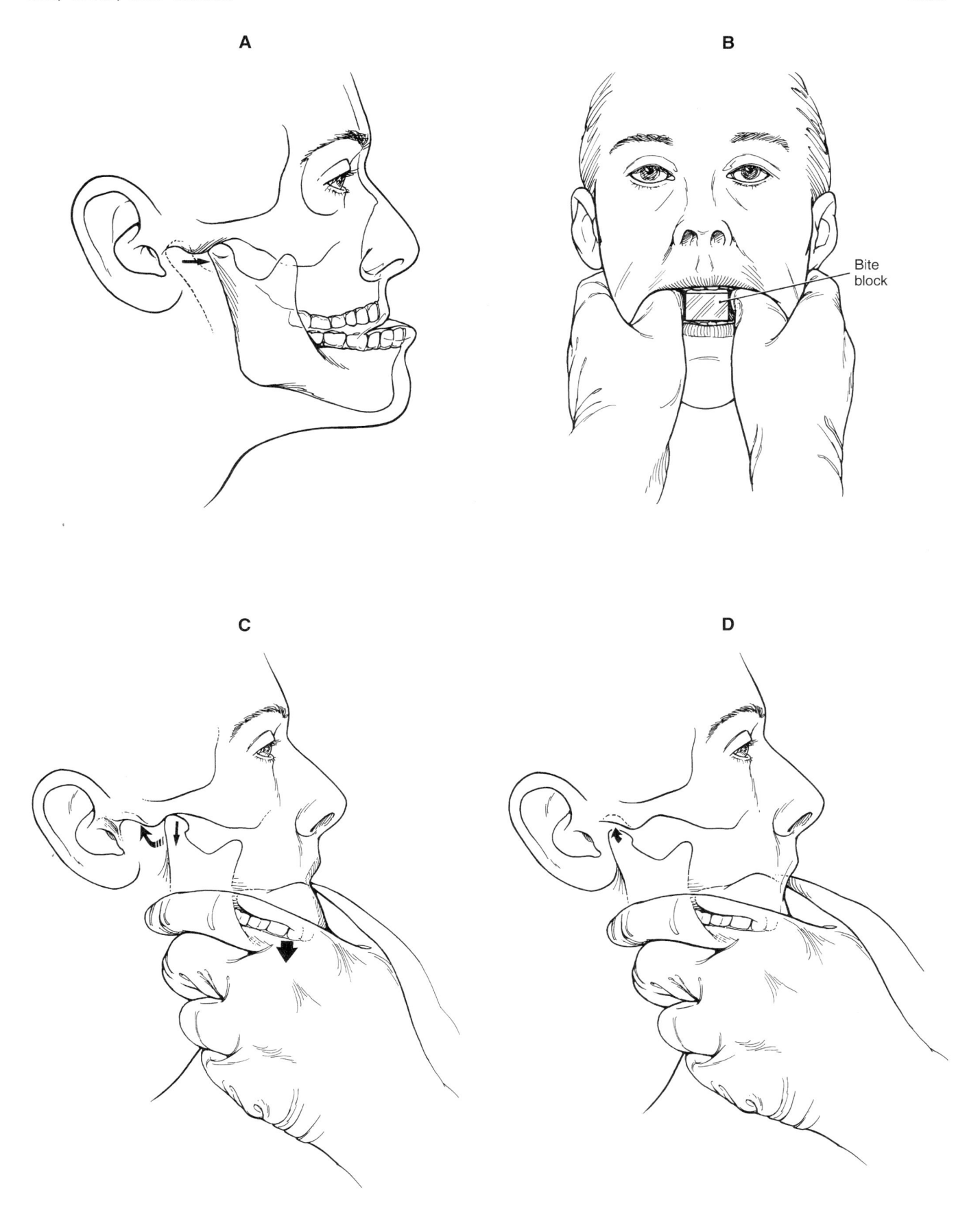

A

B

Bite block

C

D

CHAPTER 10

SKIN AND SUBCUTANEOUS TISSUE

Interrupted and Running Suture • BARRY C. SIMON

Indications
- Interrupted suture
  - Routine laceration repair
  - Repair of jagged wounds that require meticulous reapproximation
- Running suture
  - Long, relatively straight lacerations

Contraindications
- Standard contraindications to wound repair based on assessment of risk for complications, including infection; factors include wound location, contamination, and delay in seeking care
- Complex wounds

Equipment
- Anesthetic agent (lidocaine, bupivacaine), syringe, and needles
- Normal saline solution
- Wound irrigation and cleansing device or large syringe and 18-gauge angiocatheter
- Standard emergency department suture kit with minimum of:
  - Hypodermic needles (18 to 27 gauge)
  - Drapes
  - Iris scissors, straight
  - Needle holder
  - Pickups
  - Gauze sponges
- Appropriate suture material with curved needle

Procedure

1. Prepare skin surrounding the wound in sterile fashion.
2. Anesthetize the wound as indicated (by either local subcutaneous infiltration around wound edges or nerve block).
3. Cleanse, irrigate, and debride the wound as indicated.

Interrupted Wound Suture (A)
1. Closure involves the placement of single sutures tied separately.
2. Grasp curved suture needle at two thirds proximal from tip with needle holder.
3. Insert the suture needle into the skin near the edge of the wound at a 90° angle to the skin. Drive the needle through the skin, and exit into the open wound edge. Reinsert the needle on the opposite side of the wound at a depth similar to the wound exit site. Drive the needle through, and exit the skin adjacent to the wound at a point the same distance from the wound as the original skin insertion site. Pickups can be used to facilitate passage of the needle.
4. Tie the two loose ends of the suture together by looping the free end of suture around the needle holder (still holding the needle end of the suture) and pulling the needle holder through the two loops to form the first locked stitch. Pull the ends of suture so that the stitch approximates the wound edge without excessive tension on the wound.
5. Use the loose end of the suture to wrap around the needle driver once to form subsequent stitches. This should be performed approximately three times after the first locked stitch.
6. Make sure that the wound edges are well approximated without excessive tension from the sutures and that the skin everts at the edges.

Running Wound Suture (B)
1. Place a single interrupted stitch that is tied after being placed so that the needle end of the suture is left long.
2. With the needle end of the suture, take the next bite at the site of the original knot and cross subcutaneously at a 45° angle to the wound direction, exiting the skin on the other side of the wound.
3. Reenter the skin directly across from the point the needle emerged (on the side of the wound of the original needle insertion) so that the visible suture is oriented 90° to the wound direction.
4. Repeat this procedure down the length of the wound.
5. When the needle enters the skin for the last time, it crosses the wound at a 90° angle (rather than 45°), exiting the tissue near the exit site of the previous bite.
6. Leave the loop of suture on this final bite loose to act as a free end for knot tying. Tie the needle end of the suture to the loop of suture to form the final knot.

Complications
- Bleeding
- Infection
- Wound separation

Discussion
- For large lacerations the first interrupted sutures should be placed at midpoints of the laceration so that sutures can be evenly spaced throughout the laceration.

Skin and Subcutaneous Tissue

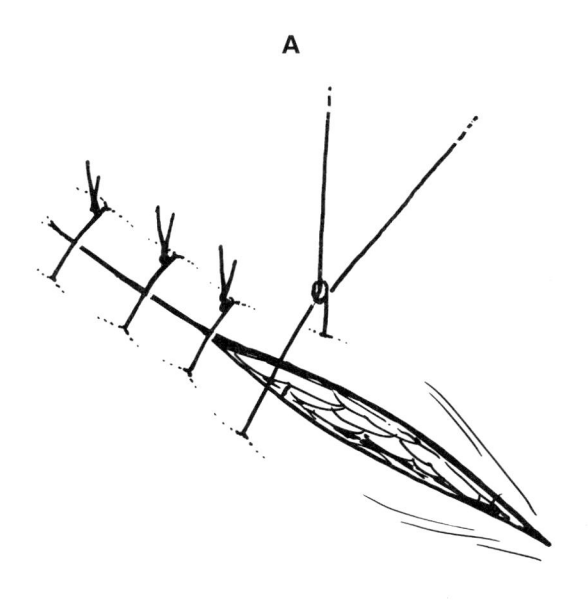

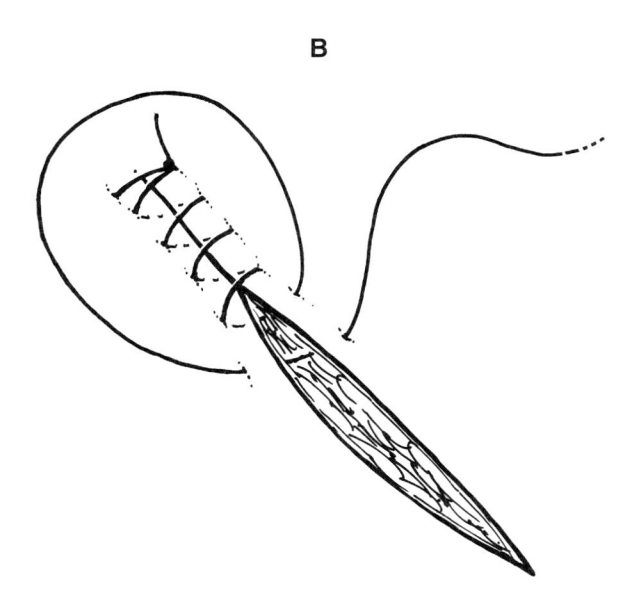

A

B

- Running sutures approximate tissue quickly and adequately for straight, simple lacerations but do not provide a great deal of strength. Regions that require strength, such as over joint surfaces, require interrupted sutures.
- If the wound becomes infected, the entire running suture must be removed, opening the length of the wound.

Bibliography

Battle R: *Plastic surgery*, Boston, 1964, Butterworth, pp 7, 45.
Lammers RL: Soft tissue procedures. In Hedges R (ed): *Clinical procedures in emergency medicine*, Philadelphia, 1991, WB Saunders, pp 515-565.
Trott AT: *Wounds and lacerations*, St Louis, 1997, Mosby, pp 154-205, 248-264.

Mattress Suture ■ BARRY C. SIMON

Indications
- Minimize and disperse tension on skin edges (horizontal mattress).
- Close potential tissue dead space in deep laceration wounds (vertical mattress).
- Improve wound edge eversion (horizontal and vertical mattress).

Contraindications
- Standard contraindications to wound repair based on assessment of risk for complications, including infection; factors include wound location, contamination, and time delay in seeking care

Equipment
- Anesthetic agent (lidocaine, bupivacaine), syringe, and needles
- Normal saline solution
- Wound irrigation and cleansing device or large syringe and 18-gauge angiocatheter
- Standard emergency department suture kit with minimum of:
  - Hypodermic needles (18 to 27 gauge)
  - Drapes
  - Iris scissors, straight
  - Needle holder
  - Pickups
  - Gauze sponges
- Appropriate suture material with curved needle

Procedure

1. Interrupted suture wound closure involves the placement of single sutures tied separately.
2. Prepare the skin surrounding the wound in sterile fashion.
3. Anesthetize the wound as indicated (by either local subcutaneous infiltration around wound edges or nerve block).
4. Cleanse, irrigate, and debride the wound as indicated.
5. Horizontal mattress:
   a. Initially, pass the needle through the wound in similar manner to interrupted suture.
   b. On exiting the skin, reintroduce the needle approximately 0.5 cm adjacent to the exit point along the wound edge *(A)*.
   c. Pass the needle back through the wound so that the needle emerges 0.5 cm from the initial insertion point.
   d. Tie the suture to form the horizontal mattress stitch.
   e. Continue the same mattress stitch as needed down the length of the wound *(B)*.
6. Vertical mattress:
   a. The vertical mattress suture has superficial and deep components.
   b. Introduce the needle at a 90° angle about 1 cm from the wound margin.
   c. Pass the needle through the depth of the wound until it emerges on the opposite side, 1 cm from the laceration margin at a 90° angle. This pass forms the deep component of the stitch *(C)*.
   d. Reintroduce the needle 1 to 2 mm from the wound epidermal edge (on the same side as the prior exit point), and pass the needle through the wound to a similar point on the opposite wound edge (the same side as the original insertion point). This pass forms the superficial component of the stitch.
   e. Tie the loose ends of the suture together to form the vertical mattress suture and approximate the wound *(D)*.

Complications
- Bleeding
- Infection

Discussion
- Both the horizontal mattress stitch and the vertical mattress stitch improve wound edge eversion.
- The horizontal mattress disperses excess skin tension and is useful for large, gaping lacerations in areas of minimal skin mobility. This stitch is also useful in cases of thin, fragile skin (such as with elderly patients) or in lacerations with significant tissue loss from injury or debridement.
- The vertical mattress closes potential spaces in large, gaping lacerations. This stitch is useful in areas of lax skin tension where maximum skin mobility is needed, such as over joint surfaces.
- For the horizontal mattress, each bite is always the same distance from the wound margin and moves down the length of the wound. For the vertical mattress, each bite is at the same perpendicular level to the wound edge, but bites are at different distances from the edge.

Bibliography
Battle R: *Plastic surgery,* 1964, Boston, Butterworth, pp 7, 45.
Lammers RL: Soft tissue procedures. In Hedges R (ed): *Clinical procedures in emergency medicine,* Philadelphia, 1991, WB Saunders, pp 515-565.
Trott AT: *Wounds and lacerations,* St Louis, 1997, Mosby, pp 154-205, 248-264.

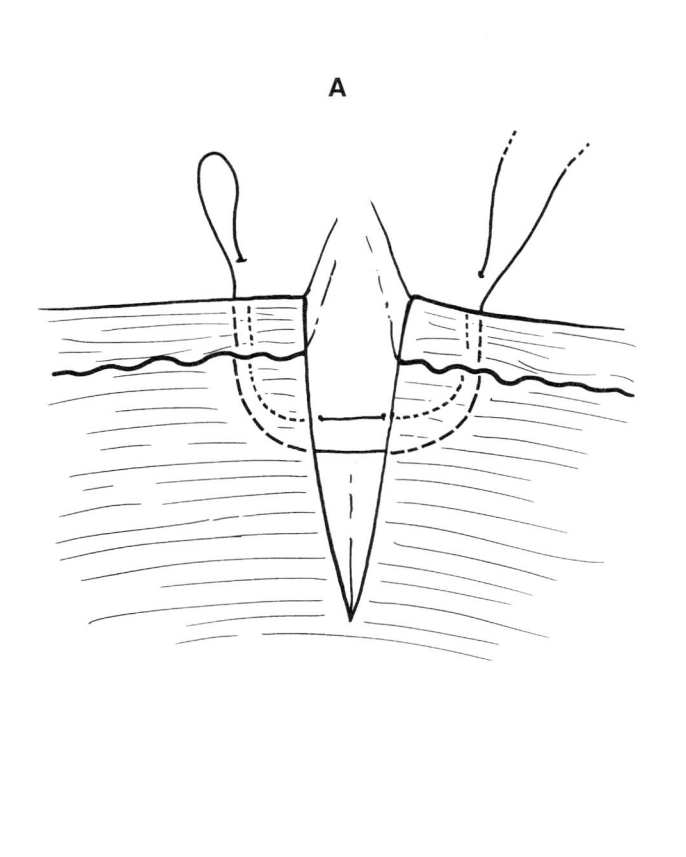

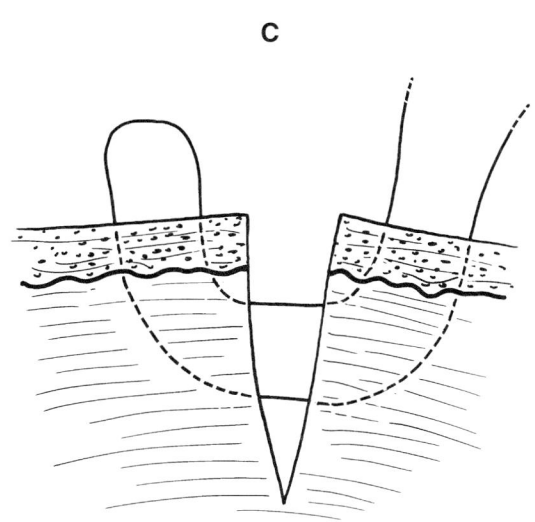

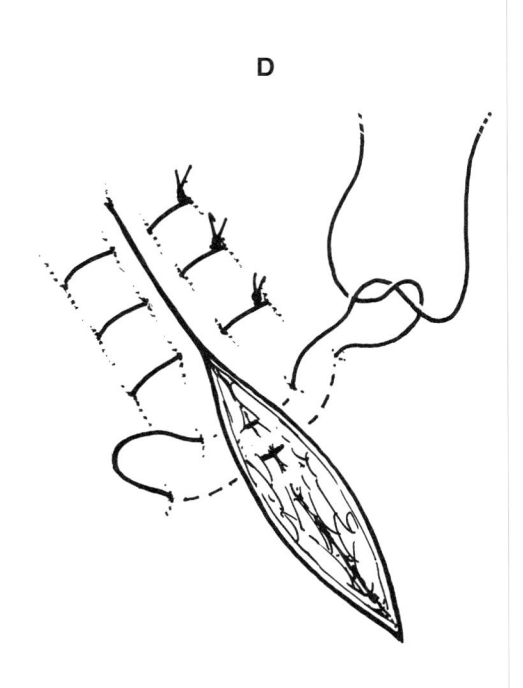

Skin and Subcutaneous Tissue

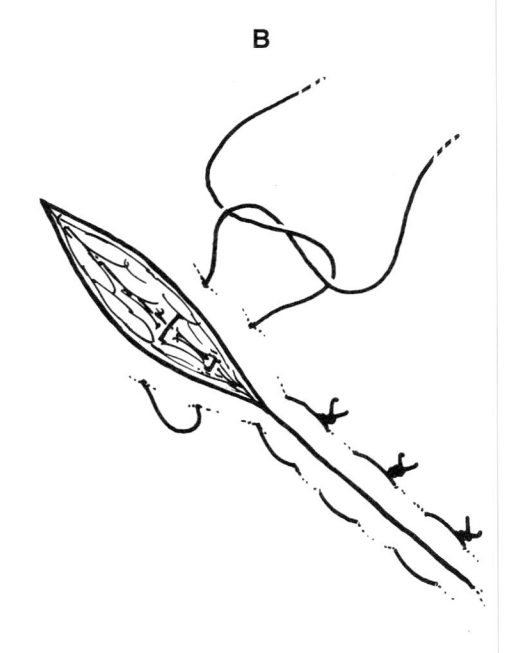

A

B

C

D

Intradermal (Buried) Suture ▪ BARRY C. SIMON

Indications
- Placing cutaneous sutures in wounds under tension can lead to ischemia of the wound margin and an unsightly scar. Proper placement of buried intradermal sutures will help to approximate dermal margins and reduce wound edge tension.

Contraindications
- Standard contraindications to wound repair based on assessment of risk for complications, including infection; factors include wound location, contamination, and delay in seeking care

Equipment
- Anesthetic agent (lidocaine, bupivacaine), syringe, and needles
- Normal saline solution
- Wound irrigation and cleansing device or large syringe and 18-gauge angiocatheter
- Standard emergency department suture kit with minimum of the following:
  - Hypodermic needles (18 to 27 gauge)
  - Drapes
  - Iris scissors, straight
  - Needle holder
  - Pickups
  - Gauze sponges
- Appropriate absorbable suture material with curved needle

Procedure

1. Prepare the skin surrounding the wound in sterile fashion.
2. Anesthetize the wound as indicated (by either local subcutaneous infiltration around wound edges or nerve block).
3. Cleanse, irrigate, and debride the wound as indicated.
4. Introduce the needle deep in the wound in the subcutaneous tissue, and direct the needle out the wound at the dermis below the skin surface *(A)*.
5. Reintroduce the needle into the dermis on the opposite wound margin, and direct the needle out the subcutaneous tissue at the same level on the opposite side *(B)*.
6. Tie and secure the knot so that it remains buried deep below the skin surface *(C, D)*.

Complications
- Wound separation
- Scarring

Discussion
- Placement of buried sutures differs from traditional suturing because of the need to bury the knot deep to the dermis. Failure to do this can interfere with dermal healing and leave a small lump under the skin surface.

Bibliography
Battle R: *Plastic surgery,* Boston, 1964, Butterworth, pp 7, 45.
Lammers RL: Soft tissue procedures. In Hedges R (ed): *Clinical procedures in emergency medicine,* Philadelphia, 1991, WB Saunders, pp 515-565.
Trott AT: *Wounds and lacerations,* St Louis, 1997, Mosby, pp 154-205, 248-264.

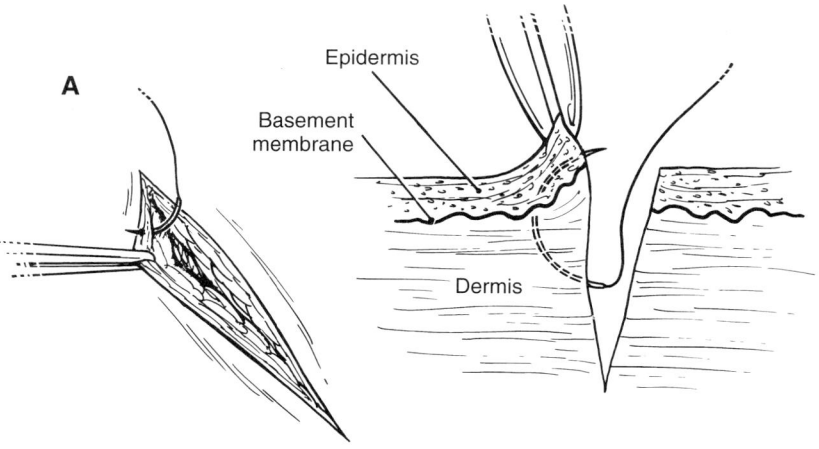

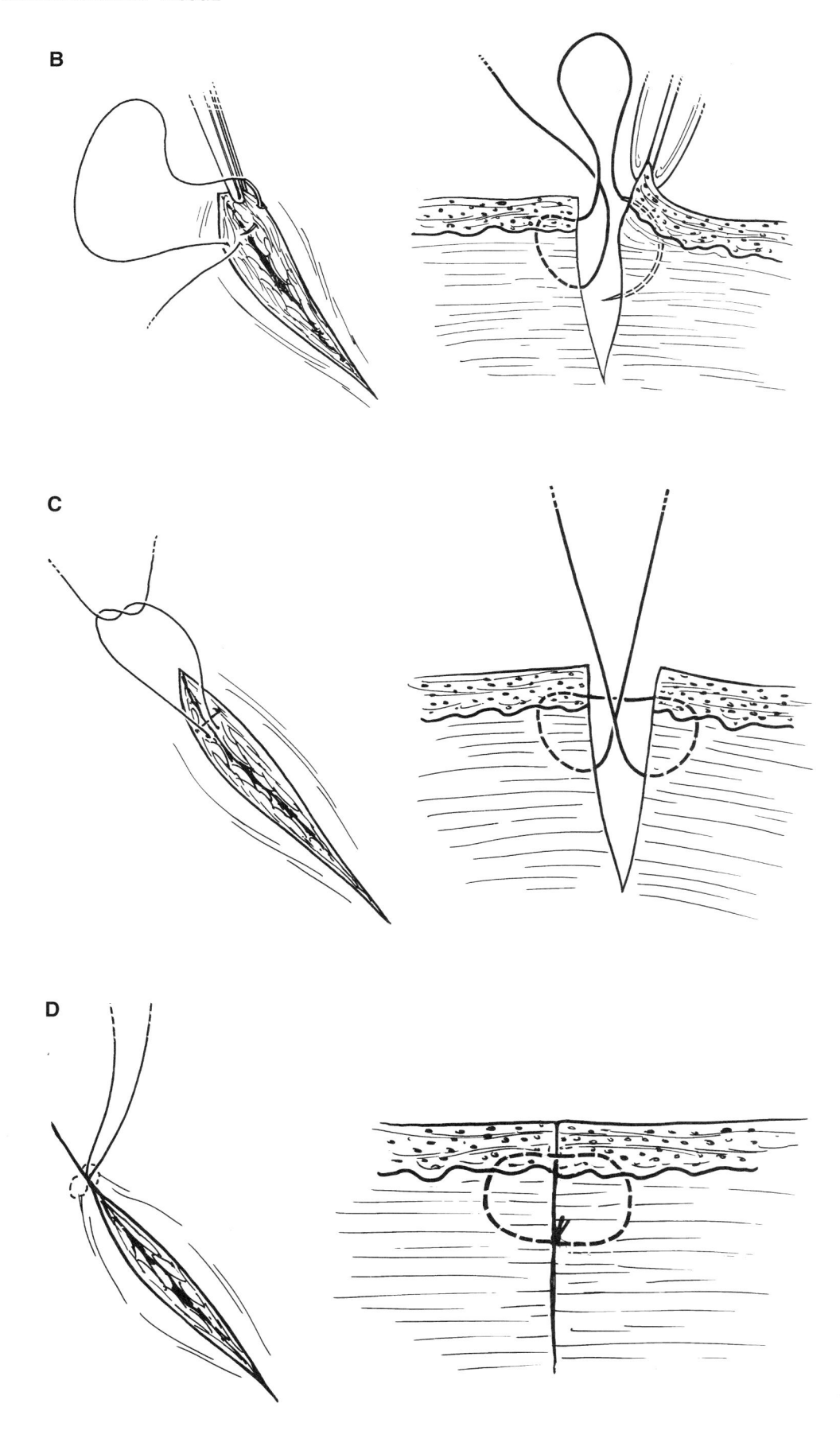

Skin and Subcutaneous Tissue

B

C

D

Scalp Laceration Repair • BARRY C. SIMON

Indications
- Staples are ideal for the skin closure of simple linear scalp lacerations.

Contraindications
- Standard contraindications to wound repair based on assessment of risk for complications, including infection; factors include wound location, contamination, and delay in seeking care
- Staples produce artifact on a computed tomographic (CT) scan and optimally should not be used before a scan is obtained. However, if they are used, the CT scan can still provide useful information. Staples may move during magnetic resonance imaging (MRI) and should not be placed if MRI is being considered.

Equipment
- Anesthetic agent (lidocaine, bupivacaine), syringe, and needles
- Normal saline solution
- Wound irrigation and cleansing device or large syringe and 18-gauge angiocatheter
- Staple device (a number of lightweight stapling devices are on the market; most come preloaded with five or more staples and are easy to use)
- If using suture, a standard emergency department suture kit with minimum of the following:
  - Hypodermic needles (18 to 27 gauge)
  - Drapes
  - Iris scissors, straight
  - Needle holder
  - Pickups
  - Gauze sponges
  - Appropriate suture material with curved needle

Procedure
1. Prepare skin surrounding the wound in sterile fashion.
2. Anesthetize the wound as indicated (by either local subcutaneous infiltration around wound edges or nerve block).
3. Cleanse, irrigate, and debride the wound as indicated.
4. Clip or trim hair that impedes closure (A).
5. Explore the wound to assess depth and complexity. Close a defect in the galea with 3-0 or 4-0 absorbable suture. Jagged or macerated lacerations may require some debridement and horizontal mattress sutures.
6. Uncomplicated scalp lacerations may be closed with staples.
7. To initiate stapling, pinch the adjacent skin margins together with fingers or forceps, attempting to evert the wound margins. Place the "mouth" of the stapler gently on the skin surface, taking care not to indent the skin (B).
8. Carefully squeeze the handle of the stapler to eject the staple into the tissue. Ideally the staple closely approximates the wound margins without indenting the surface of the skin (C).
9. To release the staple, cock your wrist back to disengage the staple from the last staple.
10. Staple removal is easy, especially if the wound is clean and free of dried secretions. The dual prongs on the disposable staple remover slide under the staple cross bar. As the handle is squeezed and the horizontal aspect of the staple is depressed, the sharp edges are eased out of the tissue for removal (D).

Complications
- Failure to repair the galea, which may lead to a cosmetic deformity related to frontalis muscle function

Discussion
- Anesthesia with epinephrine may help control bleeding.
- If staples are not available, uncomplicated scalp lacerations may be closed with separate simple interrupted monofilament nylon sutures. Absorbable polyglycolic acid sutures can be used in children and in adults who may not return for suture removal.

Bibliography
Battle R: *Plastic surgery*, Boston, 1964, Butterworth, pp 7, 45.
Lammers RL: Soft tissue procedures. In Hedges R (ed): *Clinical procedures in emergency medicine*, Philadelphia, 1991, WB Saunders, pp 515-565.
Trott AT: *Wounds and lacerations*, St Louis, 1997, Mosby, pp 154-205, 248-264.

Skin and Subcutaneous Tissue

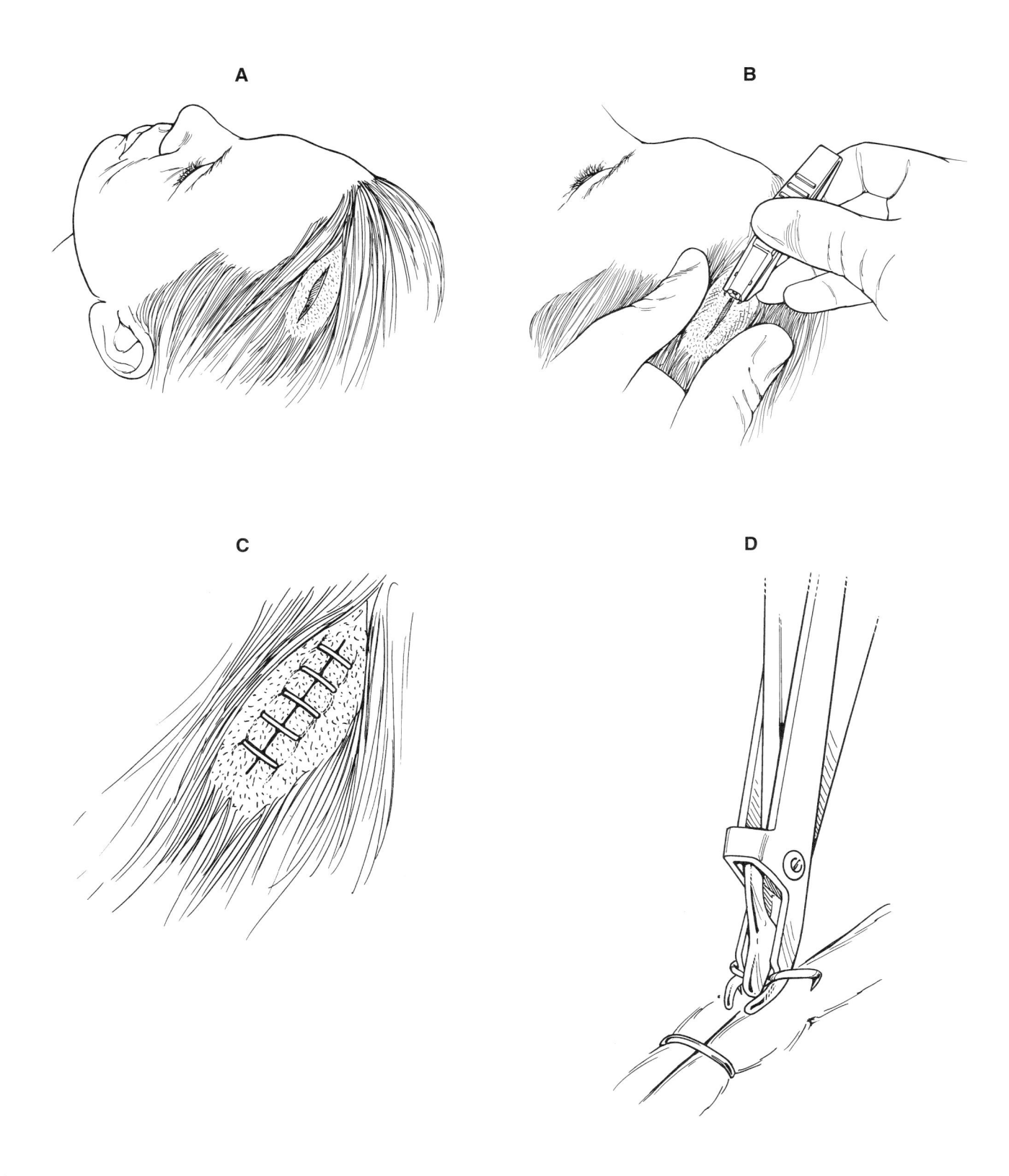

A

B

C

D

Corner Stitch (Half-Buried Horizontal Mattress)
■ BARRY C. SIMON

Indications
- Jagged and triangular wounds that create corners difficult to repair *(A)*

Contraindications
- None

Equipment
- Anesthetic agent (lidocaine, bupivacaine), syringe, and needles
- Normal saline solution
- Wound irrigation and cleansing device or large syringe and 18-gauge angiocatheter
- Standard emergency department suture kit with minimum of the following:
  - Hypodermic needles (18 to 27 gauge)
  - Drapes
  - Iris scissors, straight
  - Needle holder
  - Pickups
  - Gauze sponges
- Appropriate suture material with curved needle

Procedure

1. Prepare skin surrounding the wound in sterile fashion.
2. Anesthetize the wound as indicated (by either local subcutaneous infiltration around wound edges or nerve block).
3. Cleanse, irrigate, and debride the wound as indicated.
4. Introduce the needle percutaneously through the nonflap side of the wound a few millimeters from the corner of the wound.
5. Pass the needle horizontally through the dermis of the flap *(B)*.
6. Pass the needle into the dermis of the nonflap aspect of the wound a few millimeters from the opposite side of the corner. Be sure to take equal depth bites with each pass of the needle *(C)*.
7. Lead the suture out through the epidermis and tie it.
8. Once the corner has been repaired, close the remaining two sides of the wound with simple interrupted or running suture technique *(D)*.

Complications
- Bleeding
- Infection
- Wound separation

Discussion
- The suture should not be placed directly in the tip of the flap. This practice may stretch the tissue and further compromise blood flow to the wound margin. The corner stitch allows optimum tissue approximation with minimal tension.
- This technique can also be used to encompass multiple flaps either individually or collectively if the tips happen to be adjacent to one another.
- The most difficult but important aspect of the corner stitch is to take equal depth bites with each pass of the needle. Failure to do so will result in a wound in which the opposing sides do not lie flat. This will leave a more obvious scar.

Bibliography

Battle R: *Plastic surgery*, Boston, 1964, Butterworth, pp 7, 45.

Lammers RL: Soft tissue procedures. In Hedges R (ed): *Clinical procedures in emergency medicine*, Philadelphia, 1991, WB Saunders, pp 515-565.

Trott AT: *Wounds and lacerations*, St Louis, 1997, Mosby, pp 154-205, 248-264.

Skin and Subcutaneous Tissue

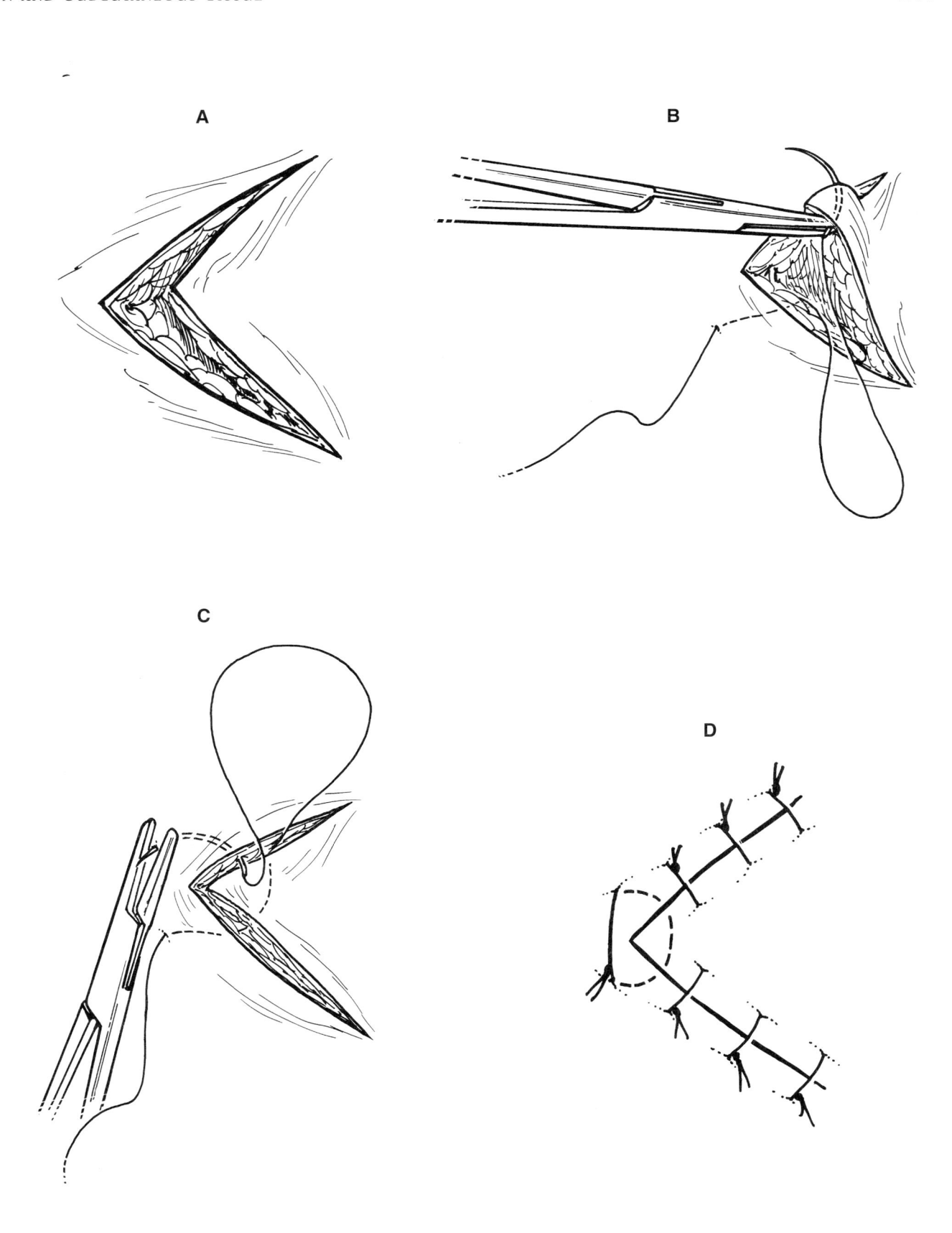

A

B

C

D

Dog Ear Repair ▪ BARRY C. SIMON

Indications
- Laceration in which one edge is longer than the other
- Curvilinear laceration

Contraindications
- Standard contraindications to wound repair based on assessment of risk for complications, including infection; factors include wound location, contamination, and time delay in seeking care

Equipment
- Anesthetic agent (lidocaine, bupivacaine), syringe, and needles
- Normal saline solution
- Wound irrigation and cleansing device or large syringe and 18-gauge angiocatheter
- Standard emergency department suture kit with minimum of the following:
  - Hypodermic needles (18 to 27 gauge)
  - Drapes
  - Iris scissors, straight
  - Needle holder
  - Pickups
  - Gauze sponges
- Appropriate suture material with curved needle
- Scalpel with No. 15 blade
- Tissue forceps

Procedure
1. Prepare and cleanse the wound in sterile fashion.
2. Perform standard repair of the wound up to approximately the final centimeter of the wound.
3. Using the No. 15 blade, make a 1-cm incision, extending the laceration at a 45° angle toward the side with redundant tissue (the long side of the wound) to create the "dog ear" *(A)*.
4. Undermine and excise the subcutaneous tissue beneath the dog ear to mobilize the skin *(B)*.
5. Gently lift the redundant tissue with the tissue forceps, and excise the small triangular piece of excess tissue in a line parallel to the original incision performed *(C)*.
6. Repair the wound in standard fashion along the length of the laceration and incision *(D)*.

Complications
- Bleeding
- Infection
- Unsightly repair and scarring
- Skin and soft tissue necrosis from excessive tissue undermining and excision

Discussion
- Incision, undermining, and excision of tissue can be difficult. Limited experience in the procedure can lead to complications, including unsightly scarring and tissue necrosis.

Bibliography
Battle R: *Plastic surgery,* Boston, 1964, Butterworth, pp 7, 45.
Lammers RL: Soft tissue procedures. In Hedges R (ed): *Clinical procedures in emergency medicine,* Philadelphia, 1991, WB Saunders, pp 515-565.
Trott AT: *Wounds and lacerations,* St Louis, 1997, Mosby, pp 154-205, 248-264.

Skin and Subcutaneous Tissue

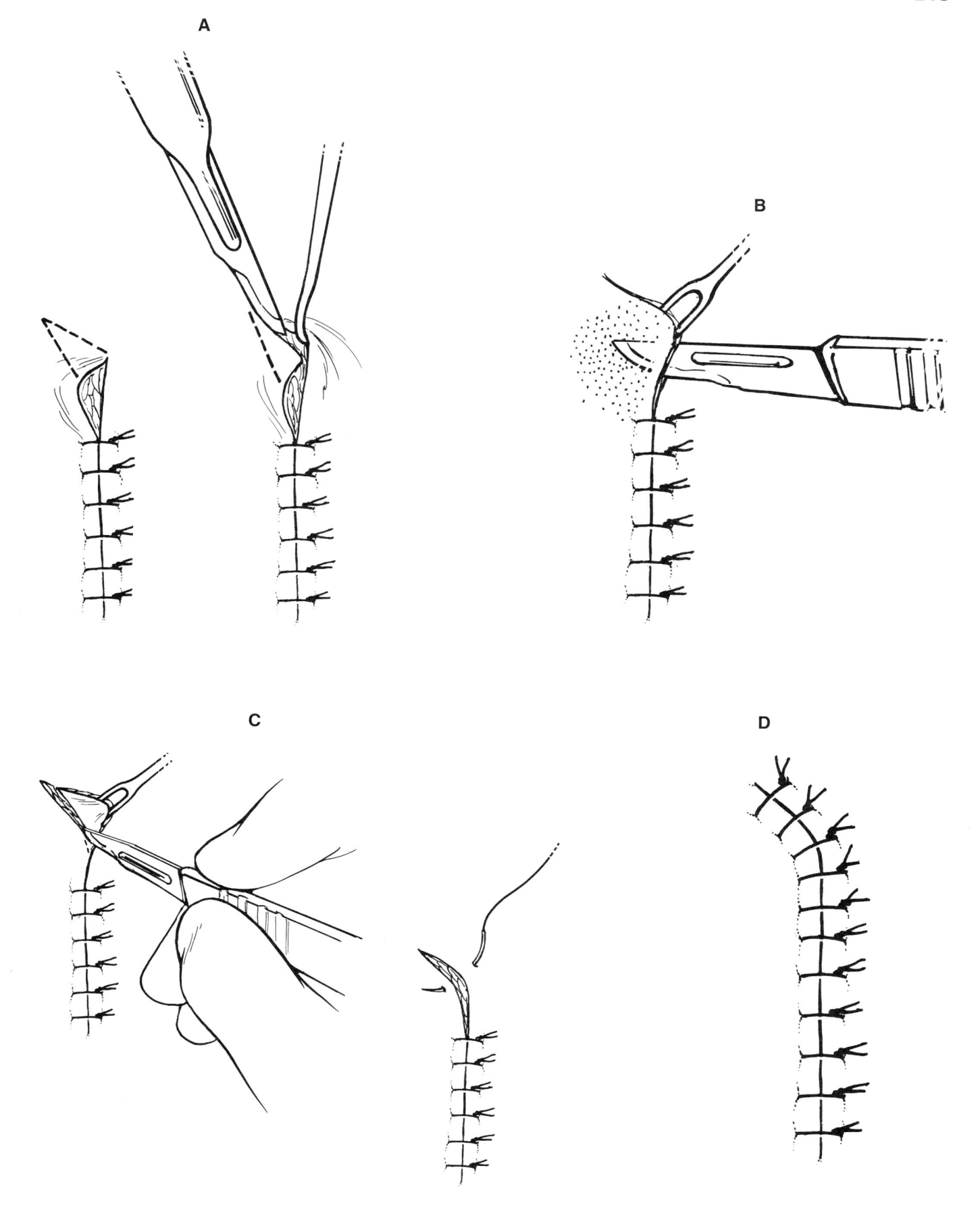

A

B

C

D

V-Y Closure ■ BARRY C. SIMON

Indications
- Closure of V-shaped wound with tissue loss or nonviable margins

Contraindications
- Standard contraindications to wound repair based on assessment of risk for complications, including infection; factors include wound location, contamination, and delay in seeking care

Equipment
- Anesthetic agent (lidocaine, bupivacaine), syringe, and needles
- Normal saline solution
- Wound irrigation and cleansing device or large syringe and 18-gauge angiocatheter
- Standard emergency department suture kit with minimum of the following:
  - Hypodermic needles (18 to 27 gauge)
  - Drapes
  - Iris scissors, straight
  - Needle holder
  - Pickups
  - Gauze sponges
- Appropriate suture material with curved needle

Procedure
1. Prepare and cleanse the wound as indicated.
2. Trim and debride nonviable tissue with iris scissors *(A, B)*.
3. Close the bottom of the V-shaped laceration with simple interrupted percutaneous stitches *(C)*.
4. Closing this portion will create a new tissue corner closer to the tip of the flap, revising the V shape into a Y-shaped laceration.
5. Secure the tip of the flap to this new tissue corner with a corner stitch *(D)*.
6. Close the remaining two limbs of the Y shape with standard simple interrupted stitches *(E)*.

Complications
- Bleeding
- Infection
- Unsightly repair and scarring

Discussion
- V-Y closures can be difficult. Limited experience in the procedure can lead to complications, including unsightly scarring.

Bibliography
Battle R: *Plastic surgery*, Boston, 1964, Butterworth, pp 7, 45.
Lammers RL: Soft tissue procedures. In Hedges R (ed): *Clinical procedures in emergency medicine*, Philadelphia, 1991, WB Saunders, pp 515-565.
Trott AT: *Wounds and lacerations*, St Louis, 1997, Mosby, pp 154-205, 248-264.

Skin and Subcutaneous Tissue

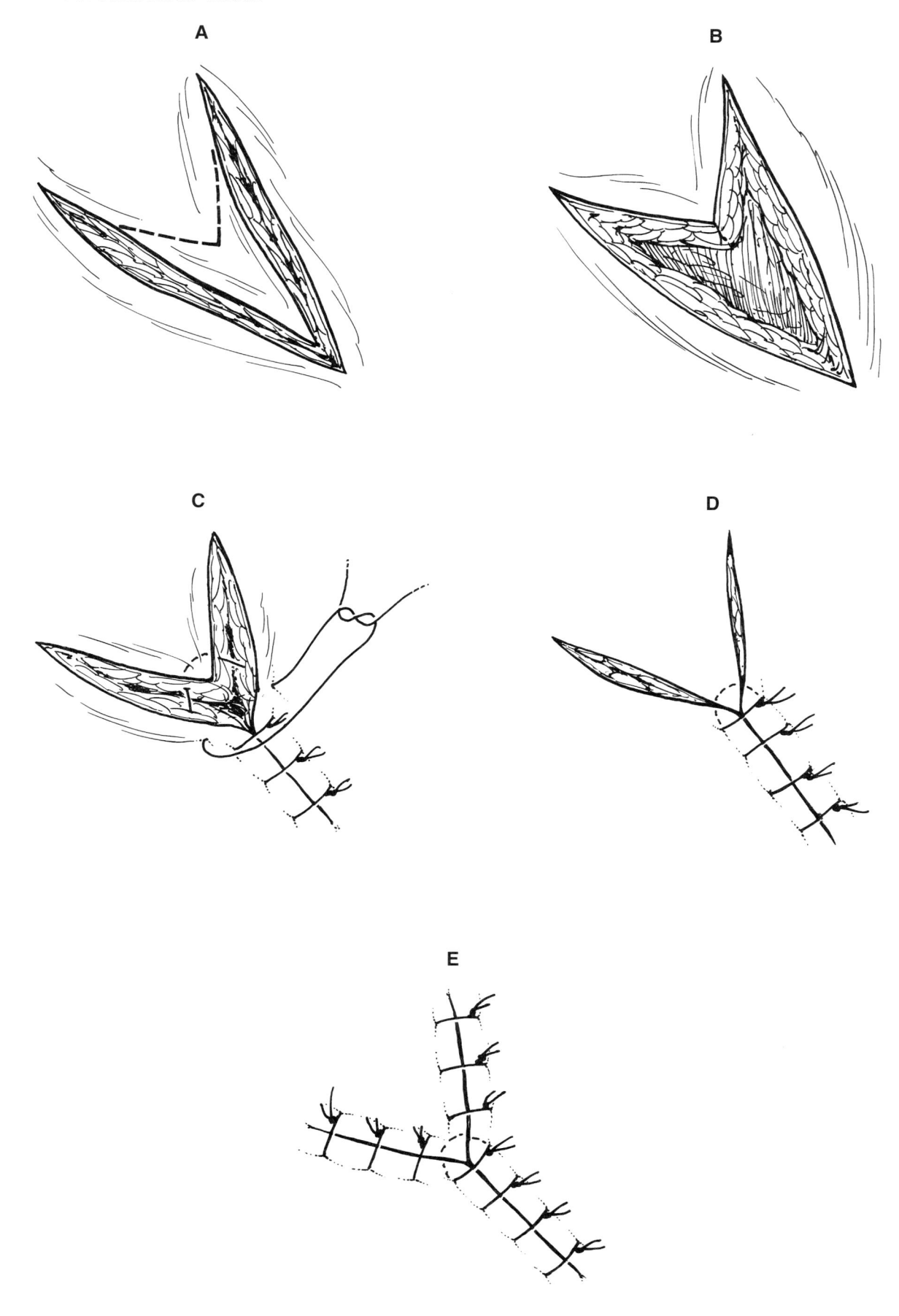

221

A

B

C

D

E

Abscess Incision and Drainage
■ HARVEY W. MEISLIN AND SAMUEL M. KEIM

Indications
- Cutaneous abscess requiring drainage *(A)*

Contraindications
- Only cellulitis present with no evidence of fluctuance
- Cosmetically important area (repeated aspiration may be preferable to incision and drainage)
- Sepsis or severe immunocompromise, necessitating delay in incision and drainage until antibiotic concentrations in the bloodstream are adequate

Equipment
- Local anesthesia (lidocaine), syringe, and needles
- Scalpel with No. 11 blade
- Sterile drapes and gloves
- Betadine antiseptic solution
- Irrigating syringe (30 ml) and plastic catheter (large bore)
- Irrigating solution (sterile water or saline solution)
- Packing tape (usually $1/8$ or $1/4$ inch, plain or with iodoform)
- Small forceps or Kelly clamp
- Adequate lighting
- Equipment stand

Procedure

1. Prepare and drape the area in sterile fashion.
2. Apply a local anesthetic agent to the area of fluctuance. Other techniques include injection of the anesthetic agent circumferentially around the abscess base, regional anesthesia, or use of the Bier block *(B)*.
3. Using a No. 11 scalpel blade, make an incision over the maximal area of fluctuance. A single incision or an elliptical removal of the roof of the abscess is indicated. The incision must extend into the abscess cavity. The depth will vary *(C)*.

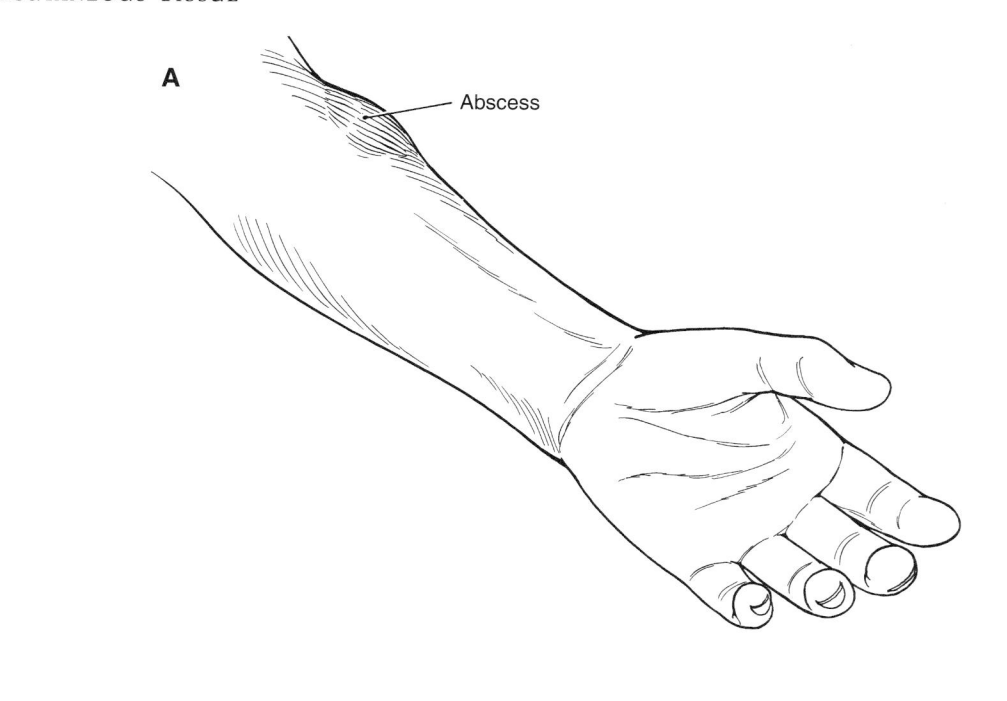

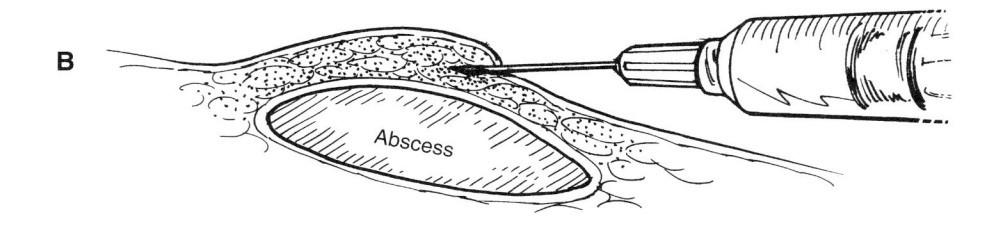

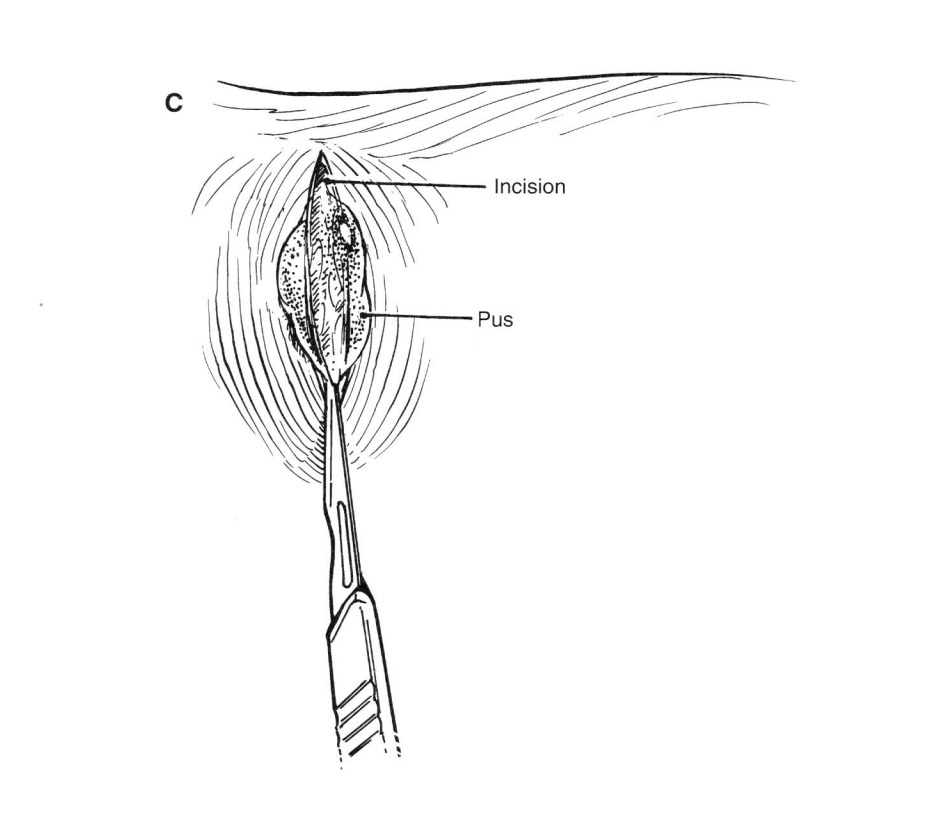

Skin and Subcutaneous Tissue

A
Abscess

B
Abscess

C
Incision
Pus

4. Using a digit or a curved hemostat, gently probe the wound and free all loculated tissue *(D)*.
5. Copiously irrigate the abscess cavity to remove any purulence, foreign body, or necrotic tissue *(E)*.
6. Ensure adequate hemostasis.
7. Gently pack the wound. The packing should be only long enough to reach the depth of the abscess cavity and extend a few centimeters out through the skin surface *(F)*.
8. Apply a dry sterile dressing.
9. Advise the patient to soak the involved area in warm water for 10 to 15 minutes three or four times a day for 2 or 3 days. Antibiotics are not indicated.
10. Rechecking is necessary to remove packing or if signs of persistent inflammation or infection occur. The packing should be removed in 48 hours except in cosmetically important areas such as the face, where removal may be accomplished in 24 hours. Repacking is necessary only if purulence continues to be present.

Complications

- Cellulitis
- Fasciitis
- Myositis
- Septicemia
- Meningitis
- Neurovascular injury to surrounding tissues, including nerves, vessels, muscles, tendons, and bone
- Reaccumulation of abscess

Discussion

- Since the incision and drainage procedure is unavoidably painful for some patients, provision of systemic analgesia or sedation may be needed beforehand.
- For most abscesses, antibiotics, Gram's stain, and culture are not indicated. For immunosuppressed or high-risk patients, cultures and antibiotics should be used. The choice of antibiotics is guided by the anatomic site involved and whether the abscess extends from mucous membranes (oral or rectal opening).
- Recurrent abscesses may be evidence of systemic disease. Fistulas may form in the lower abdomen and perirectal area.

Bibliography

Meislin HW, Guisto JA: Soft-tissue infections. In Rosen P, Barkin R (eds): *Emergency medicine: concepts and clinical practice*, St Louis, 1995, Mosby.

Meislin HW et al: Cutaneous abscesses: anaerobic and aerobic bacteriology and outpatient management, *Ann Intern Med* 87(2):145-149, 1977.

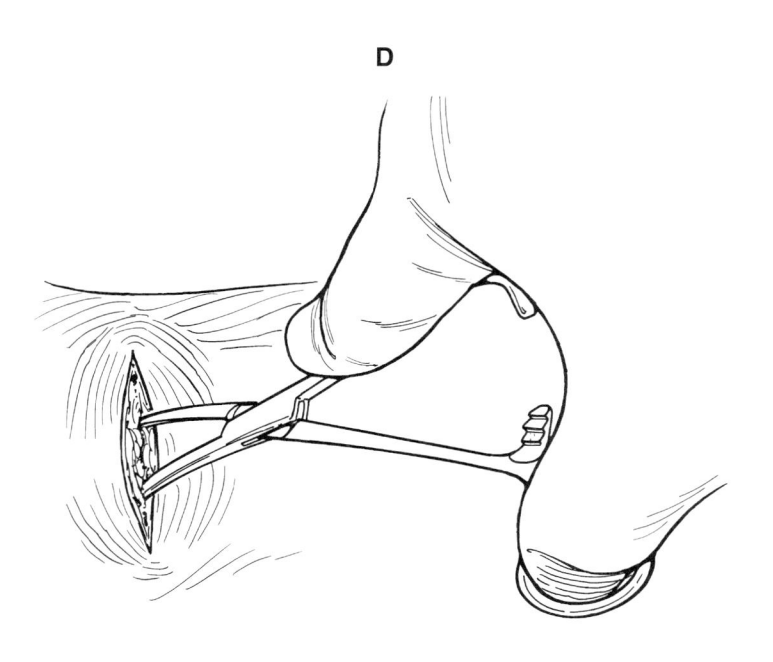

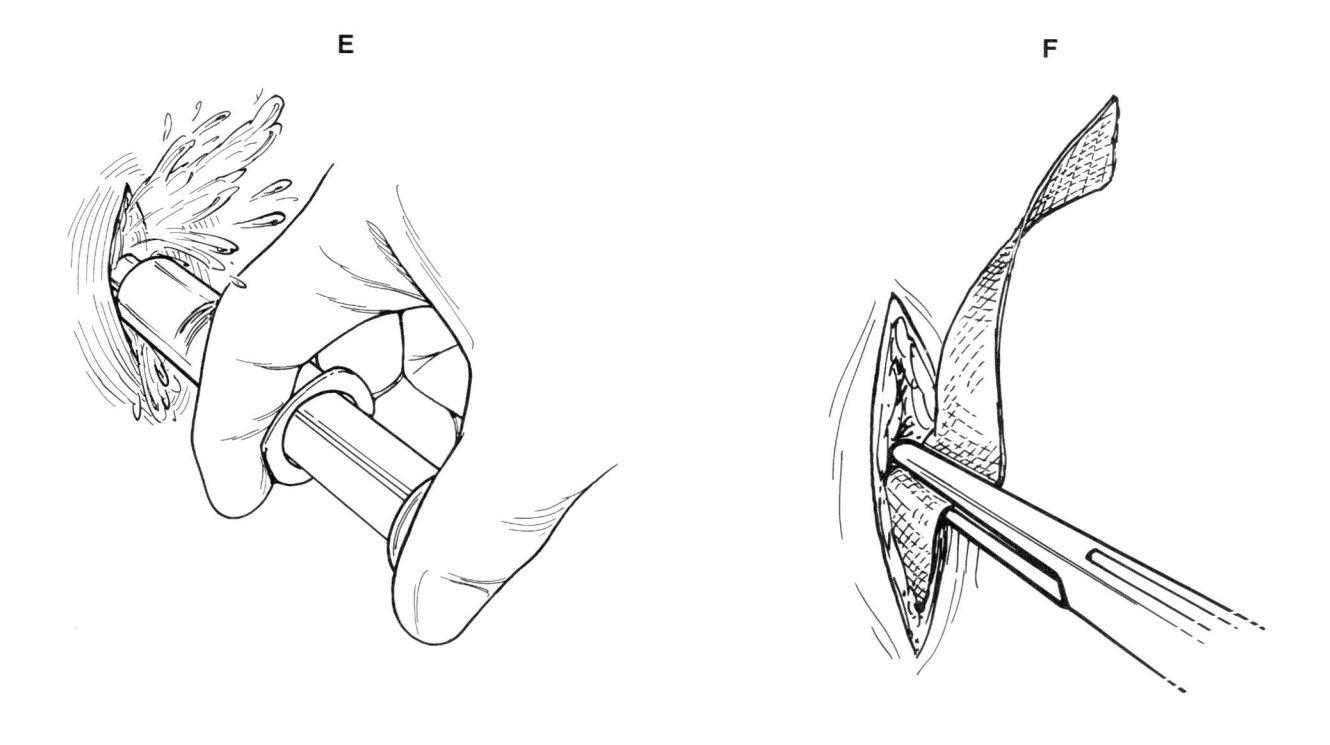

Skin and Subcutaneous Tissue

D

E

F

CHAPTER 11

EXTREMITIES

Fascial Compartment Pressure Measurement (Anterior Compartment, Lower Leg) ▪ LESLIE W. MILNE

Indications
- Extremity pain out of proportion to clinical findings
- Clinical manifestations: pressure, pain on stretch, paresis, paresthesias (with pulses and pink color)
- Extremity that has suffered fracture, vascular injury, prolonged compression, burn, crush, or overexertion and in which elevated compartment pressures are suspected
- Unresponsive patients, uncooperative patients, or patients with peripheral nerve deficits and possibly elevated pressures, although the examination is unreliable

Contraindications
- Infection at the site of introduction of the needle

Equipment
- Mercury manometer
- Two 18-gauge needles
- Two pieces of extension tubing
- Three-way stopcock
- Normal saline vial
- Betadine antiseptic solution
- Local anesthetic (1% lidocaine), syringe, and needles
- 20-ml syringe

Procedure

1. Place the patient in a supine position. Make sure no external pressures (e.g., splints, tourniquets) are being applied to the compartment.
2. Assemble tubing, needle, stopcock, syringe, and manometer as illustrated *(A)*.
3. Prepare the lower leg skin overlying the compartment in sterile fashion.
4. Anesthetize the skin with a small amount of local anesthetic (see step 9 for locating entry sites). Avoid deep injection of anesthetic, which may falsely elevate the pressures. Consider conscious sedation in a struggling or uncooperative patient, since physical restraint on the extremity may raise tissue pressures.
5. Insert the 18-gauge needle into the vented vial of saline solution. Turn the stopcock so that it is OFF to the manometer *(A)*.
6. Aspirate saline solution into tubing until it reaches halfway between the vial and stopcock. Avoid allowing bubbles into tubing.
7. Turn the stopcock so that it is OFF to the vial to avoid losing saline solution from the tubing as the needle is removed from the vial *(B)*. Remove the syringe from the stopcock, and pull back the plunger so that 15 cc of air is in the syringe. Reattach the syringe to the three-way stopcock.
8. Remove the needle from the vial, and insert it into the muscle compartment *(C)*. Turn the stopcock so that the syringe is open to both sets of tubing *(D)*.

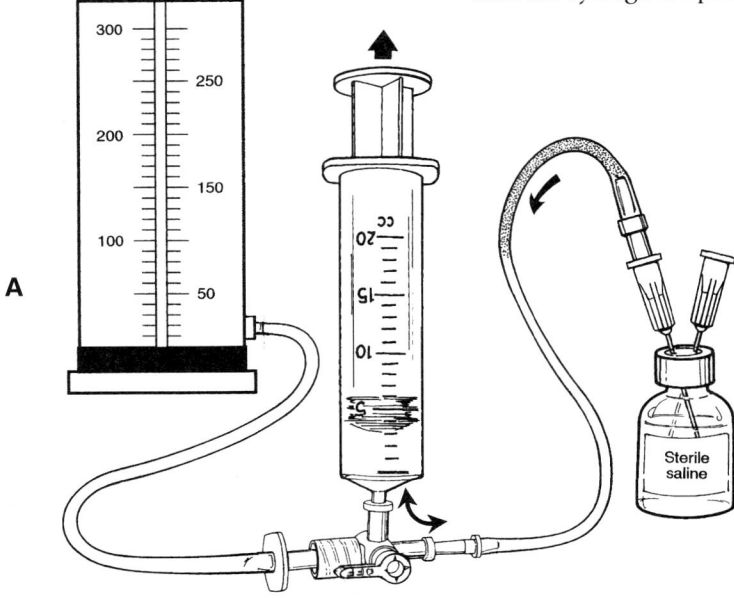

EXTREMITIES 229

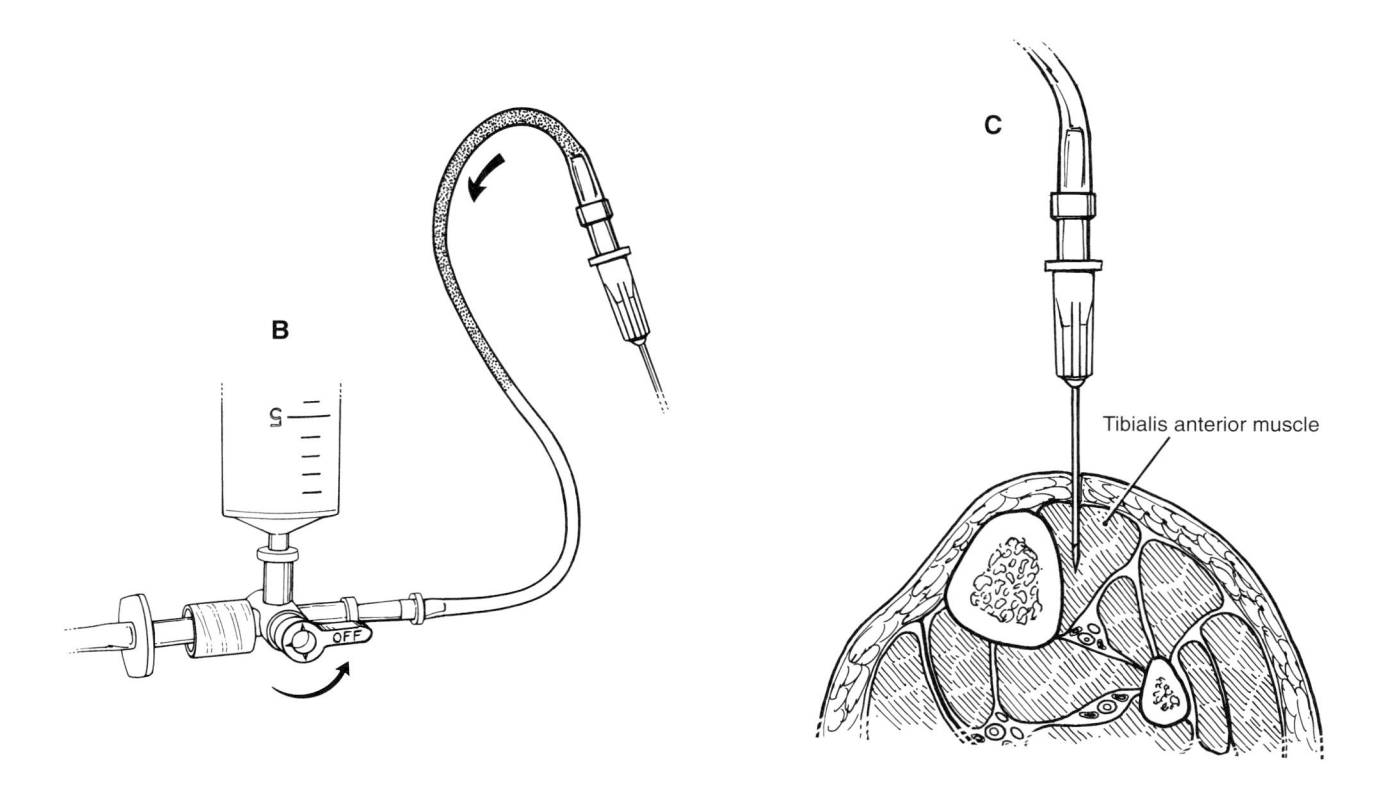

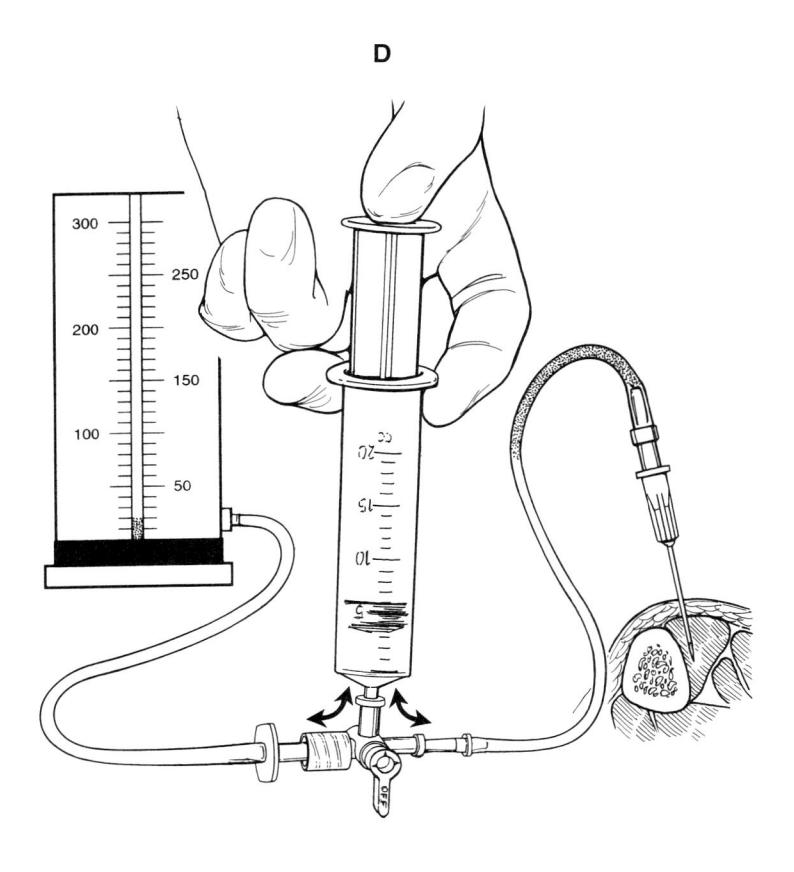

B

C

Tibialis anterior muscle

D

9. All lower leg compartments are entered in the area at the junction of the proximal and middle thirds of the lower leg *(E)*. The compartments are located as follows *(F)*:
    a. Anterior: Find the junction of the proximal and middle thirds of the tibia anteriorly, and enter the compartment 1 cm lateral to the border of the anterior tibia. Enter perpendicular to the skin, to a depth of 1 to 3 cm. To confirm placement, squeeze the anterior compartment or plantar flex and dorsiflex the foot and observe for a rise in pressure on the manometer.
    b. Deep posterior: Elevate the leg slightly off the bed. Palpate the medial border of the tibia, and enter just posterior to this site. Aim toward the posterior border of the fibula, and advance 2 to 4 cm. Confirm placement by everting the ankle and extending the toes and watching for a pressure rise on the manometer.
    c. Lateral: Elevate the leg slightly off the bed. Palpate the posterior border of the fibula at the junction of the proximal and middle thirds of the lower leg. Enter the muscle compartment just anterior to the posterior fibular border. Advance 1 to 1.5 cm perpendicular to skin and toward the fibula. Withdraw slightly if bone is struck. Confirm placement by compressing the lateral compartment and inverting the foot.
    d. Superficial posterior: Place the patient in a prone position. Locate the junction of the proximal and middle thirds of the lower leg posteriorly, and enter perpendicular to the skin in this area. Aim toward the center of the leg compartment just above or below the needle site, and dorsiflex the foot.
10. With the stopcock positioned to keep the syringe open to both pieces of tubing (to patient and to manometer), *slowly* depress the plunger on the syringe while observing the saline solution column in the tubing *(D)*. The saline solution will move into the muscle compartment when the pressure in the tubing system exceeds the pressure in the tissue. The manometer reading should be noted at the time the saline solution moves. This is recorded as the tissue pressure in millimeters of mercury.
11. Remove the needle and obtain a second reading by reinserting the needle into the compartment and repeating steps 7, 8, and 10. Check the needle for blood or tissue before reinserting.

Complications

- Pain
- Inaccurate readings
- Exacerbation of a compartment syndrome by injecting fluid

Discussion

- Whereas this technique is useful in the emergency department, it is considered less accurate and less reproducible than the Stryker intracompartmental monitor and the arterial line system.
- The most important part of the procedure is to depress the plunger slowly to allow the mercury column to rise accurately and reflect the compartment pressure.
- The plunger should not be pulled back with the system open to tissue because this could cause a tissue plug in the needle.
- Exact numbers for significantly elevated tissue pressures remain controversial. A pressure of 25 to 30 mm Hg is abnormal, and fasciotomy should be considered. Consultation with an orthopedist is recommended.

Bibliography

Moed BR, Thorderson PK: Measurement of intracompartmental pressure: a comparison of the slit catheter, side-ported needle, and simple needle, *J Bone Joint Surg [Am]* 75:231, 1993.

Netter FH: *The CIBA collection of medical illustrations. Vol 8. Musculoskeletal. Part III. Trauma, evaluations, and management*, West Caldwell, NJ, 1993, Ciba-Geigy, pp 13-18.

EXTREMITIES

E

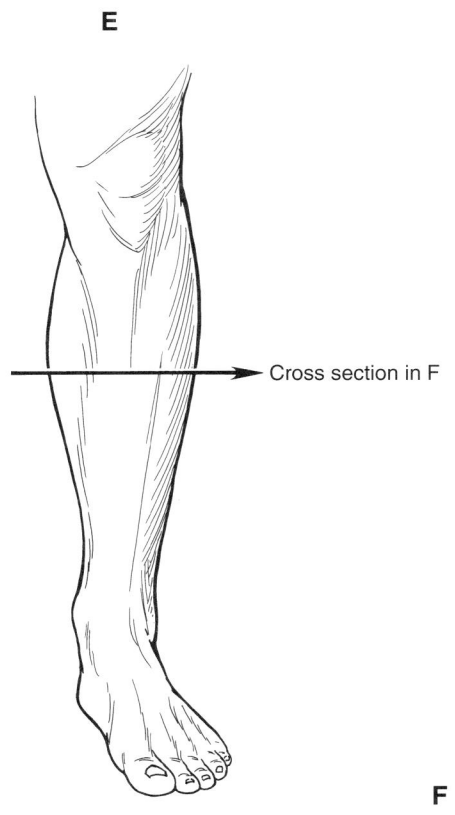

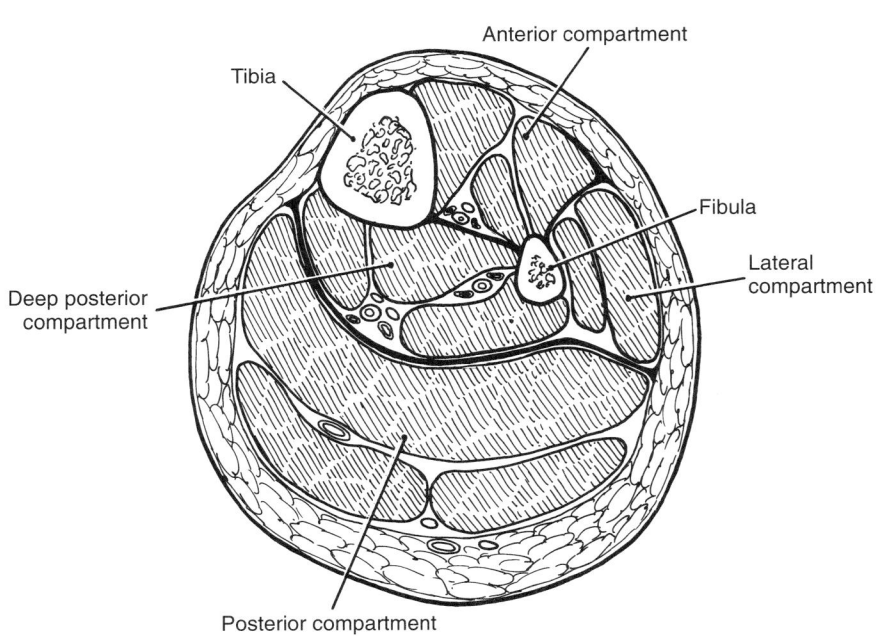

Cross section in F

F

Tibia
Anterior compartment
Fibula
Lateral compartment
Deep posterior compartment
Posterior compartment

Arthrocentesis of the Knee ■ LESLIE W. MILNE

Indications
- Diagnosis uncertain
- Infection suspected
- Pain relief and increase in range of motion
- Removal of hemarthrosis

Contraindications
- Absolute contraindication:
  - Skin infection over entry site
- Relative contraindications:
  - Uncorrected coagulopathy, bleeding diatheses
  - Joint prosthesis (consult orthopedist)
  - Bacteremia

Equipment
- Sterile gloves and drapes
- Local anesthetic (lidocaine 1% to 2%, with or without epinephrine), syringe, and needles
- 18- or 19-gauge needle
- 10-ml or larger syringe
- Betadine antiseptic solution
- Towel roll (optional)
- Slide and tubes for laboratory studies

Procedure

1. Place the patient in a supine position with the knee in extension or in slight flexion with a towel roll behind the knee *(A)*.
2. Identify an area at the intersection of the proximal pole of the patella and either the medial or the lateral edge of the patella.
3. Locally infiltrate the area selected with 4 to 10 ml of local anesthetic. Do not hit the bone with the needle.
4. Prepare and drape the entire patellar area (medially and laterally) in sterile fashion.
5. Enter the skin with the 18-gauge needle attached to the syringe, holding the needle parallel to the gurney. Be careful not to strike the underside of the patella when entering. Aspirate gently on the syringe while advancing the needle *(B)*.
6. Stop advancing when there is easy flow into the syringe. Leaving the needle in place, switch to a larger syringe to remove the remaining volume. Do not place excessive negative pressure on the syringe because this will pull the synovium over the needle bevel and prevent flow.
7. For traumatic hemarthroses, optionally inject up to 15 ml of 0.25% bupivacaine into the joint area before removing the needle. This may provide short-term pain control in an acute tear of the anterior cruciate ligament.
8. Remove the needle. Send the aspirate for Gram's staining, culture and sensitivity tests, cell count, and crystal analysis if infection or inflammation is suspected.
9. Apply a compression dressing if a large effusion was drained.

Complications
- Introduction of infection
- Damage to the articular surface of the patella
- Hemarthrosis if underlying coagulopathy is present
- Vasovagal reaction

Discussion
- The operator should ensure that the effusion is in the joint (posterior to the patella) and *not* simply a prepatellar bursitis that causes swelling anterior to the patella.
- The suprapatellar pouch extends well above the patella and communicates with the joint space. Direct passage under the patella should be avoided because striking the articular cartilage with the needle causes unnecessary trauma and later arthritic changes. If the effusion is very small, the operator may have to pass the needle directly under the patella but should aim upward toward the suprapatellar pouch.
- If aspiration of fluid is difficult while the needle is clearly in the joint space, the operator may be exerting too much force on the syringe, causing synovium to obstruct the needle. Options are to switch to a smaller syringe and apply less tension or simply to remove the syringe (leaving the needle in the joint) and "milk" the knee on the side away from the needle, allowing the joint fluid to drain by gravity.
- A small amount of aspirate should be placed in an emesis basin or other container to look for fat globules floating to the surface. This suggests possible fracture, such as of the tibial plateau, and in the case of a traumatic knee injury additional studies are warranted.
- An anterior approach can be used with the patient sitting up and the knee flexed to 90°. The needle is inserted below the patellar pole and to the side of the patellar tendon, which is midline. The needle is directed parallel to the tibial plateau.

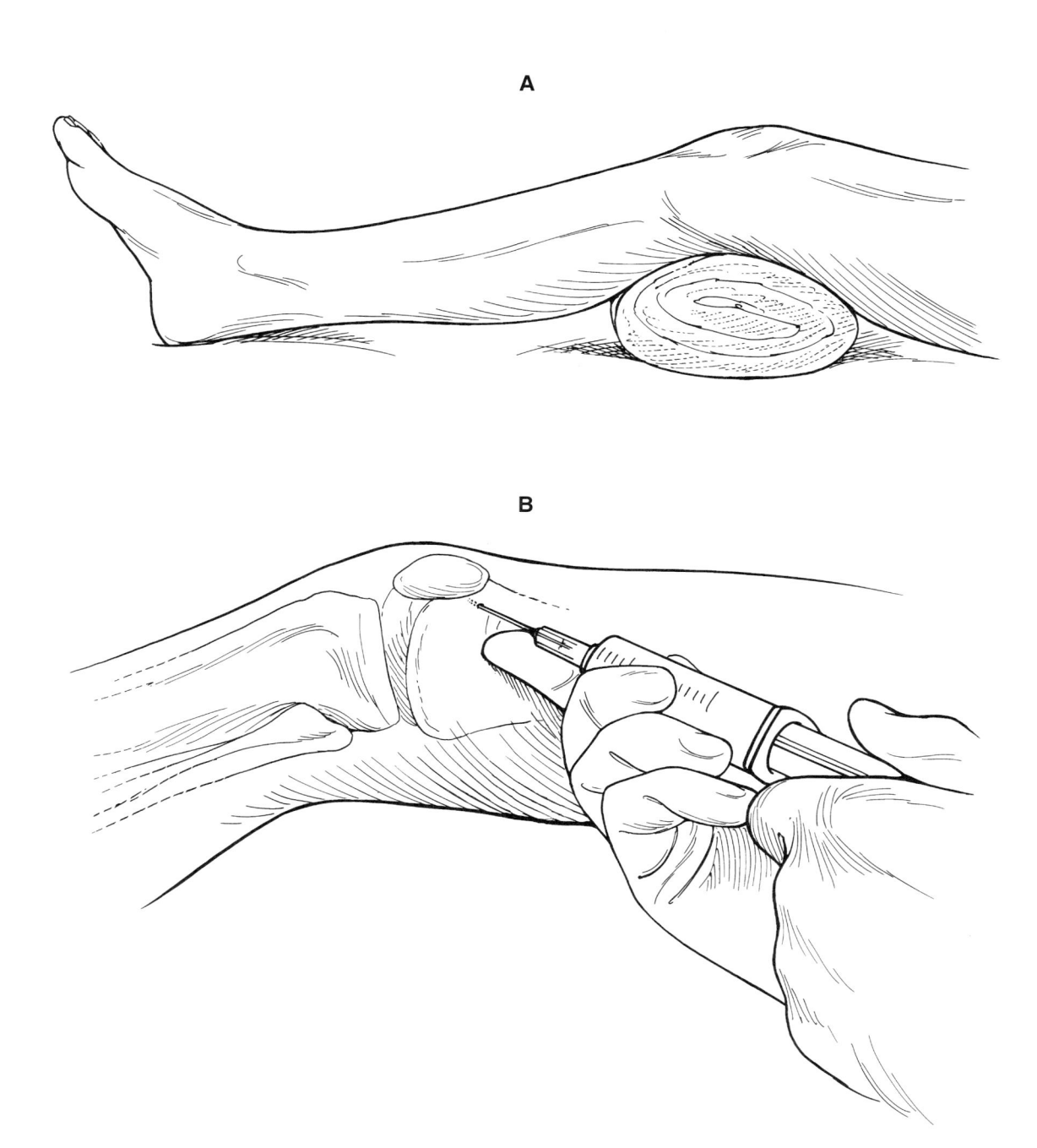

- Having an assistant apply pressure from the opposite side of the knee, as well as proximal and distal to the patella, may channel the fluid toward the aspirating needle.

Bibliography

Doherty M et al: *Rheumatology examination and injection techniques,* London, 1992, WB Saunders, pp 86-88, 121-123.

Kelley WN et al: *Textbook of rheumatology, vol 1,* ed 4, Philadelphia, 1993, WB Saunders, p 554.

Roberts NW et al: Dry taps and what to do about them: a pictoral essay on failed arthrocentesis of the knee, *Am J Med* 100(4):461-464, 1996.

Arthrocentesis of the Ankle ▪ LESLIE W. MILNE

Indications
- Uncertain diagnosis
- Suspected infection

Contraindications
- Absolute contraindication:
  - Skin infection over entry site
- Relative contraindications:
  - Uncorrected coagulopathy, bleeding diatheses
  - Joint prosthesis (consult orthopedist)
  - Bacteremia

Equipment
- Sterile gloves and drapes
- Local anesthetic (lidocaine 1% to 2% with or without epinephrine), syringe, and needles
- 20-gauge needle
- 10-ml syringes
- Betadine antiseptic solution
- Slide and tubes for laboratory studies

Procedure

1. Locate the tibialis anterior tendon anteriorly. The tendon can be easily identified by dorsiflexion of the foot. Also identify the joint line between the tibia and talus. Entry into the joint will be between the tibialis anterior tendon and the extensor hallucis longus tendon *(A)*.
2. Place the foot in a moderate amount of plantar flexion with the patient supine.
3. Prepare the anterior ankle in sterile fashion. Locally anesthetize the skin with lidocaine.
4. Insert the 20-gauge aspirating needle from an anterior approach tangential to the curve of the talus. Apply gentle aspiration on the syringe as the needle is advanced 2 to 3 cm. To avoid scraping the talus, do not direct the needle downward toward the heel *(B)*.
5. Remove as much fluid as possible from the joint. Leave the needle in place, and change syringes if the volume exceeds syringe capacity.
6. Send the aspirate for a Gram's stain, culture and sensitivity tests, cell count with differential, and crystal analysis if infection or inflammation is suspected.

Complications
- Introduction of infection
- Damage to the articular surface of the tibia or talus
- Hemarthrosis if underlying coagulopathy is present
- Vasovagal reaction

Discussion
- The ankle is the joint most likely to become infected after injection and aspiration, so particular attention should be paid to aseptic technique.
- Traction on the foot may enlarge the target area when the operator is attempting to enter the joint.
- The joint space may also be entered just medial to the tibialis anterior tendon.
- If infection is suspected and only a few drops of joint fluid are aspirated, the laboratory study of choice is the Gram's stain.

Bibliography
Doherty M et al: *Rheumatology examination and injection techniques*, London, 1992, WB Saunders, pp 103, 121-123.
Kelley WN et al: *Textbook of rheumatology, vol 1*, ed 4, Philadelphia, 1993, WB Saunders, pp 554-555.
Vander Salm TJ et al: *Atlas of bedside procedures*, ed 2, Boston, 1988, Little, Brown, pp 452-453, 462-463.

EXTREMITIES

A

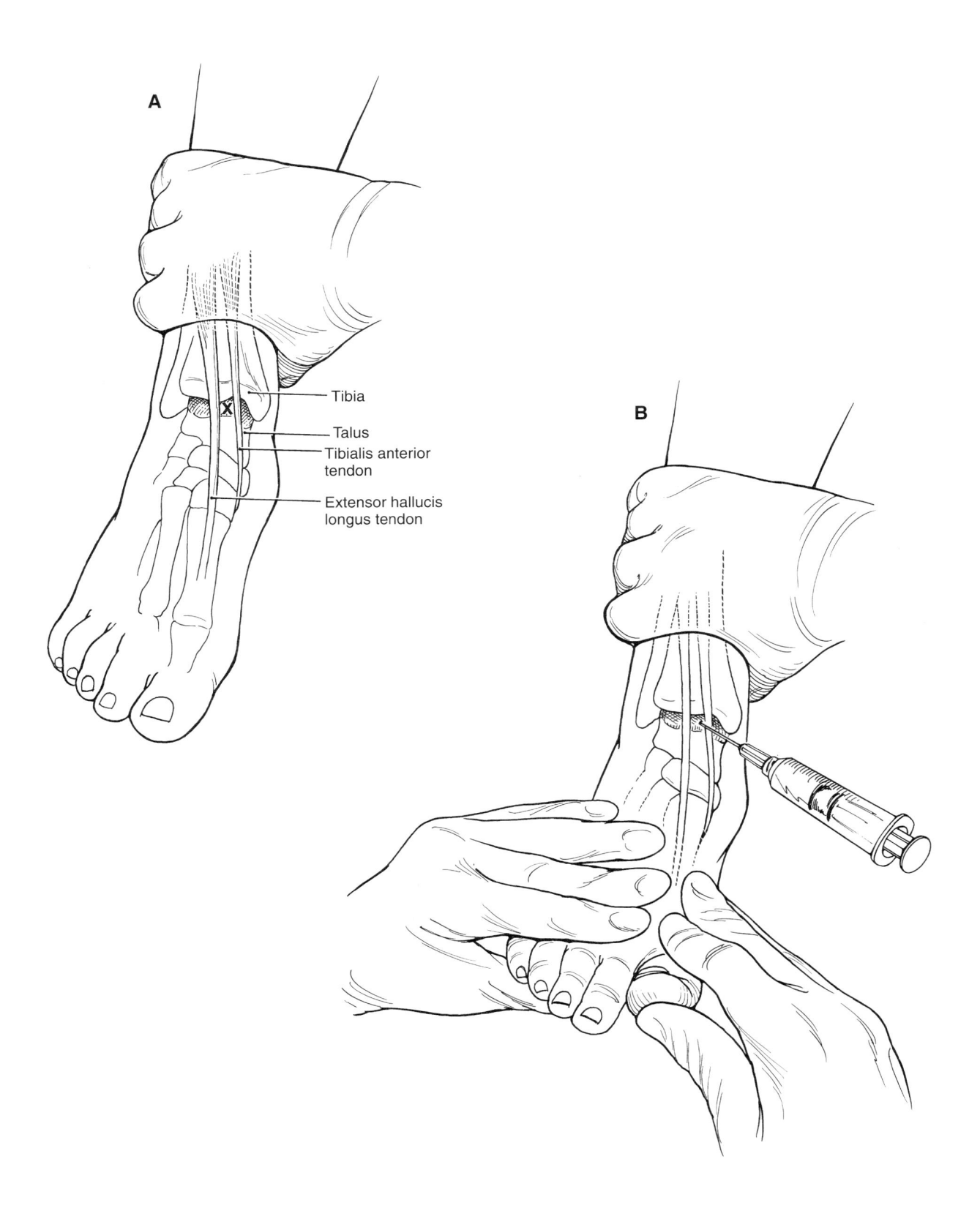

- Tibia
- Talus
- Tibialis anterior tendon
- Extensor hallucis longus tendon

B

Arthrocentesis of the Metatarsophalangeal Joint
■ LESLIE W. MILNE

Indications
- Uncertain diagnosis
- Suspected infection
- Pain relief with anesthetic or corticosteroid administration

Contraindications
- Absolute contraindication:
  - Skin infection over entry site
- Relative contraindications:
  - Uncorrected coagulopathy, bleeding diathesis
  - Joint prosthesis (consult orthopedist or podiatrist)
  - Bacteremia

Equipment
- Sterile gloves and drapes
- Local anesthetic (lidocaine 1% to 2% without epinephrine), syringe, and needles
- 22- or 23-gauge, $1/2$- to 1-inch needle
- 3-ml syringe
- Betadine antiseptic solution
- Tubes for laboratory studies

Procedure
1. Locate the extensor tendon by extending the toes. This structure should be avoided *(A)*.
2. Identify the joint space by palpating the distal portion of the metatarsal and the proximal portion of the proximal phalanx.
3. Place the patient supine, and prepare the foot and toe in sterile fashion. Local infiltration with lidocaine is optional.
4. Flex the toe 15° to 20°. Apply traction to the toe to increase the target area and facilitate joint entry.
5. Enter the metatarsophalangeal joint with a 22- or 23-gauge needle, on a 3-ml syringe, that is inserted either medial or lateral to the extensor tendon *(B)*. Aspirate gently while advancing the needle.
6. Since the volume will be minimal, Gram's stain is the most important laboratory test.

Complications
- Introduction of infection
- Damage to articular surfaces
- Hemarthrosis if underlying coagulopathy is present
- Vasovagal reaction

Discussion
- Extensor surfaces are generally preferred for arthrocentesis because neurovascular structures tend to be located on the flexor surfaces.
- If the condition is thought to be inflammatory (e.g., gout, arthritis) and not infectious, a small amount of triamcinolone (up to 5 mg) may be injected into the joint after the aspiration. It can be mixed with a small amount of lidocaine.
- Corticosteroid solutions should never be injected into a joint that might be infected.
- If corticosteroids are injected into the joint, warn the patient about a painful "steroid flare" 24 hours after the procedure. Place the patient on 2-day course of antiinflammatory medication unless a contraindication exists. Have the patient rest the joint for 24 to 48 hours and avoid participating in sports for 5 days.

Bibliography
Doherty M et al: *Rheumatology examination and injection techniques,* London, 1992, WB Saunders, pp 56, 121-123.
Kelley WN et al: *Textbook of rheumatology, vol 1,* ed 4, Philadelphia, 1993, WB Saunders, p 556.
Vander Salm TJ et al: *Atlas of bedside procedures,* ed 2, Boston, 1988, Little, Brown, pp 452-453, 462-463.

A

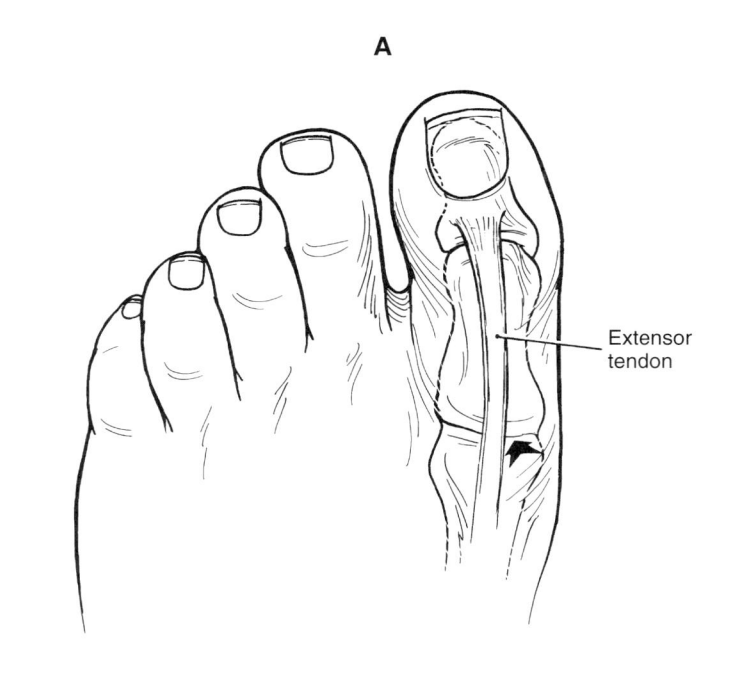

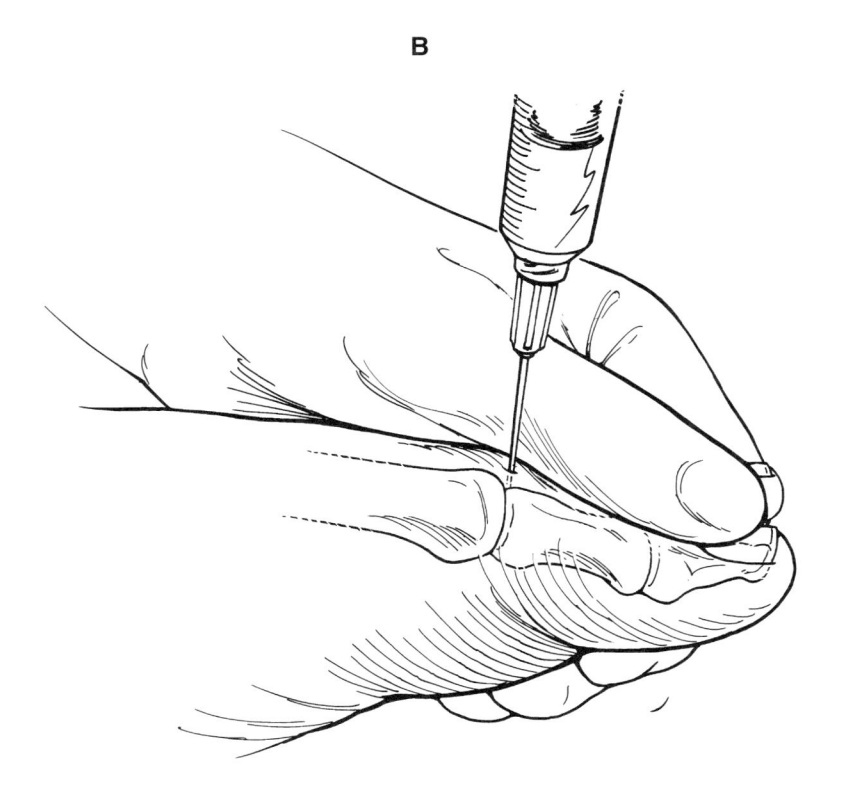

Extensor tendon

B

Aspiration of the Shoulder ▪ LESLIE W. MILNE

Indications
- Uncertain diagnosis
- Suspected infection
- Removal of blood or local anesthetic injection after a shoulder dislocation

Contraindications
- Absolute contraindication:
  - Skin infection over entry site
- Relative contraindications:
  - Uncorrected coagulopathy, bleeding diathesis
  - Joint prosthesis (consult orthopedist)
  - Bacteremia

Equipment
- Sterile gloves and drapes
- Local anesthetic (lidocaine 1% to 2% with or without epinephrine), syringe, and needles
- 20- or 22-gauge, 1½-inch needle
- 5- and 10-ml syringes
- Betadine antiseptic solution
- Slides and tubes for laboratory studies

Procedure

1. Place the patient in a sitting position with the shoulder externally rotated.
2. Prepare the anterior shoulder area in sterile fashion.
3. Locate the humeral head anteriorly. Entry will be just medial to this and just lateral and inferior to the coracoid process.
4. Locally anesthetize the entry site.
5. Direct the 20- or 22-gauge needle from an anterior approach. It should be aimed in a posterior, lateral, and slightly superior direction until the joint space is entered. If bone is struck, pull back and redirect the needle. Apply traction on the syringe plunger as the needle is advanced *(A)*.
6. Collect joint aspirate, and send for Gram's staining, culture and sensitivity tests, cell count with differential, and crystal analysis.

Complications
- Introduction of infection
- Damage to the articular surface of the glenoid fossa or humerus
- Hemarthrosis if underlying coagulopathy is present
- Vasovagal reaction

Discussion

- The true shoulder joint (glenohumeral joint) is moderately difficult to enter and is rarely aspirated or injected. More commonly it is entered to administer local anesthetic (1% lidocaine 20 ml) before relocation after dislocation. In this case the joint capsule is disrupted and can easily be entered laterally by inserting the needle 2 cm lateral and inferior to the acromion process and directing it caudad.
- Atraumatic shoulder pain thought to be caused by rotator cuff tendinitis or bursitis often responds well to injection of local anesthetic with or without corticosteroid into the subacromial space (*not* the glenohumeral joint). The area is entered posteriorly by following the scapular spine laterally. At a point 1 cm inferior to where it turns to become the acromion process is a large space that will easily accommodate a 20-gauge needle with anesthetic (1% lidocaine 4 ml and 0.25% bupivacaine 4 ml) and corticosteroid (triamcinolone 40 mg). The needle is advanced 2 to 4 cm, slightly superiorly, staying underneath the acromion process. Fluid should flow easily as it is injected. Corticosteroids should not be injected if infection is suspected or the rotator cuff is thought to be torn. For 2 days after corticosteroid injection the shoulder should be rested and nonsteroidal antiinflammatory drugs should be given to prevent painful "steroid flare." No sporting activity should be permitted for 5 days.

Bibliography

Doherty M et al: *Rheumatology examination and injection techniques*, London, 1992, WB Saunders, pp 36-38, 121-123.

Kelley WN et al: *Textbook of rheumatology, vol 1*, ed 4, Philadelphia, 1993, WB Saunders, pp 554-555.

Matthew D et al: Intraarticular lidocaine vs. intravenous analgesic for reduction of acute shoulder dislocation: a prospective randomized study, *Am J Sports Med* 23(1):54, 1995.

Trimmings NP: Hemarthrosis aspiration in treatment of anterior dislocations of the shoulder, *J R Soc Med* 78(12):1023, 1986.

A

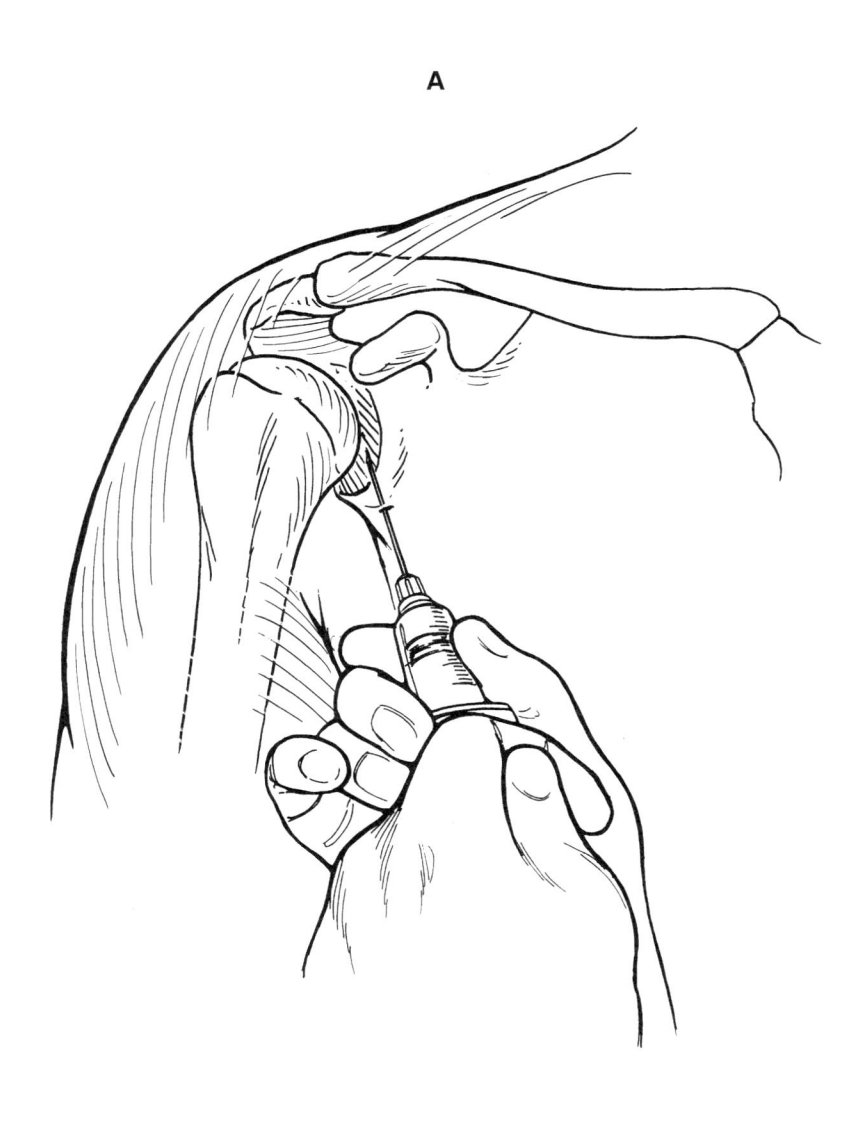

Arthrocentesis of the Elbow
■ LESLIE W. MILNE

Indications
- Uncertain diagnosis
- Suspected infection
- Drainage of hemarthrosis and improvement of range of motion
- Pain relief with anesthetic injection after aspiration of effusion

Contraindications
- Absolute contraindication:
  - Skin infection over entry site
- Relative contraindications:
  - Uncorrected coagulopathy, bleeding diathesis
  - Joint prosthesis (consult orthopedist)
  - Bacteremia

Equipment
- Sterile gloves and drapes
- Local anesthetic (lidocaine 1% to 2% with or without epinephrine), syringe, and needles
- 21- or 22-gauge needle
- 10-ml syringes
- Betadine antiseptic solution
- Slide and tubes for laboratory studies

Procedure

1. Place the arm along a firm surface with the elbow flexed to 90° and thumb up. The same elbow position with the forearm pronated is also acceptable.
2. Palpate the radial head by passively supinating and pronating the forearm.
3. Once the joint line is located, palpate just below this area to a small hollow between the radial head and lateral epicondyle of the humerus. This area can also be located by extending the elbow and feeling the small gap between these two bones. This will be the entry site *(A)*.
4. Prepare the area in sterile fashion
5. Enter the site from a lateral approach with the needle and syringe. Aspirate gently on the syringe as the needle enters *(B)*. Avoid forcing the needle deeply between the two bones.
6. Aspirate as much fluid as possible. Change syringes while keeping the needle in the joint if the effusion is large. If infection or inflammation is suspected, send samples for Gram's staining, culture and sensitivity tests, cell count with differential, and crystal studies.

Complications
- Introduction of infection
- Damage to the articular surface
- Hemarthrosis if underlying coagulopathy is present
- Vasovagal reaction

Discussion
- The operator should make sure the effusion is in the joint and should not be fooled by an olecranon bursitis that causes swelling between the olecranon and the skin.
- A posterior approach can also be used. The arm is positioned as described above with the elbow flexed to 90°. After palpating the olecranon process posteriorly, the operator moves slightly superiorly and laterally to this area and inserts the needle into the olecranon fossa.
- If the volume of aspirate is minimal and infection is suspected, Gram's stain is the priority laboratory study.
- Leaving the needle in place and simply changing syringes, the operator may inject a small amount (1 to 2 ml) of 0.25% bupivacaine after the procedure for the treatment of traumatic effusions. This will provide short-term pain relief.

Bibliography
Doherty M et al: *Rheumatology examination and injection techniques,* London, 1992, WB Saunders, p 47.
Kelley WN et al: *Textbook of rheumatology,* vol 1, ed 4, Philadelphia, 1993, WB Saunders, p 556.
Vander Salm TJ et al: *Atlas of bedside procedures,* ed 2, Boston, 1988, Little, Brown, pp 452-453, 456-457.

EXTREMITIES 241

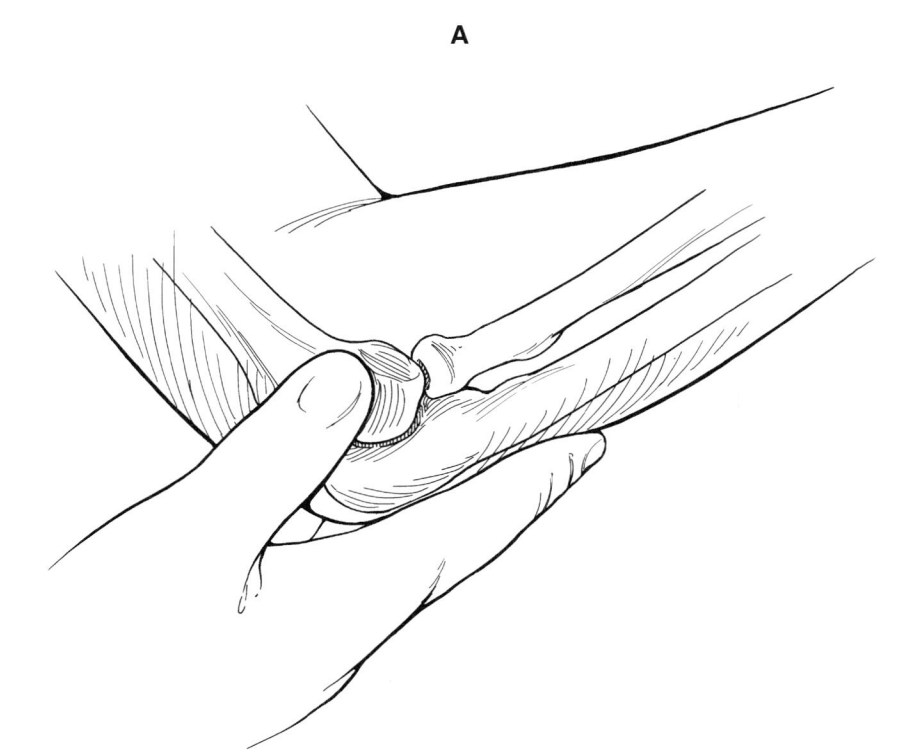

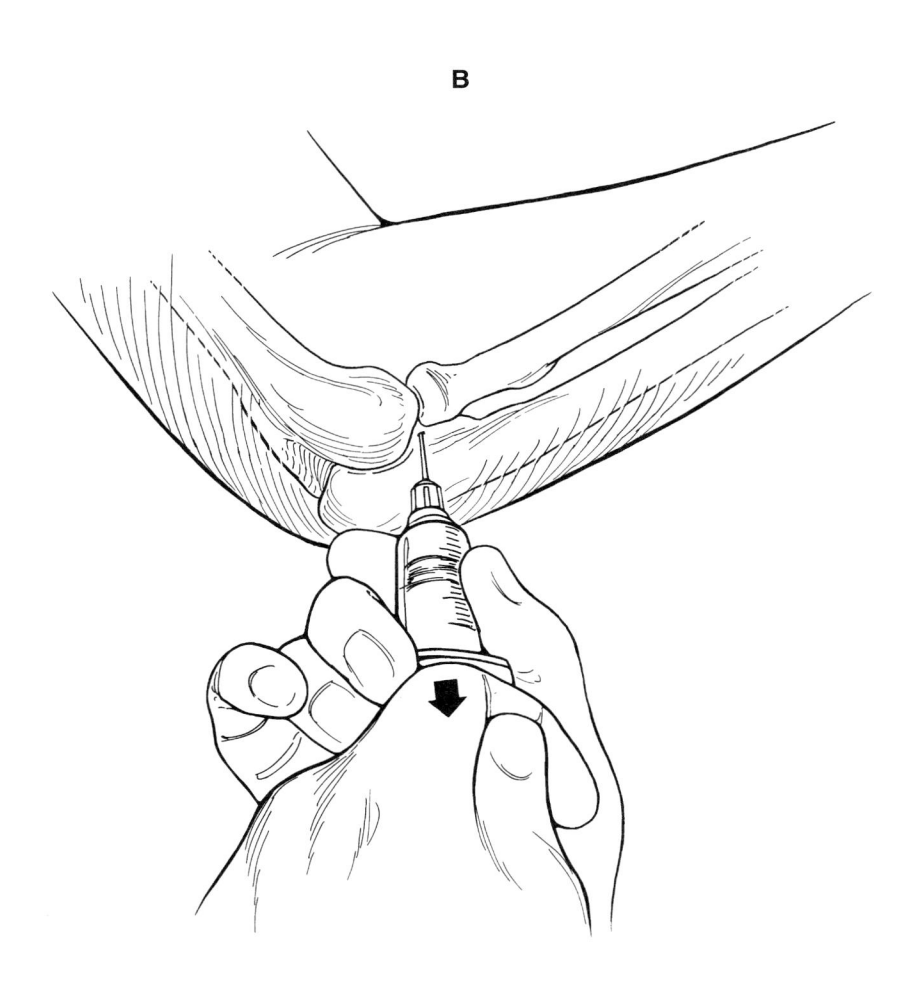

A

B

Arthrocentesis of the Wrist ▪ LESLIE W. MILNE

Indications
- Suspected infection
- Uncertain diagnosis

Contraindications
- Absolute contraindication:
  - Skin infection over entry site
- Relative contraindications:
  - Uncorrected coagulopathy, bleeding diathesis
  - Joint prosthesis (consult orthopedist)
  - Bacteremia

Equipment
- Sterile gloves and drapes
- Local anesthetic (lidocaine 1% to 2% with or without epinephrine), syringe, and needles
- 22-gauge needle
- 3- or 5-ml syringe
- Betadine antiseptic solution
- Slide and tubes for laboratory studies

Procedure
1. Place the patient in a supine position.
2. Identify the entry site on the dorsal surface of the wrist by flexing and extending the wrist. Entry can be achieved at the radiocarpal junction, in the hollow just distal and ulnar to Lister's tubercle (bump on dorsal distal radius). The site can also be located by moving ulnarly to the origin of the extensor pollicis longus. Avoid the anatomic snuffbox area.
3. Prepare the wrist in sterile fashion, and anesthetize the skin locally with lidocaine.
4. Hold the wrist in 20° of flexion and slight ulnar deviation while applying traction to the hand. Insert the 22-gauge needle perpendicular to the skin surface, and advance it into the joint while gently aspirating *(A)*.
5. Send fluid for Gram's staining and other studies as volume allows.

Complications
- Most joints should be entered from the extensor side to avoid the neurovascular structures found on the flexor surface.
- The joint may also be entered just to the radial side of the ulnar styloid.
- If the joint is clearly uninfected and the diagnosis is inflammatory disease, up to 20 mg of triamcinolone may be injected into the painful joint. The patient should be warned about a "steroid flare" causing pain at 24 hours, and prophylactic antiinflammatory medication for 2 days should be prescribed if no contraindications exist. The joint should be splinted for 48 hours, and sports participation should be avoided for at least 5 days.

Bibliography
Doherty M et al: *Rheumatology examination and injection techniques,* London, 1992, WB Saunders, pp 57, 121-123.
Kelley WN et al: *Textbook of rheumatology,* vol 1, ed 4, Philadelphia, 1993, WB Saunders, pp 554-555.

EXTREMITIES

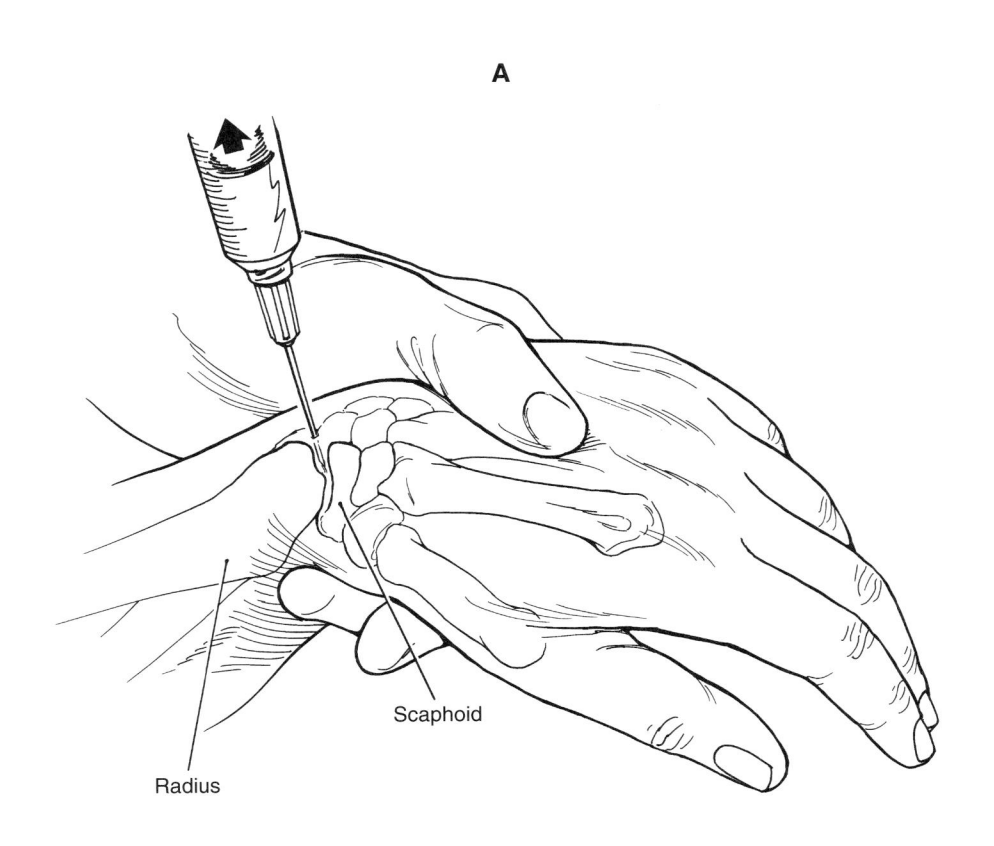

A

Scaphoid

Radius

Hand

Felon Drainage SAMUEL M. KEIM AND HARVEY W. MEISLIN

Indications
- Felon (closed space infection with abscess in the pulp of a distal phalanx)

Contraindications
- Superficial infection of the distal fingerpad (may require only elevation, antibiotics, and warm soaks)

Equipment
- Sterile drapes and gloves
- Sterile gauze packing
- Betadine antiseptic solution
- Anesthetic agent (buffered lidocaine), syringe, and needles
- Scalpel with No. 11 blade

Procedure
1. Prepare the entire affected hand proximal to the wrist crease in sterile fashion.
2. Have the patient place the hand, palmar space down, on a sterile drape. Typically the procedure can be performed on a working stand next to the patient's bed with the patient lying supine or sitting upright.
3. Apply a digital anesthetic block to the proximal base of the affected finger.
4. Using the scalpel, make a high lateral incision dorsal to the neurovascular bundle on the ulnar aspect of digits 1 to 4 and the radial aspects of digits 1 and 5 to avoid the greatest pincher surfaces *(A, B)*.
5. Irrigate the wound, and insert a loose gauze pack to prevent the wound from closing and allow drainage. Place the digit within a tube dressing and splint.
6. Prescribe antistaphylococcal antibiotics, elevation, and follow-up in 48 hours for packing removal.

Complications
- Abscess extension, necrosis, and osteomyelitis caused by inadequate drainage
- Damage to digital nerves, vessels, fat pad, flexor sheath, or skin caused by incorrect incision placement

Discussion
- Early drainage of felons is important to prevent ongoing tissue destruction and eventual ischemic necrosis, extension of the infection into the flexor sheath, osteomyelitis, and septic arthritis of the distal interphalangeal (DIP) joint.
- Drainage can also be accomplished by an incision made across the pad of the finger at a level below the neurovascular bundle that crosses all septa. After copious irrigation a gauze wick can be pulled through the incision to prevent closure *(C, D)*.
- Another technique, advocated by Kilgore, uses a palmar longitudinal incision. Regardless of technique, the incision should *not* cross the DIP flexion crease because this would result in contracture.

Bibliography
Canales FL et al: The treatment of felons and paronychias, *Hand Clin* 5(4):515-523, 1989.
Hausman MR, Lisser SP: Hand infections, *Orthop Clin North Am* 23(1):171, 1992.
Kilgore E et al: Treatment of felons, *Am J Surg* 130:195, 1975.
Mann R: *Infections of the hand*, Philadelphia, 1988, Lea & Febiger, p 3.
Milford L: Infections of the hand. In Crenshaw AH et al (eds): *Campbell's operative orthopaedics*, vol 1, ed 8, St Louis, 1992, Mosby.

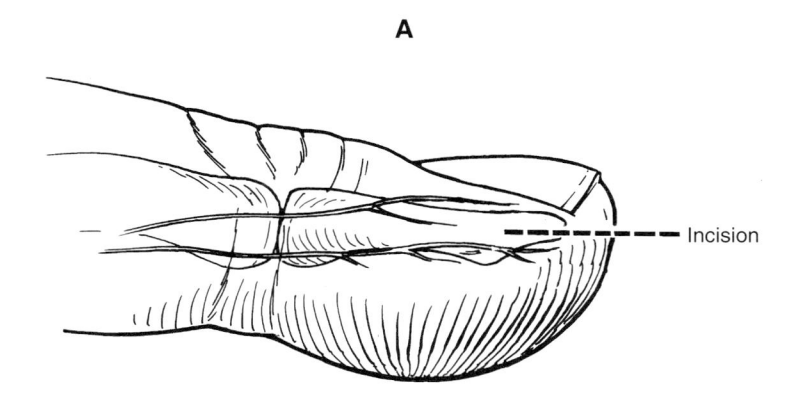

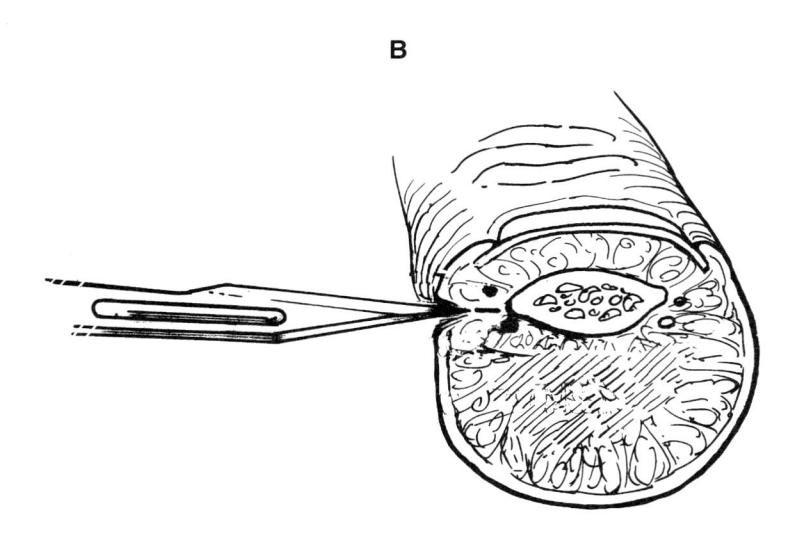

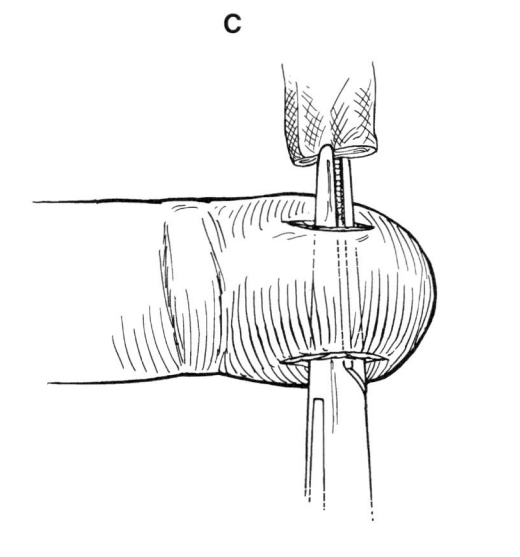

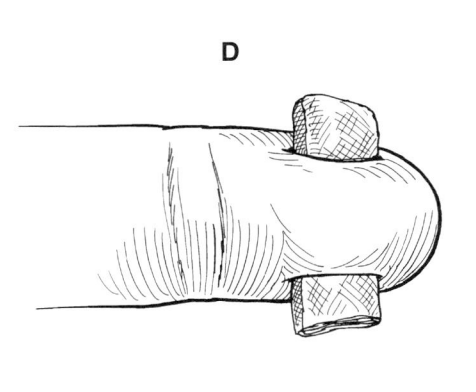

EXTREMITIES 245

A

------- Incision

B

C

D

Paronychia Drainage SAMUEL M. KEIM AND HARVEY W. MEISLIN

Indications
- Paronychia (infection and abscess between the lateral nail fold and nail plate) *(A)*
- Eponychia (infection and abscess between proximal nail fold and nail plate)

Contraindications
- Chronic paronychia, which may be infected by atypical mycobacteria and *Candida albicans;* the patient should be referred to a hand surgeon or a dermatologist

Equipment
- Sterile drapes and gloves
- Sterile gauze packing
- Betadine antiseptic solution
- Local anesthetic (buffered lidocaine), syringe, and needles
- Scalpel with No. 11 blade

Procedure

1. Prepare the entire affected hand distal to the wrist crease in sterile fashion.
2. Place a sterile drape around the hand on the workstand to expose the affected finger.
3. Apply a digital anesthetic block at the proximal base of the affected finger.
4. Insert the tip of the No. 11 blade into the swollen sulcus of the lateral nail fold or eponychium. This should result in liberation of a small amount of pus *(B)*.
5. Irrigation and placement of a strip of fine gauze packing into the sulcus of a large paronychia for 24 to 48 hours may promote continued drainage.
6. If pus has accumulated beneath the nail, remove a small section of nail to allow adequate drainage. Insert a small piece of gauze into the sulcus of the eponychium to prevent adherence of the fold.
7. Antistaphylococcal antibiotics, elevation, and immobilization should be instituted. The patient should have close follow-up to ensure continued improvement and detect complications.

Complications
- Osteomyelitis of the distal phalanx
- Damage to tissue, digital arteries, nerves, and nail matrix from inappropriate incision
- Chronic paronychia

Discussion
- Any violation of the contact between nail fold and nail plate may result in infection (paronychia or eponychia) manifested as an extremely tender swelling of the space immediately adjacent to the nail. Early in the course the drainage procedure may not liberate any pus. However, it is better to err on the aggressive side than to miss an early abscess. A simple small paronychia may be drained without digital anesthesia by elevating the nail cuticle with an 18-gauge needle or No. 11 blade scalpel tip.

Bibliography

Canales FL et al: The treatment of felons and paronychias, *Hand Clin* 5(4):515-523, 1989.

Lee TC: The office treatment of simple paronychias and gangliones, *Med Times* 109(9):49-51, 54-55, 1981.

A

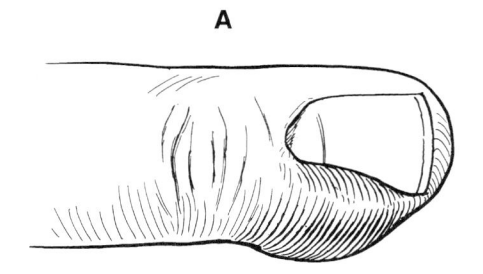

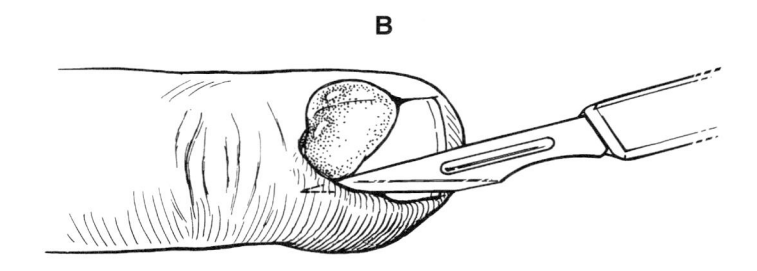

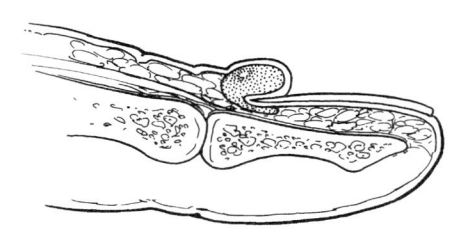

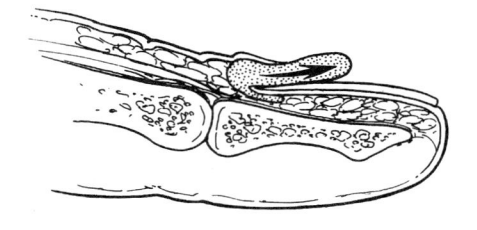

B

Ring Removal — Samuel M. Keim and Harvey W. Meislin

Indications
- Difficulty removing a ring when edema may lead to distal ischemia *(A)*

Contraindications
- Severely traumatized finger (i.e., complex laceration or partial amputation) when manipulation may lead to significant worsening of the injury

Equipment
- Ring cutter if available, or the following:
  - Latex or flexible phlebotomy tourniquet
  - Large-caliber suture or ⅛-inch umbilical tape
  - Hemostat or paperclip

Procedure

1. Wrap the flexible latex tourniquet in a spiraling fashion from the fingertip proximally to partially exsanguinate the finger and reduce swelling.
2. If this is not enough to facilitate removal of a stubborn ring, work a sturdy suture material, such as 0 silk or umbilical tape, beneath the ring *(B)*.
3. Wrap the suture circumferentially in a spiraling fashion beginning at the ring and working distally *(C)*.
4. Pull the end of the suture proximal to the ring upward gradually, moving the ring distally *(D, E)*. Be careful not to put too much torque on the suture, which might break.

EXTREMITIES 249

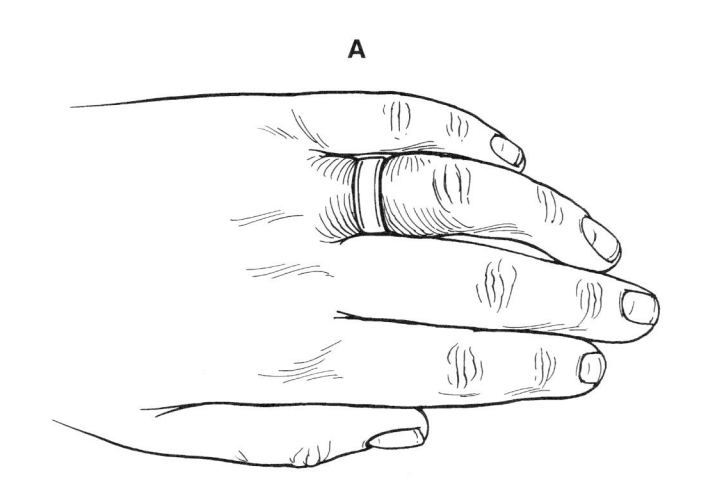

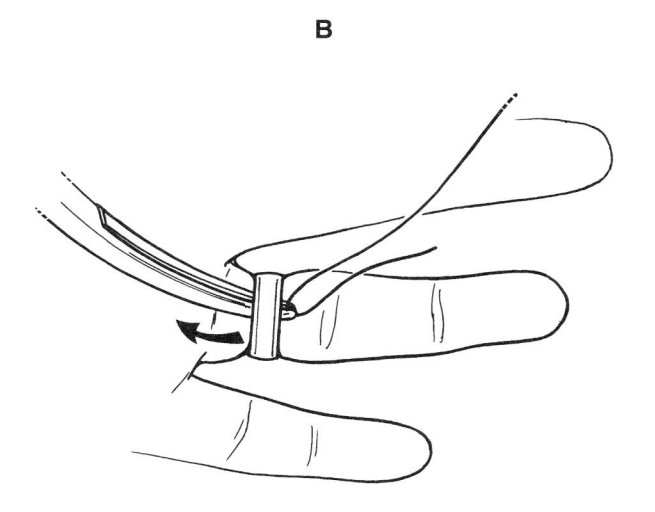

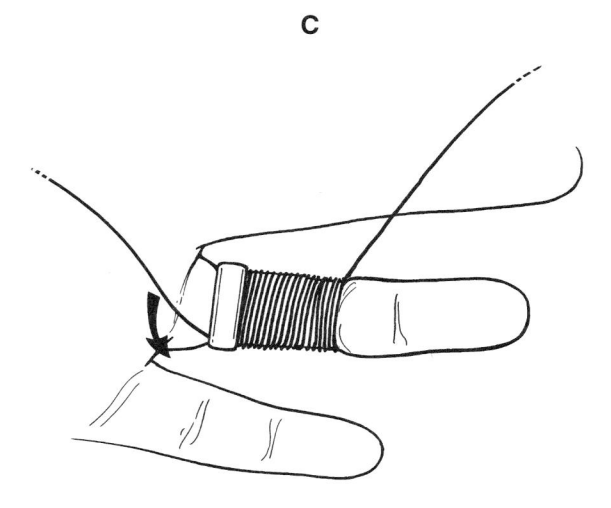

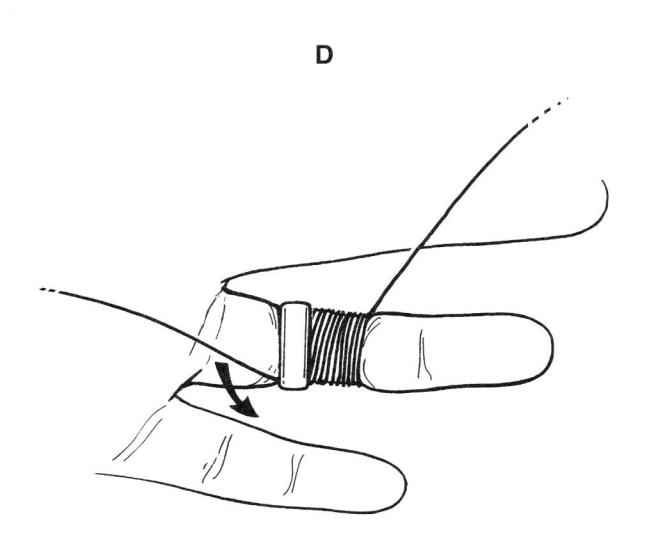

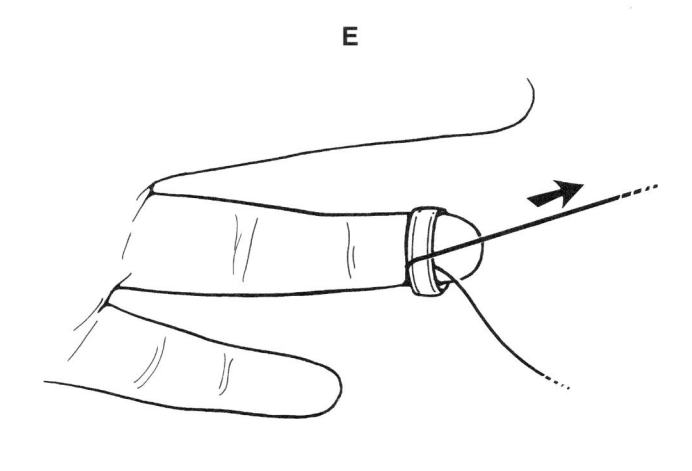

A

B

C

D

E

Complications

- Ischemic compromise and compartment syndrome from failure to remove a ring from a grossly edematous digit
- Further complication to traumatic injuries of the digit because the stubborn ring is impeding vascular return.

Discussion

- Many emergency departments have commercially available ring cutters (F) that make removal easy. The decision of whether to remove the ring intact or cut it should be discussed with the patient.

Bibliography

Fasano FJ Jr, Hansen RH: Foreign body granuloma and synovitis of the finger: a hazard of ring removal by the sawing technique, *J Hand Surg* 12(4):621-623, 1987.

Mizrahi S, Lunski I: A simplified method for ring removal from an edematous finger, *Am J Surg* 151(3):412-413, 1986.

Rubman MH, Taylor K: A rapid method for emergency ring removal, *Am J Orthop* 25(1):42-44, 1996.

Thilagarajah M: An improved method of ring removal, *J Hand Surg [Br]* 24(1):118-119, 1999.

F

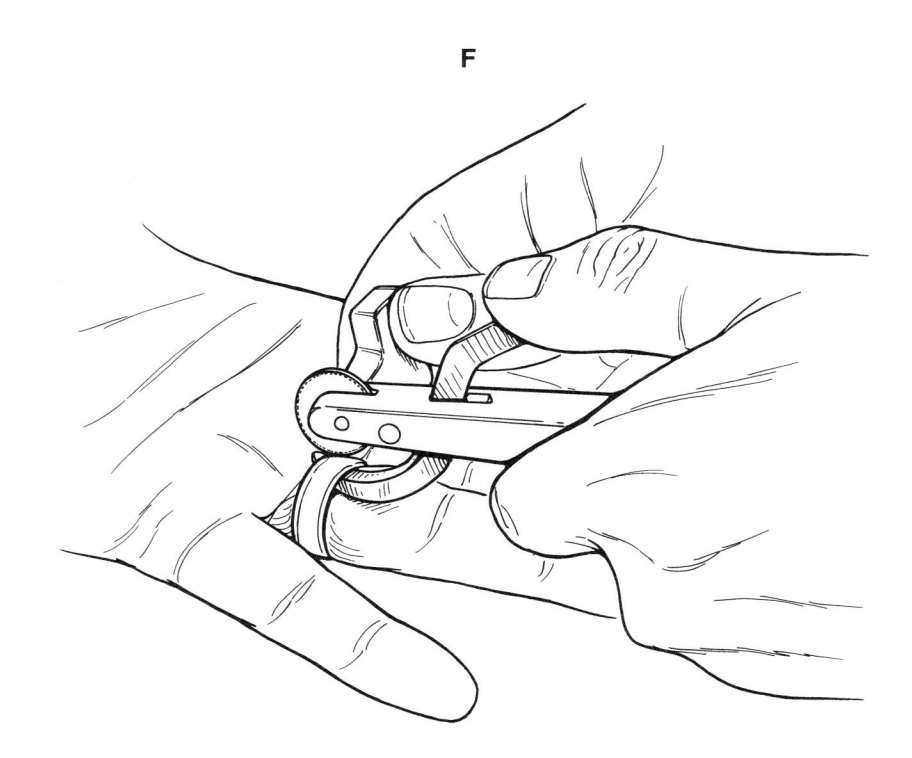

Nail Removal   Harvey W. Meislin and Samuel M. Keim

Indications
- Nail infection (bacterial or fungal)
- Nail trauma with laceration or separation of the nail bed
- Partial nail removal to gain access to the nail bed in order to drain a paronychia
- Ingrown nail

Contraindications
- Drainage of subungual abscess or hematoma (can be accomplished by nail fenestration)

Equipment
- Sterile drapes and gloves
- Betadine antiseptic solution
- Anesthetic for digital block (buffered 1% or 2% lidocaine without epinephrine), syringe, and needle
- Heavy scissors
- Curved and straight clamps
- Scalpel with No. 15 blade
- Bovie cautery or silver nitrate stick
- Petrolatum-impregnated gauze
- Dry sterile dressings

Procedure

1. Prepare the entire affected digit and web spaces in sterile fashion, and drape the involved area.
2. Apply a digital anesthetic block to the proximal base of the affected digit *(A)*.
3. Using blunt and sharp dissection, peel the nail off the nail bed toward the cuticle fold *(B)*.
4. Bisect the nail by cutting through its midportion from the tip down through the lunula to the nail base. Be careful not to cut the nail bed *(C)*.
5. Remove the bisected nail.
6. Apply compression or cauterization with a silver nitrate stick or a Bovie cautery to control the small blood vessel at the base of the eponychial fold.
7. If there is excessive buildup of granulation tissue along the paronychial fold, remove it *(D)*.
8. Once the nail is removed, inspect the nail bed and repair as necessary *(E)*.
9. If both halves of the nail must be removed, remove the other portion at this time.
10. Push a petrolatum-impregnated gauze or packing into the eponychial fold at the base of the nail to prevent syncytium formation and a ridged nail.
11. Apply a dry sterile dressing
12. Inspect the wound in 48 to 72 hours.

Complications
- Injury to the nail bed
- Bleeding
- Destruction of the nail matrix
- Syncytium formation and ridged nail
- Malformed nail

Discussion
- In some circumstances, especially traumatic, the nail may be removed, the nail bed drained or repaired, and the nail replaced to act as coverage for the wound.
- Although patients are often hesitant about having a nail removed, it is important to stress the benefits. Absence of the nail helps infection to resolve faster, prevents spread of infection, makes hematomas less painful, and promotes more rapid healing with a cosmetically improved appearance of the nail.

Bibliography
Greig JD et al: The surgical treatment of ingrown toenails, *J Bone Joint Surg [Br]* 73(1):131-133, 1991.

Roser SE, Gellman H: Comparison of nail bed repair versus nail trephination for subungual hematomas in children, *J Hand Surg [Am]* 24(6):1166-1170, 1999.

EXTREMITIES

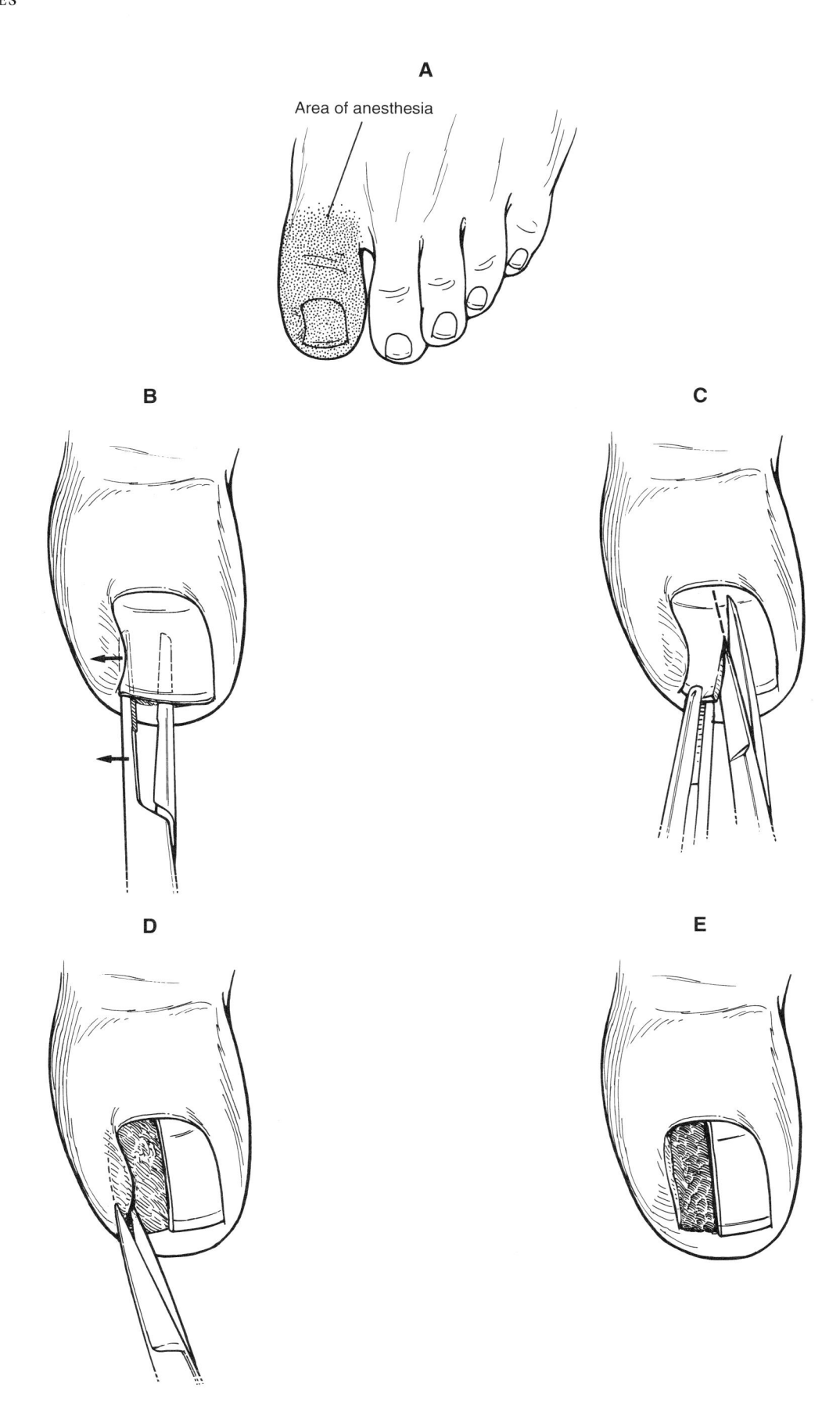

A

Area of anesthesia

B

C

D

E

Fish Hook Removal HARVEY W. MEISLIN AND SAMUEL M. KEIM

Indications
- Removal of an imbedded fish hook from the skin

Contraindications
- None

Equipment
- Large suture material (0 or larger)
- Betadine antiseptic solution

Procedure

1. Depending on the patient, the area of initial penetration may need to be anesthetized, although for most patients this is not the case. Prepare the area in sterile fashion *(A)*.
2. Using large suture, tie the sutures with several knots at the point where the hook is imbedded into the skin *(B)*.
3. Push down on the nonbarbed shank of the fish hook so that it runs parallel to the skin surface *(C)*.
4. Compress the hook that is in the tissue, forcing it to form a tighter curvature.
5. With the shank of the hook parallel to the skin and compression on either side of the entry point of the hook into the skin, pull smartly on the suture, directing it radially to the curvature of the hook *(D)*. This should free the barb portion of the hook from the skin, and the hook should be easily removed. Inspect and cleanse the wound, and dress it appropriately.

Complications
- Reentry of the hook through the tissues of the patient
- Inadvertent imbedding of the fish hook into the skin of the health care provider
- Infection

Discussion
- Another method of removing the fish hook is by pushing the hook via its natural curvature out through another opening made in the skin. This is less preferable because it creates another invasion of the skin and enhances the potential for infection. Some physicians advise making a very small incision in the skin at the point of entry so that the barb exits more freely. There is no advantage to this process.

Bibliography

Danesh J et al: Fish hook injuries—wounded anglers and string theory, *NZ Med J* 105(931):136, 1992.
David SS: Fish-hook removal, *Lancet* 338(8780):1463-1464, 1991.
Graham P: Removal of embedded fish-hook, *Aust Fam Physician* 24(4):691, 1995.

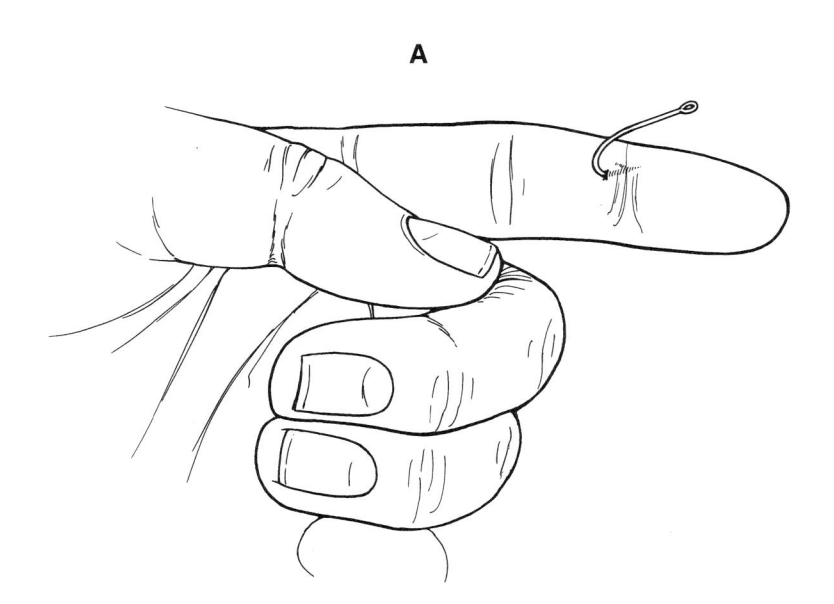

A

B

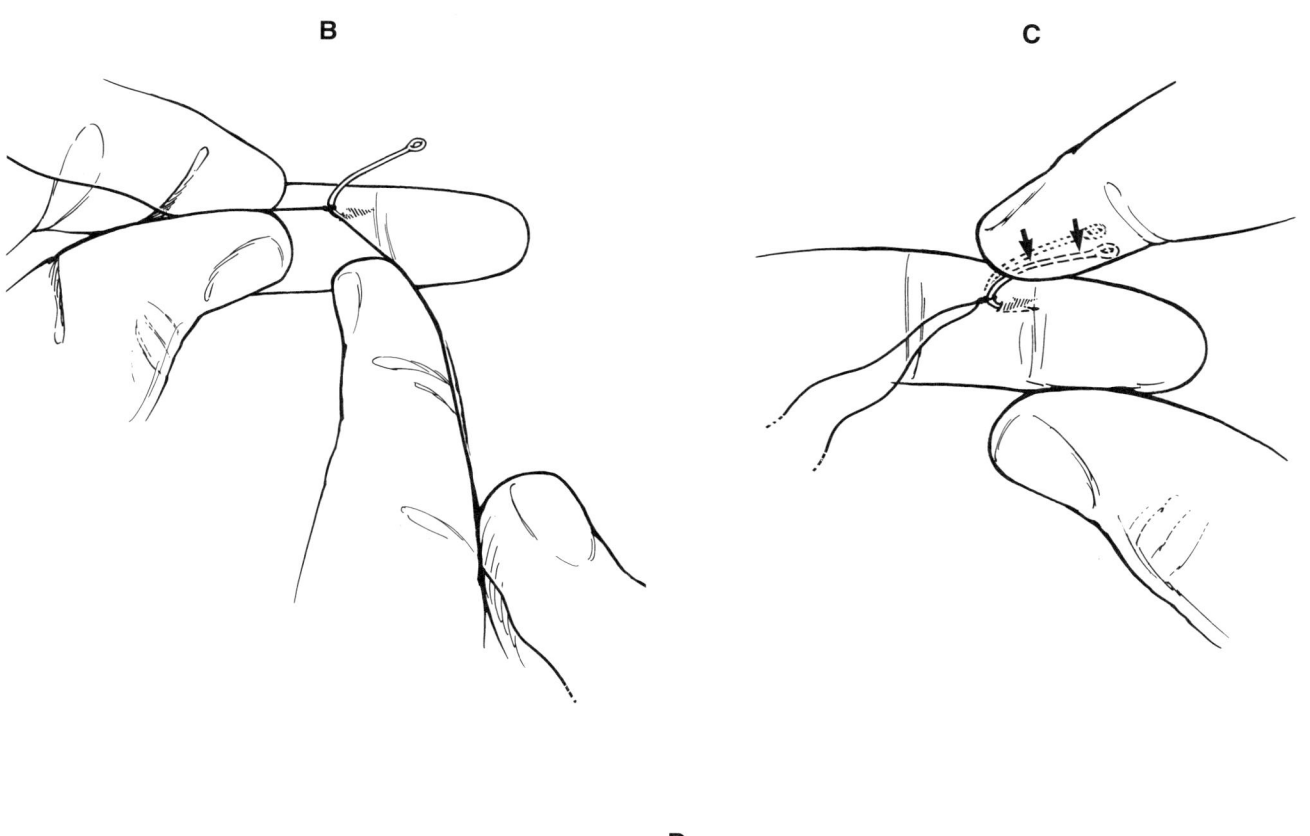

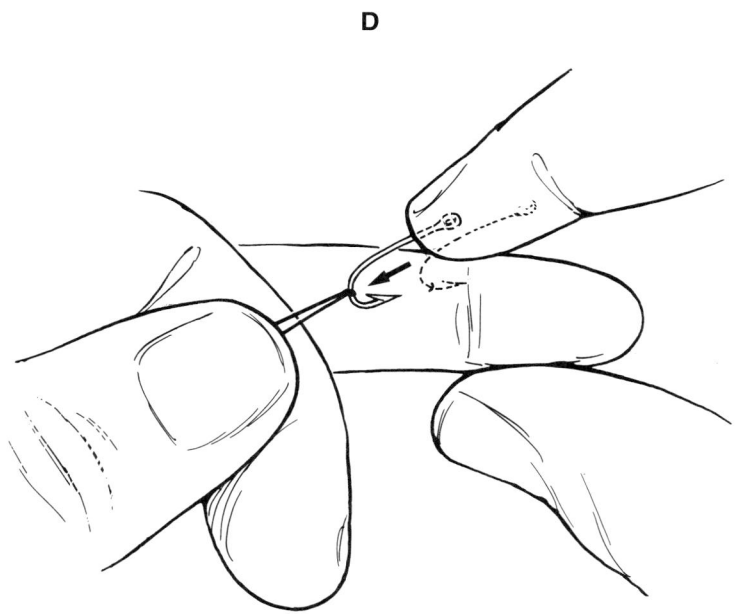

C

D

CHAPTER 12

REDUCTION AND SPLINTING

Dislocation Reduction

Closed Reduction of Anterior Shoulder Dislocations   Mary Anne Fuchs

Indications
- Acute anterior shoulder dislocation

Equipment
- Folded sheets (traction-countertraction technique)
- 5- to 10-lb weights and tape (Stimson's technique)
- IV analgesia and sedation

Procedure

Stimson's Technique with Scapular Rotation Modification

1. Position the patient prone with the affected arm hanging off the edge of the bed.
2. Have an assistant gently apply 5 to 10 lb of consistent longitudinal traction on the arm in a downward direction (weights may be used rather than pressure by assistant).
3. After 5 to 10 minutes of traction, attempt to push the inferolateral border of the scapula medially, rotating the superior aspect of the scapula laterally *(A)*. Slight external rotation while applying traction to the hanging arm may be helpful.
4. Confirm the reduction by examination, and reassess neurovascular status. Immobilize the shoulder with a sling and swath or shoulder immobilizer, and refer the patient to an orthopedist for follow-up.

External Rotation Technique

1. Position the patient supine or semiupright.
2. Support the patient's elbow with one hand, while holding the patient's wrist with the other *(B)*.
3. Adduct the shoulder, and apply longitudinal traction while holding the elbow.
4. Externally rotate the patient's arm slowly and gently, waiting for muscle relaxation if resistance or patient discomfort is encountered.
5. Once the arm is externally rotated to 90°, slowly abduct the shoulder until reduction occurs *(C)*.
6. If reduction does not occur with abduction, manipulate the upper arm and attempt to lift the humeral head into the glenoid socket. Alternatively, apply pressure with your thumbs at the anterosuperior aspect of the humeral head to push the dislocated head over the glenoid rim (modified Milch's technique)
7. Confirm the reduction by examination, and reassess neurovascular status. Immobilize the shoulder with a sling and swath or shoulder immobilizer, and refer the patient to an orthopedist for follow-up.

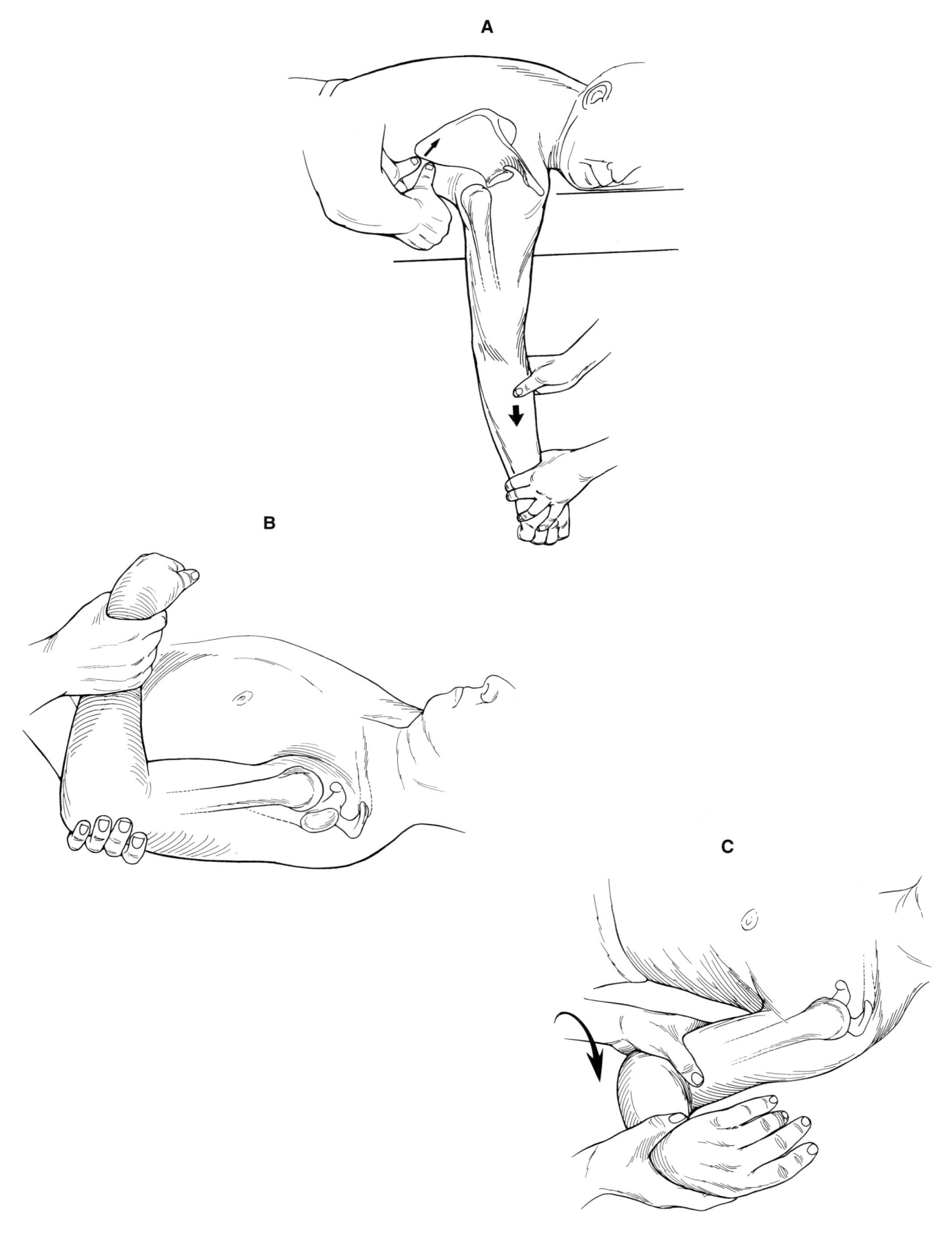

Reduction and Splinting

259

A

B

C

Traction-Countertraction Technique

1. Position the patient supine with a folded sheet wrapped under the affected axilla and around the chest.
2. Apply gentle, steady traction along the axis of the humerus with the shoulder at approximately 45° of abduction. Have an assistant simultaneously provide countertraction by holding the ends of the sheet on the side of the patient opposite the dislocation *(D)*. It may take several minutes or more of steady traction before muscle relaxation is sufficient.
3. If necessary, rock the humerus from internal to external rotation to help disengage the humeral head from the glenoid rim and facilitate reduction. Use of another sheet wrapped around the patient's flexed elbow and the physician's waist so that the operator can lean back to apply traction will free the operator's hands to control internal or external rotation. Gentle lateral traction to the proximal humerus may also be helpful.
4. Confirm the reduction by examination, and reassess neurovascular status. Immobilize the shoulder with a sling and swath or shoulder immobilizer, and refer the patient to an orthopedist for follow-up.

Complications

- Nerve injury (usually axillary nerve neurapraxia)
- Further joint capsule damage
- Soft tissue entrapment (generally preventing closed reduction)

Discussion

- A patient self-reduction technique (Aronen's technique) has been described. The patient sits upright in bed or on the floor with the ipsilateral knee flexed. The patient interlocks the fingers, clasps the hands together, and loops them around the knee *(E)*. The patient then slowly leans back until the elbows are straight. With steady pressure the patient simultaneously lean backs and extends the hip, creating gentle traction and countertraction to reduce the shoulder.
- If examination reveals evidence of a neurovascular injury, prompt reduction is the priority. Leverage techniques, which may worsen the injury, should be avoided. Elbow flexion will reduce tension on the neurovascular structures.
- Closed reduction can be attempted with most anterior shoulder dislocations that have associated simple fractures. Adequate analgesia and muscle relaxation are essential, and simple traction methods are advisable. Fractures of the greater tuberosity are often reduced into a more anatomic position with shoulder reduction.
- Shoulder dislocations lasting more than 1 or 2 days are considered chronic. These dislocations are generally difficult to reduce with closed reduction because of muscle spasm and contracture. They are also more susceptible to complications during reduction.
- Immediate reduction generally requires less force and can often be accomplished without medication. Early reduction minimizes the stretching of neurovascular structures and the damage of the humeral articular surface. Gentle reduction can be attempted in the field if the clinical diagnosis is certain, the patient cooperative, the examination otherwise benign, and the transport time long. Gentle traction techniques are recommended.

Bibliography

Aronen JG, Chronister RD: Anterior shoulder dislocations: easing reduction by using linear traction techniques, *Phys Sports Med* 23:65-69, 1995.

Gleeson AP: Anterior glenohumeral dislocations: what to do and how to do it, *J Accid Emerg Med* 15:7-12, 1998.

Riebel DB, McCabe JB: Anterior shoulder dislocation: a review of reduction techniques, *Am J Emerg Med* 9:180-188, 1991.

Simon RR, Keonigsknecht SJ: *Emergency orthopedics: the extremities*, ed 3, Norwalk, Conn, 1996, Appleton & Lange.

Zahiri CA et al: Anterior shoulder reduction technique—revisited, *Orthopedics* 20:515-521, 1997.

Reduction and Splinting

D

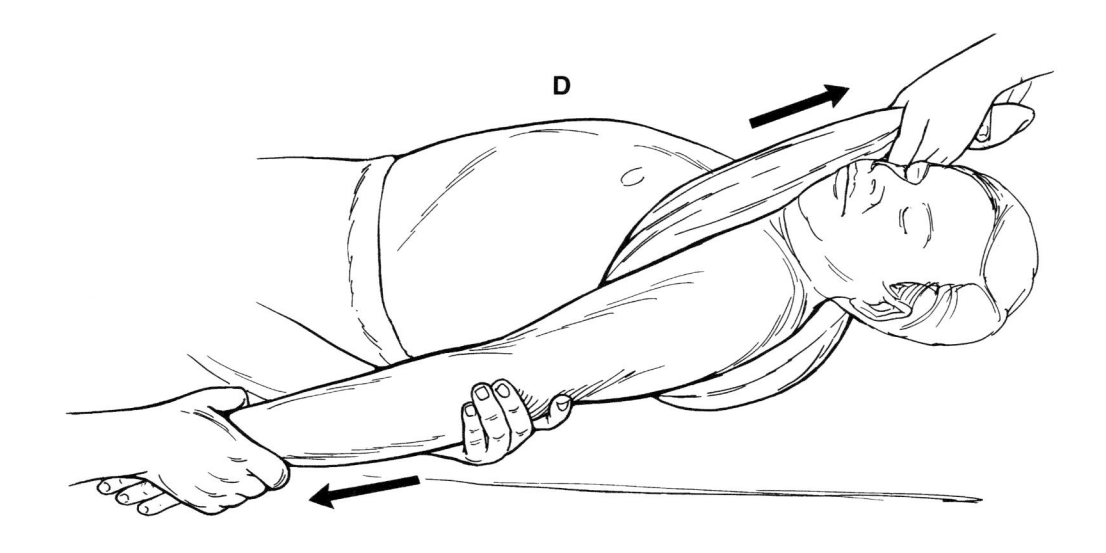

E

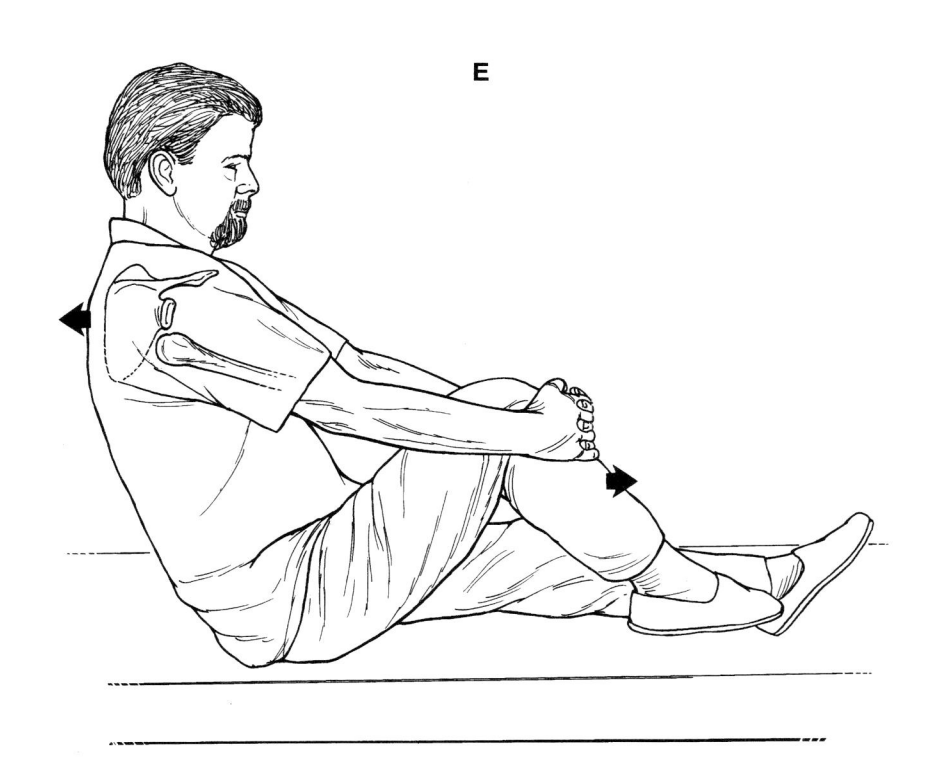

Posterior Elbow Dislocation Reduction with the Puller Technique
MARY ANNE FUCHS

Indications
- Acute posterior dislocation of the elbow joint

Equipment
- Equipment for IV sedation and analgesia (usually needed)

Procedure

1. Perform careful neurovascular examination before and after manipulation.
2. Obtain sufficient analgesia and muscle relaxation with IV medications.
3. In the puller technique, pulling force is applied directly to the anterior aspect of the proximal forearm *(A)*.
4. Position the patient supine or sitting.
5. Holding the patient's wrist with one hand, apply steady traction to the supinated forearm (along the axis of the forearm) with the elbow flexed. Have an assistant hold the patient's upper arm to apply countertraction.
6. With the other hand, gently apply downward pressure (along the axis of the upper arm) on the patient's proximal forearm to unlock the coronoid process.
7. If reduction does not occur by traction and downward pressure alone, gently flex and extend the elbow while maintaining traction to unlock the coronoid process.
8. Perform a careful neurovascular examination.
9. Immobilize the extremity by applying a posterior splint or sling with the elbow in 90° flexion. Close orthopedic follow-up is recommended.

Complications
- Peripheral neurovascular injuries and associated fractures
- Median nerve entrapment
- Delayed circulatory compromise
- Compartment syndrome

Discussion

- The assistant applying countertraction on the upper arm can use the thumbs to simultaneously "push" the olecranon forward into position (modified pusher technique). In younger children, Lavine's push-off technique, in which the child sits in the parent's lap, has been described. With one hand, traction is applied on the forearm (along its axis) with the elbow flexed. Countertraction is applied on the upper arm with the other hand, and the thumb is used to push the olecranon into position.
- An alternative technique has the patient prone with the elbow flexed and the forearm hanging over the side of the bed. Gentle traction is applied downward on the forearm by the operator or with the use of weights. The operator's thumbs are then used to push the olecranon over the humeral head and into position.

Bibliography

Kumar A, Ahmed M: Closed reduction of posterior dislocation of the elbow: a simple technique, *J Orthop Trauma* 13(1):58-59, 1999.

Rockwood CA, Wilkins KE: *Fractures in children*, Philadelphia, 1996, Lippincott-Raven.

Royle SG: Posterior dislocation of the elbow, *Clin Orthop Rel Res* 269:201-204, 1991.

Simon RR, Keonigsknecht SJ: *Emergency orthopedics: the extremities*, ed 3, Norwalk, Conn, 1996, Appleton & Lange.

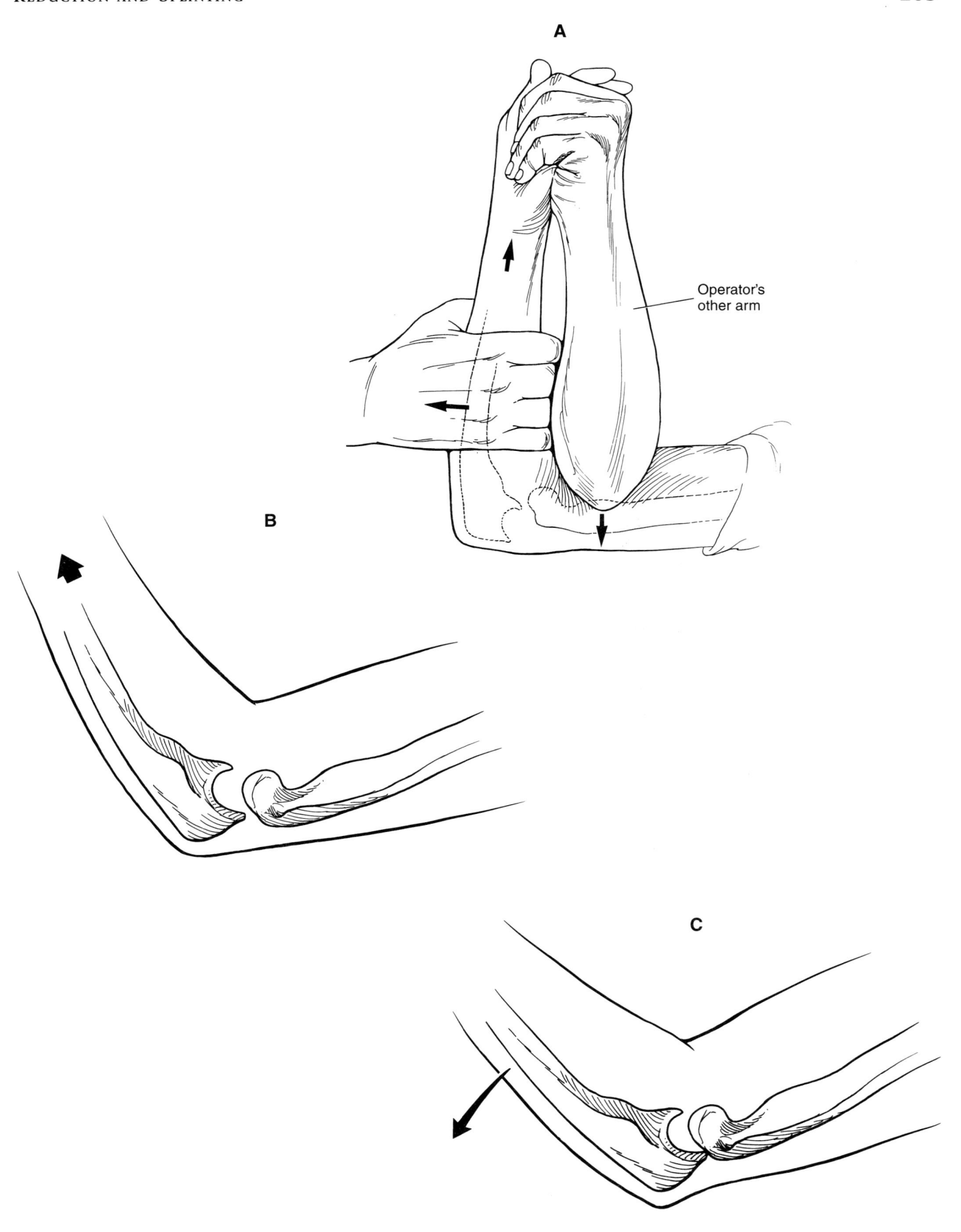

REDUCTION AND SPLINTING   263

A

Operator's other arm

B

C

Radial Head Subluxation Reduction by the Flexion-Supination Method
Mary Anne Fuchs

Indications
- Acute radial head subluxation in children

Equipment
- None

Procedure

1. With one hand cupping the affected elbow, apply pressure with the thumb over the area of the radial head *(A)*.
2. Hold the child's wrist with the other hand, and simultaneously flex the elbow and supinate the forearm slowly *(B, C)*.
3. An audible or palpable click and sudden release of resistance are usually noted with reduction.
4. After reduction the child is usually pain free and moves the arm easily. No immobilization is required. If the child can use the arm but the pain persists, immobilize the arm in a posterior splint and sling and recheck within 24 hours. If the child does not use the arm in a normal manner in 15 to 30 minutes, either reduction has not been accomplished or another diagnosis should be suspected.

Complications
- Recurrence

Discussion

- Radiographs are not indicated. Reduction is confirmed when the child begins to use the arm without apparent pain.
- An alternative extension-pronation method has been described. Pressure is applied over the area of the radial head with one hand while the other hand slowly extends and pronates the elbow. Slight longitudinal traction during elbow extension may be helpful. This method has been reported to have a higher success rate.

Bibliography

Graeme KA, Jackimczyk KC: The extremities and spine, *Emerg Med Clinics North Am* 15(2):365-379, 1997.

Quan L, Marcuse EK: The epidemiology and treatment of radial head subluxation, *Am J Dis Child* 139(12):1194-1197, 1985.

Schunk JE: Radial head subluxation: epidemiology and treatment of 87 episodes, *Ann Emerg Med* 19(9):1019, 1990.

Reduction and Splinting

265

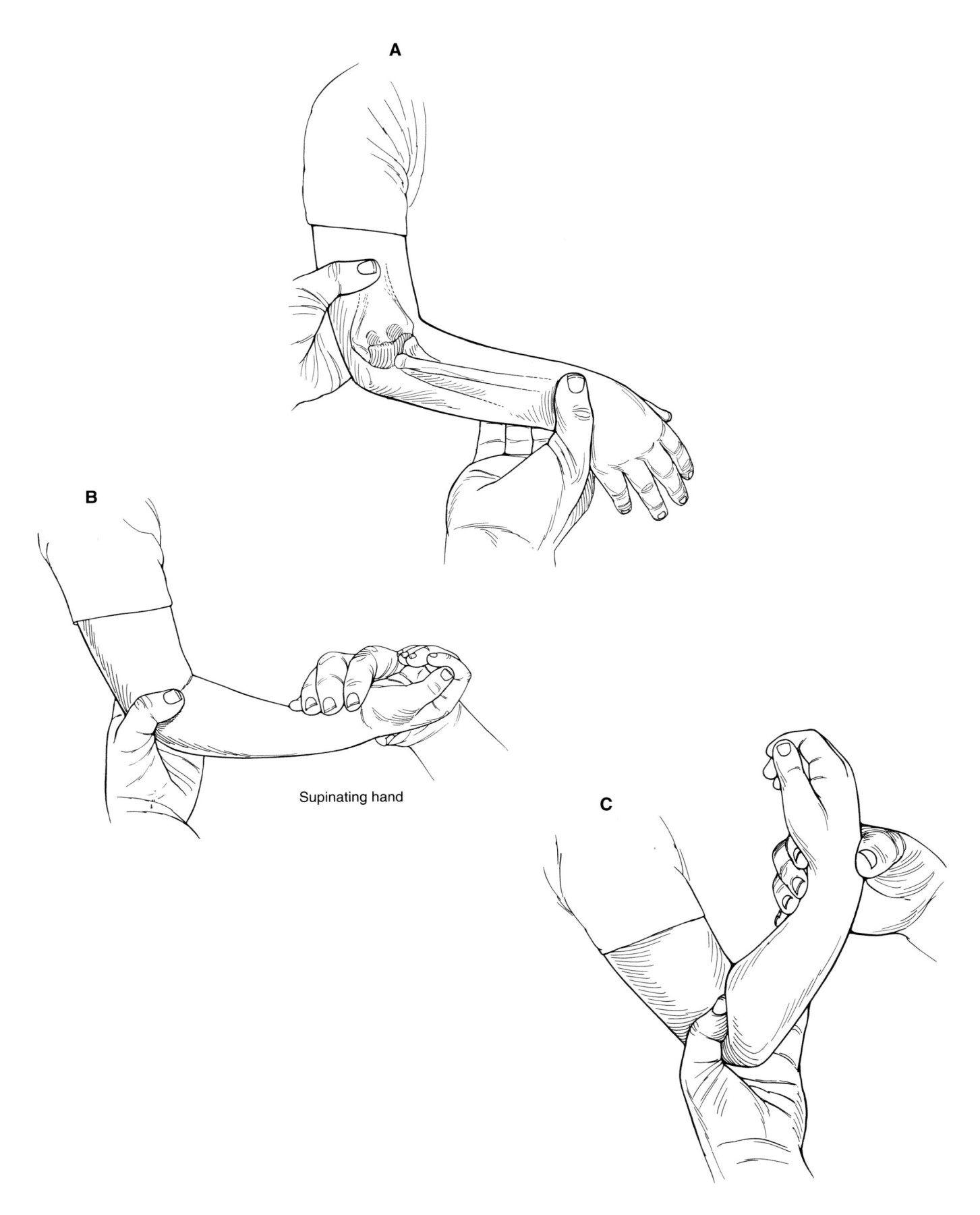

A

B

Supinating hand

C

Finger Dislocations   Mary Anne Fuchs

Indications
- Acute dislocations of the finger interphalangeal and metacarpophalangeal joints

Equipment
- Gauze for improved traction

Procedure

Distal Interphalangeal Joint Reduction
1. Apply longitudinal traction with slight exaggeration of the deformity (i.e., hyperextension for dorsal dislocations).
2. Gently manipulate the joint into its normal position.
3. For dorsal dislocations apply dorsal pressure to the base of the dislocated phalanx to facilitate reduction.
4. If the joint is stable, apply a dorsal splint in 5° to 10° of flexion for 2 to 3 weeks. If the joint is unstable or evidence of volar plate disruption is found, apply a dorsal splint in 30° of flexion and arrange prompt referral to a specialist.

Proximal Interphalangeal Joint Reduction (A, B)
1. Apply longitudinal traction with slight exaggeration of the deformity (i.e., hyperextension for dorsal dislocations).
2. Gently manipulate the joint into its normal position.
3. For a dorsal dislocation apply dorsal pressure to the base of the dislocated phalanx to facilitate reduction.
4. For a stable dorsal dislocation, splint the finger in 15° to 30° flexion for 1 week followed by 3 weeks of dynamic splinting via "buddy taping" to the adjacent finger. For an unstable dorsal dislocation, splint the finger with the proximal interphalangeal (PIP) joint in 15° of flexion and arrange for orthopedic follow-up within the week. For a volar dislocation immobilize the PIP joint in extension and refer the patient for possible surgical repair of the volar plate or central slip detachment.

Metacarpophalangeal Reduction (C, D)
1. Flex the wrist to relax the extrinsic flexor tendons.
2. Apply firm dorsal pressure to the base of the proximal phalanx.
3. Avoid excessive hyperextension or longitudinal traction, which may cause the volar plate to become interposed within the joint space.
4. Immobilize the finger in flexion for 1 to 2 weeks followed by 3 weeks of dynamic splinting via "buddy taping."

Complications
- Irreducibility
- Persistent pain, stiffness, and swelling
- Persistent volar plate and collateral ligament instability
- Associated tendon avulsions (DIP injuries)
- Boutonniere deformity (volar PIP dislocations)

Discussion
- If dislocations of the digits are not easily reduced, the patient may have a complex "buttonholed" dislocation or soft tissue interposed in the joint, necessitating open reduction. Repeated attempts at closed reduction may lead to further damage to the soft tissues or neurovascular bundle.
- Joint stability testing, and often reduction, is best performed with the use of digital anesthesia. Active range of motion and gentle lateral stress testing (with the joint extended) should be performed. Lack of full active range of motion should not be assumed to be the result of joint pain or stiffness. Instability indicates complete and multiple ligamentous disruption, necessitating surgical repair.

Bibliography
Freiberg A et al: Management of proximal interphalangeal joint injuries, *J Trauma* 46(3):523-528, 1999.
Harrison BP, Hilliard MW: Emergency department evaluation and treatment of hand injuries, *Emerg Med Clin North Am* 17(4):793-822, 1999.
Hossfeld GE, Uehara DT: Acute joint injuries of the hand, *Emerg Med Clin North Am* 11(3):781-796, 1993.

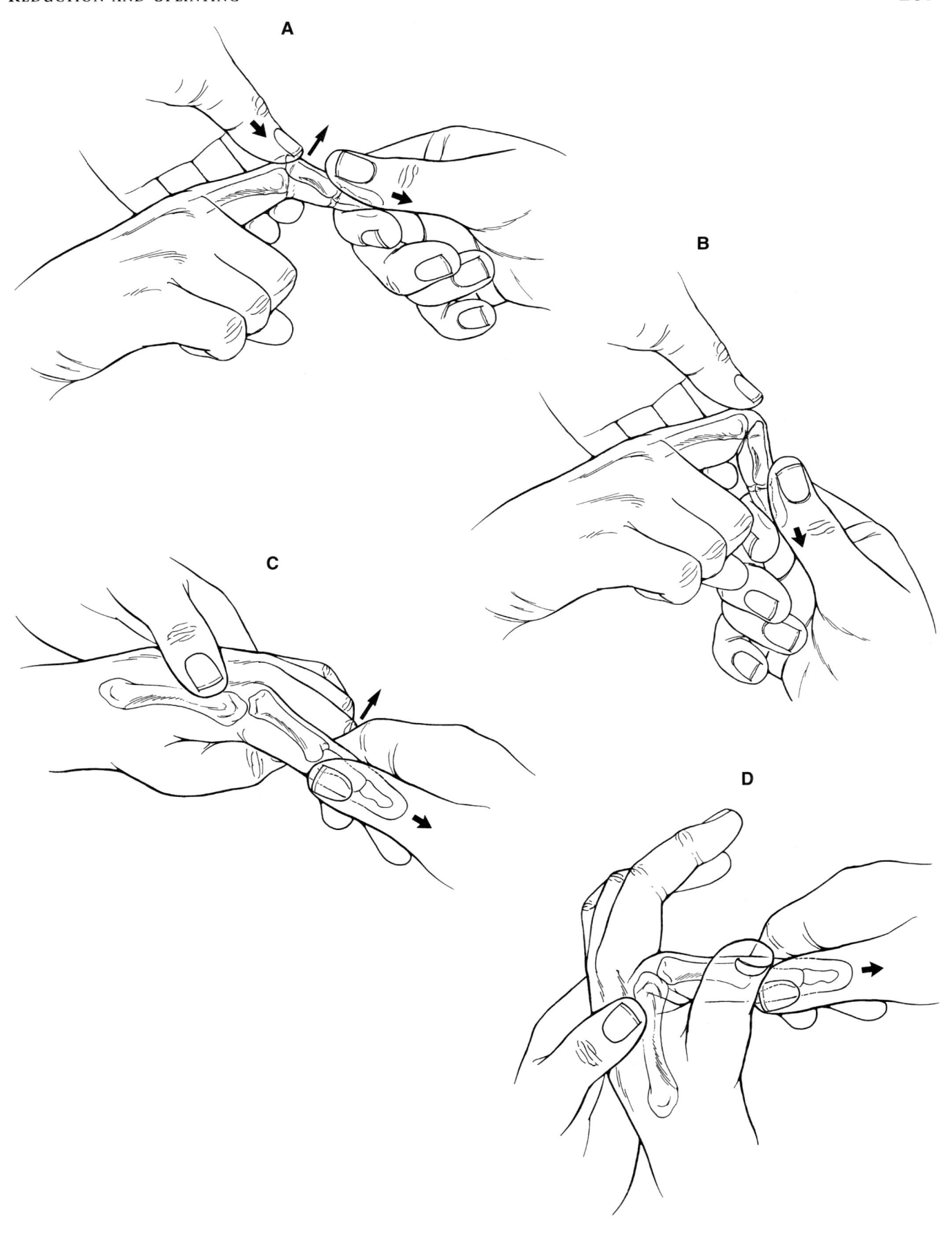

Reduction and Splinting

267

A

B

C

D

Posterior Hip Reduction by the Standard Supine (Allis) Method
MARY ANNE FUCHS

Indications
- Acute traumatic hip dislocation

Equipment
- Equipment for IV sedation and analgesia

Procedure

1. Always perform a thorough neurovascular examination before and after reduction.
2. Provide IV sedation and analgesia.
3. Place the patient supine on a firm surface
4. Have an assistant stabilize the pelvis by providing countertraction downward posteriorly on the iliac spines of the patient.
5. Standing over the patient, flex the affected hip and knee to 90°, maintaining slight adduction and internal rotation.
6. Apply steady upward traction on the proximal calf (lifting the femoral head up into the acetabulum) until reduction occurs. Gentle internal rotation may aid in reduction, but avoid forceful rotation that can cause a femoral neck fracture *(A, B)*.
7. After reduction maintain the leg in slight abduction and external rotation and place the leg in longitudinal traction. Alternatively, place a pillow between the knees to prevent adduction. Consider admission for strict non-weight-bearing and observation.

Complications

- Acetabular and femoral head, neck, or shaft fractures
- Knee injury
- Sciatic nerve contusion, laceration, or traction injury
- Traumatic arthritis

Discussion

- Most hip dislocations can be reduced by closed manipulation with IV sedation if reduction is performed within 8 to 12 hours. Irreducibility may be a result of buttonholing of the femoral head through the joint capsule or the interposition of loose bodies or soft tissue. If attempts at closed reduction are unsuccessful, open reduction is mandatory.
- The alternative Stimson's technique has the patient prone with the hips at the edge of the bed and the affected extremity hanging over the side. The hip and knee are flexed at 90° while the foot rests on the knee of the operator, who then applies steady downward traction on the proximal calf. An assistant supports the opposite leg and may also apply pressure on the greater trochanter of the affected hip to help push it anteriorly into the acetabulum.

Bibliography

Canale ST: *Campbell's operative orthopaedics*, ed 9, St Louis, 1998, Mosby, pp 2637-2641.

Paletta GA, Andrish JT: Injuries about the hip and pelvis in the young athlete, *Clin Sports Med* 14(3):591-628, 1995.

Rockwood CA, Wilkins KE: *Fractures in children*, Philadelphia, 1996, Lippincott-Raven.

Schlickewei W, Elseasser B: Hip dislocation without fracture: traction or mobilization after reduction? *Injury* 24(1):27-31, 1993.

REDUCTION AND SPLINTING 269

A

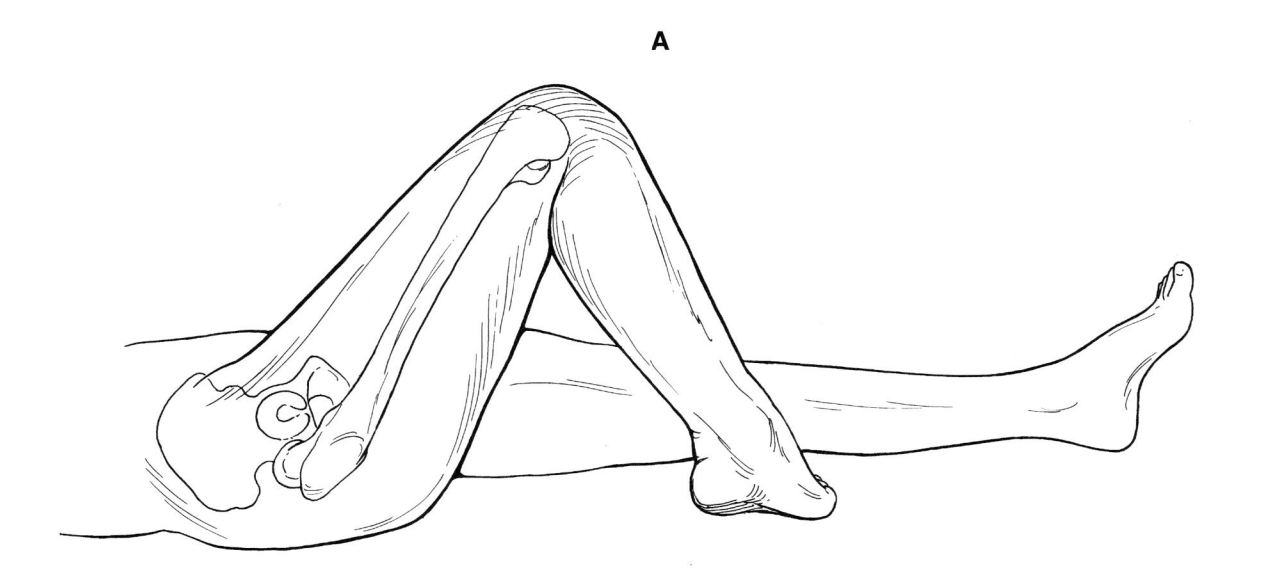

B

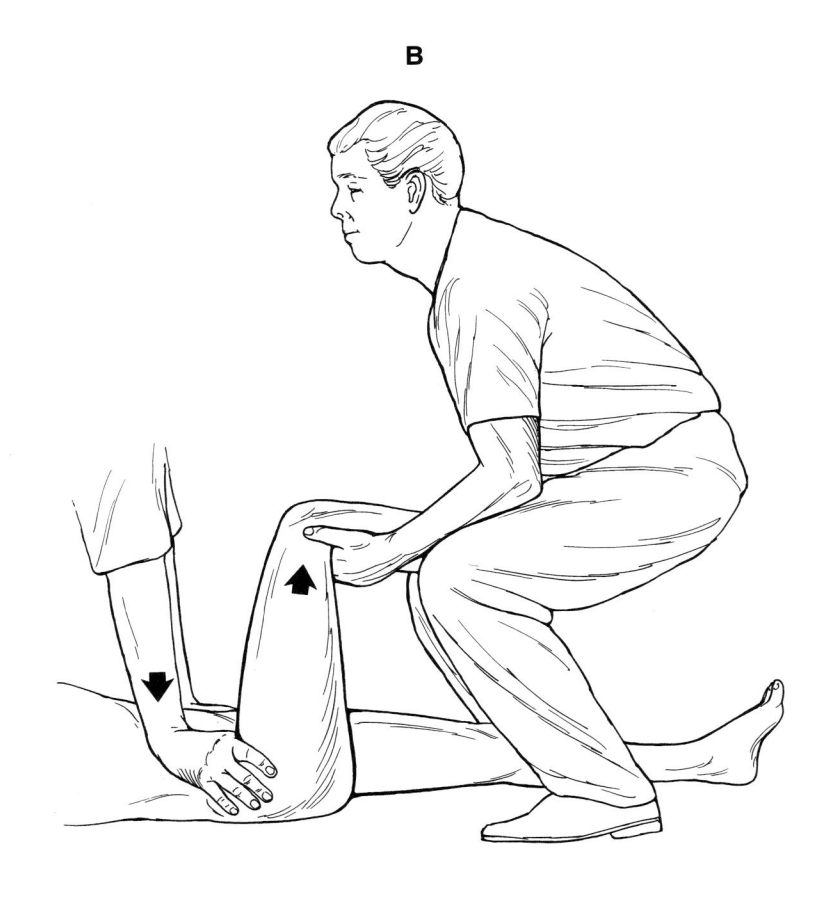

Patellar Dislocation Reduction MARY ANNE FUCHS

Indications
- Acute lateral patellar dislocation

Equipment
- Rarely, equipment for IV analgesia

Procedure

1. Position the patient supine with the knee slightly flexed and supported.
2. Gently extend the knee to 180° (may be sufficient to reduce the patella).
3. Apply gentle, medially directed pressure over the lateral aspect of the patella until the patella slides over the lateral femoral condyle into position *(A, B)*.
4. Place the affected knee in a knee immobilizer, and prescribe non-weight-bearing status. Refer the patient for orthopedic follow-up.

Complications

- Recurrent dislocations and subluxations

Discussion

- The patient with a lateral patellar dislocation typically holds the affected knee in slight flexion, unable to bear weight. The deformity is obvious, although swelling and hemarthrosis may also be present. With reduction the patient usually exhibits apprehension and has a sense of instability with lateral motion of the patella ("patellar apprehension sign").
- Although closed reduction of lateral patellar dislocations is easily accomplished, the rarer superior, medial, and intraarticular dislocations usually require operative reduction.
- Five percent of patellar dislocations have associated osteochondral fractures of the patella or lateral femoral condyle. A radiographic finding of a fat-fluid level indicates the presence of a fracture.

Bibliography

Roberts DM, Stallard TC: Emergency department evaluation and treatment of knee and leg injuries, *Emerg Med Clin North Am* 18(1):67-84, 2000.

Simon RR, Keonigsknecht SJ: *Emergency orthopedics: the extremities,* ed 3, Norwalk, Conn, 1996, Appleton & Lange.

Reduction and Splinting

A

Femur
Patella
Fibula
Tibia

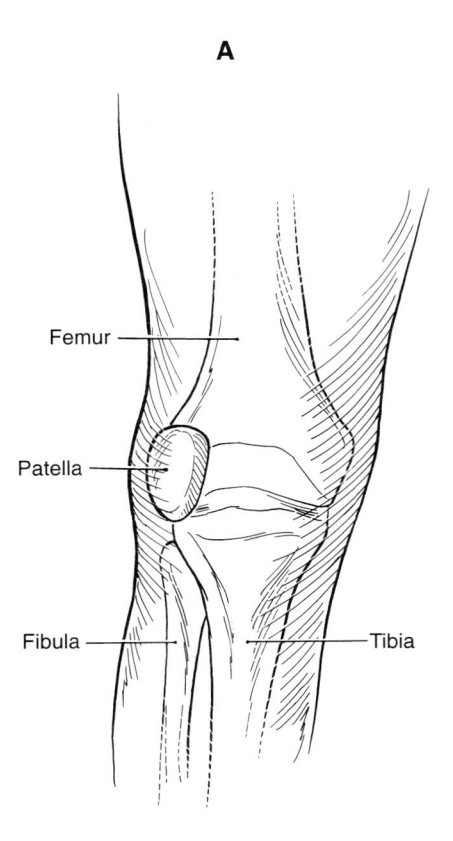

B

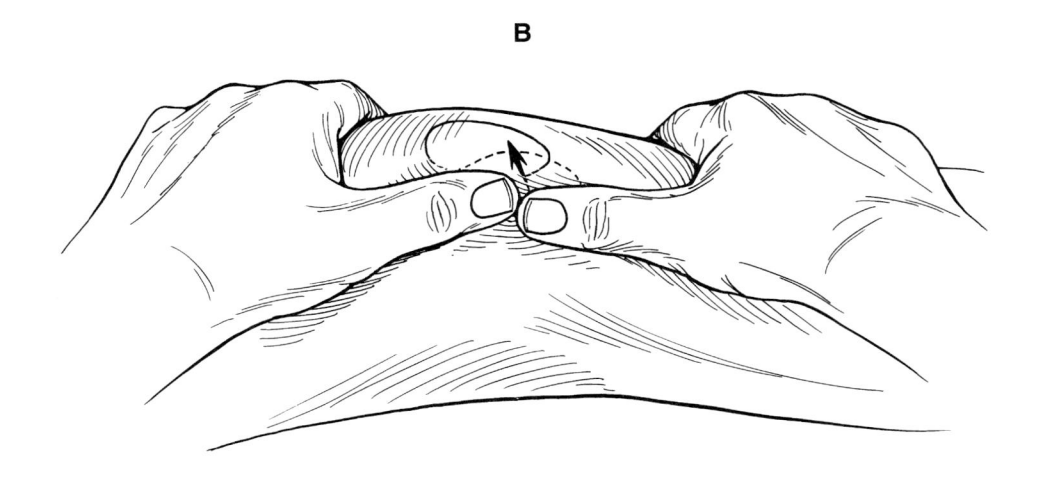

Splinting · DANIEL P. DAVIS

Indications
- Temporary immobilization of any orthopedic injury, including fractures and soft tissue injuries, until a definitive procedure is performed or immobilization device applied
- Protection of an injured extremity when occult injury is suspected although radiographs did not reveal a fracture
- Immobilization for control of pain from severe arthritis, contusions, or soft tissue injuries, including laceration repairs or nonhealing wounds

Contraindications
- Necessity for open reduction of an unstable or open fracture
- Concern for compartment syndrome in the affected extremity
- Skin at high risk for infection (i.e., with abrasions or ulcerations); caution should be used when applying a splint in this circumstance

Equipment
- Orthopedic or trauma scissors
- Standard gloves for plaster splints (special gloves are recommended for fiberglass or resin)
- Plaster slabs or rolls with the slowest setting speed available (usually in green label) in a quantity that will create 5 to 10 layers in the upper extremities and 10 to 15 layers in the lower extremities
- Webril rolls 1 inch wider than plaster in a quantity that will create three to five layers on the "skin side" of the splint and one layer on the outside of the splint, as well as extra to pad pressure points
- Alternatively, prefabricated splints in which the plaster (or synthetic resin) and padding are already supplied
- Cotton rolls covered by Webril (for bulky Jones splint)
- Bucket or basin of cool water
- Elastic bandages (such as Ace wrap)

Procedure

General Splints

1. Measure the opposite extremity, using the Webril roll, to determine the length of plaster necessary to create the splint. Plaster should be $1/2$ to 1 inch longer than measured length because some degree of contraction will occur. Lay out three to five layers of Webril, and set a single layer of the same length aside. For prefabricated splints, cut the length so that the plaster portion is $1/2$ to 1 inch longer than the measured length.

2. Roll out 5 to 10 layers of plaster for the upper extremity (10 to 15 layers for the lower extremity) on top of the Webril. The Webril should extend at least $1/2$ inch beyond the edge of the plaster on all four sides *(A)*.

3. Arrange the patient in a comfortable position, and use an assistant whenever possible. Perform any reduction as indicated at this time, and have the assistant hold the extremity in the proper position while the remainder of the splint is prepared. Place extra Webril over bony prominences to prevent pressure points.

4. Completely submerge the plaster (but not Webril) into cool water *(B)*. Squeeze the plaster and resaturate it several times. Lift the plaster out of the water, and squeeze to remove as much excess water as possible. For fiberglass or other resins do not squeeze the material after removing it from the water the last time.

5. Lay the plaster back onto the Webril, and run the heels of both hands along the plaster to remove bubbles and seal the plaster layers to each other *(C)*. Flip the plaster over, and repeat on the other side. Add the final Webril layer over the top of the plaster (this layer will face out, away from the skin).

6. Place the splint over the extremity in desired position. Have an assistant hold the splint in place while the Ace wrap is applied. The Ace wrap should be rolled from distal to proximal with the roll facing out to facilitate the "rolling" action. Overlap each layer by approximately half the width of the roll. Use as many rolls as required to entirely cover the splint. To avoid causing compartment syndrome, do not use excessive tension.

7. Once the Ace wrap covers the splint entirely, place the extremity into proper position and maintain for at least 5 to 10 minutes. Do not allow the extremity to move during this critical period, or the splint will crack and become useless. Determine which splint surfaces are most crucial for holding the extremity in proper position (i.e., the palmar and dorsal surfaces of the hand for injuries near the wrist, and the plantar surface of the foot for ankle injuries), and hold pressure on these areas for the entire setting period, using the heel of your hand to ensure a flat surface.

8. Instruct the patient not to move or "test" the splint, especially during the hour after application. The affected extremity should be elevated when possible to minimize edema formation, and the splint should be kept dry at all times, regardless of the material used.

Reduction and Splinting 273

A

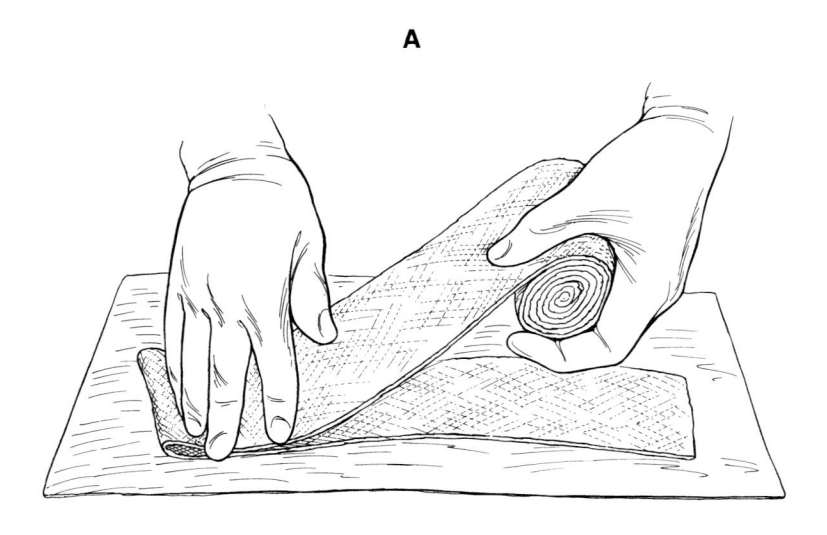

B

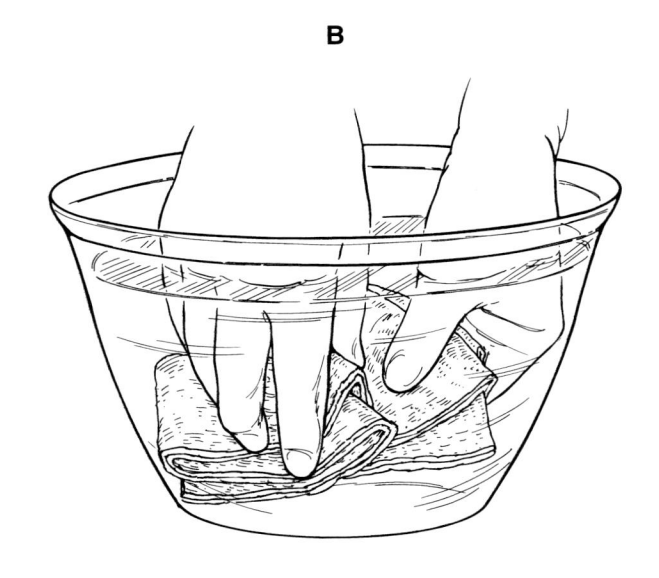

C

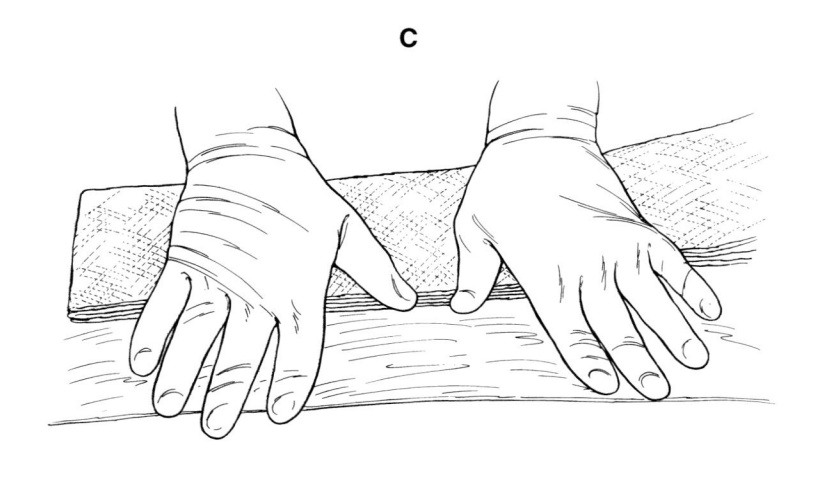

Specific Splints

Upper extremity

Volar splint

1. The volar splint is useful for protecting wrist "sprains," carpal tunnel syndrome, dorsal tendon injuries, dorsal surface lacerations, and carpal injuries (except scaphoid). It is inadequate for distal radius fractures.
2. The splint should extend from the distal palmar crease to the midforearm *(D-F)*.
3. A hole should be cut in the plaster before wetting to allow a space for the thumb.
4. To allow maximum function, the Ace wrap should not immobilize the thumb.

Ulnar gutter splint

1. The ulnar gutter splint is useful for 4th and 5th metacarpal injuries, carpal injuries on the ulnar side, isolated ulnar styloid fractures, and unstable phalangeal fractures of the ring and little fingers.
2. The splint should extend from the PIP joint (more distally for phalangeal injuries) to midforearm. The wrist should be held in 15° to 30° of extension, and the MCP joints should be held in 90° of flexion ("intrinsic plus") *(G-I)*.
3. The plaster should be wide enough to encompass the 4th and 5th metacarpals.

REDUCTION AND SPLINTING 275

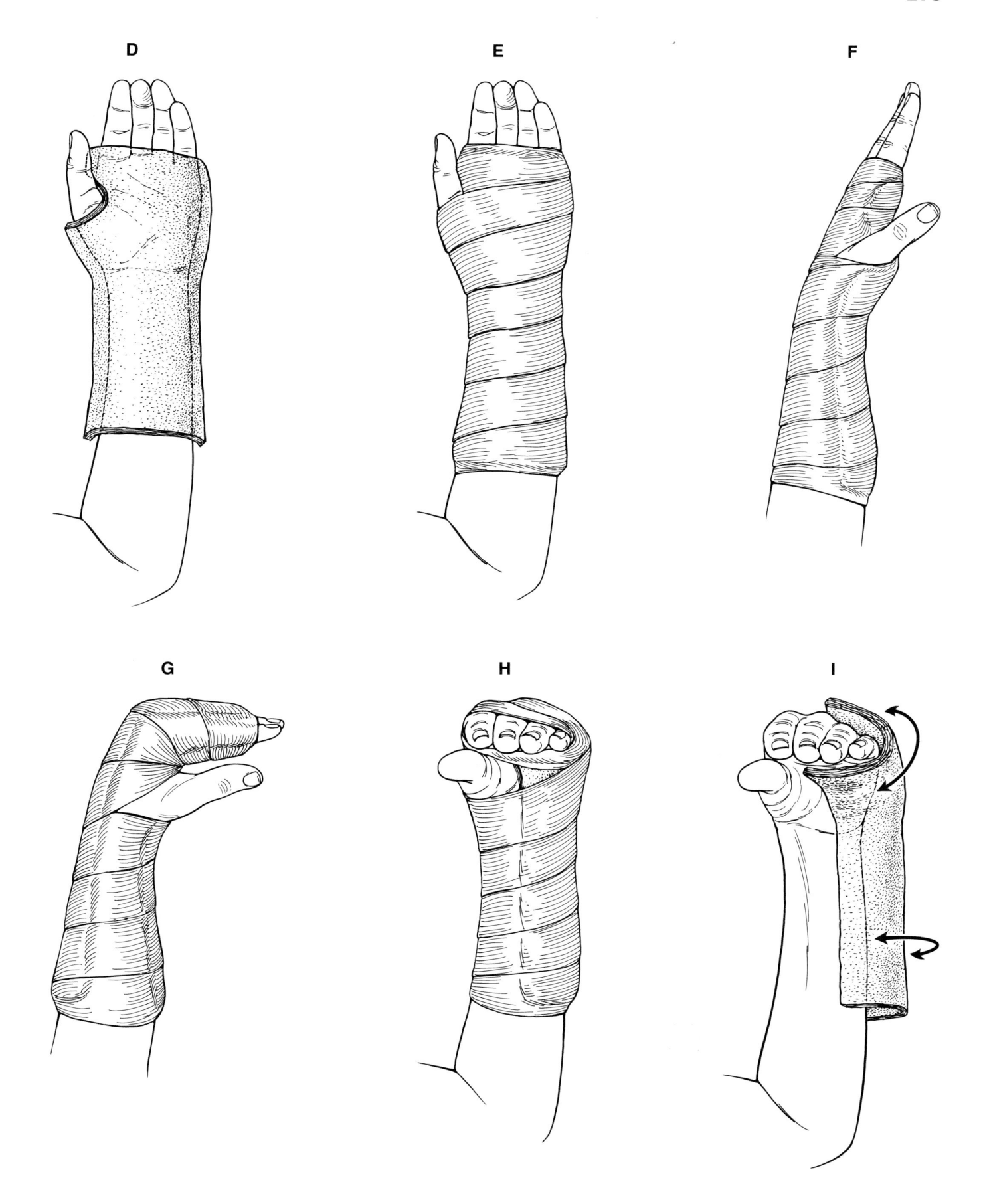

D

E

F

G

H

I

THUMB SPICA SPLINT *(J-N)*
1. The thumb spica splint is useful for gamekeeper's thumb, de Quervain's tenosynovitis, 1st metacarpal fractures, and scaphoid fractures.
2. The splint should extend from the thumb tip to midforearm, with the wrist in neutral position. The thumb should be in neutral position to allow opposition of the thumb and middle finger ("soda can position") for scaphoid and metacarpal fractures and de Quervain's tenosynovitis. Slight adduction is used for gamekeeper's thumb.

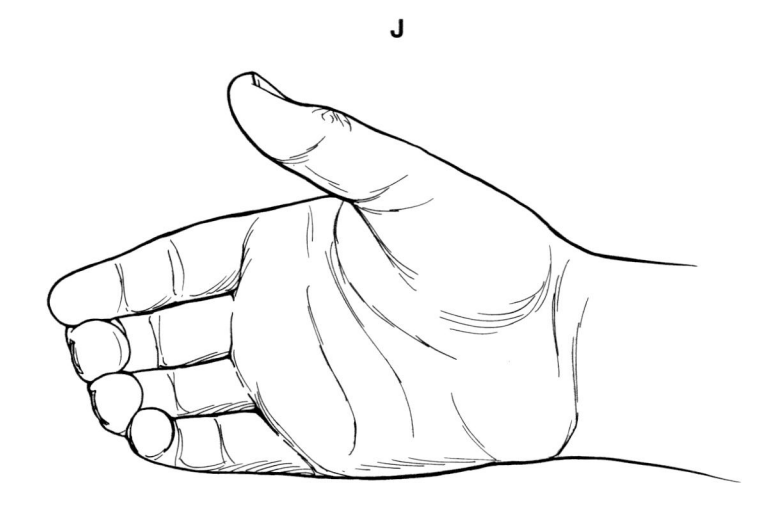

J

REDUCTION AND SPLINTING 277

K

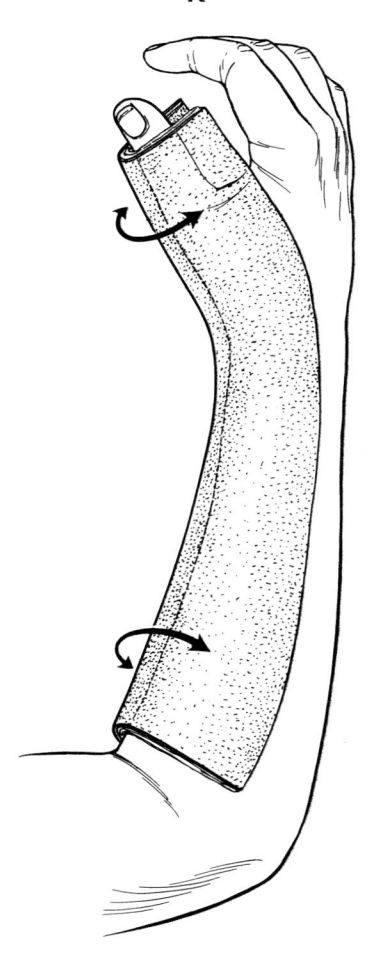

L

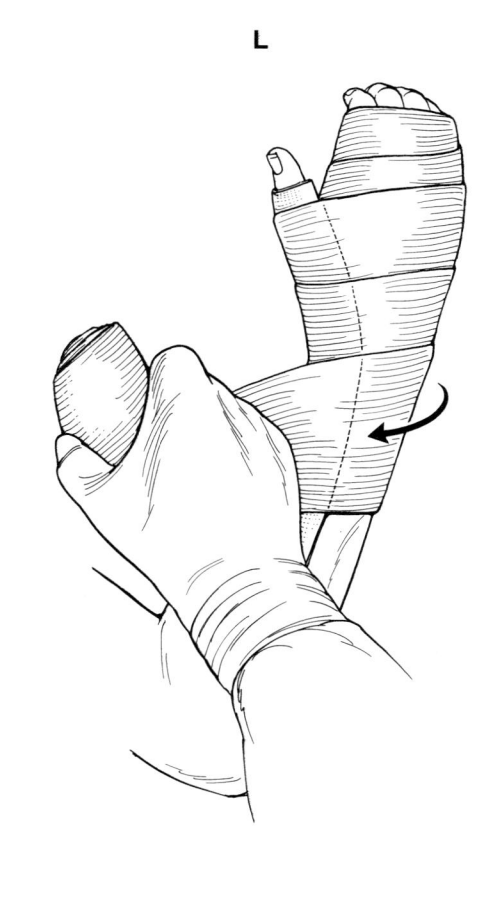

M

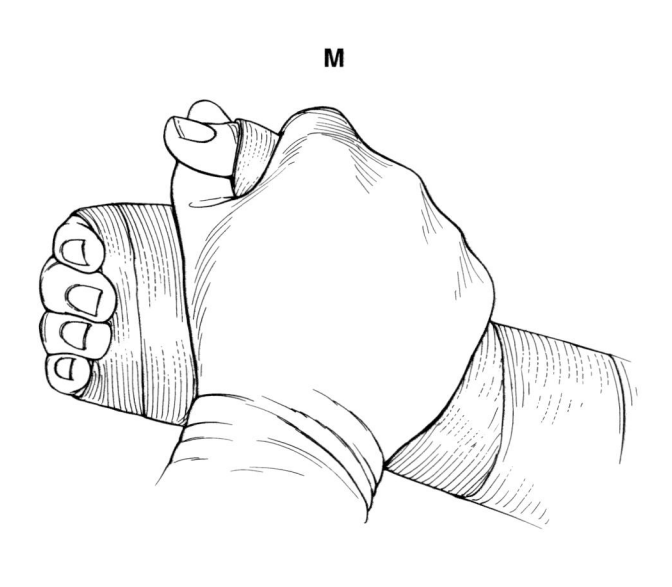

N

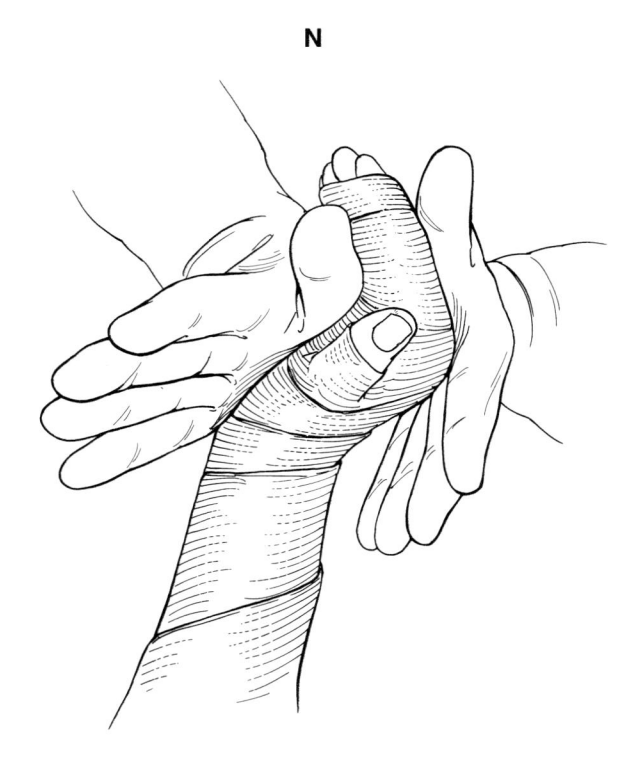

COAPTATION (SUGAR TONG) SPLINT
1. The coaptation splint is useful for any radius or ulna fractures except isolated ulnar styloid fractures (ulnar gutter splint) or radial head fractures (arm sling only).
2. The splint should extend from the palmar crease around the elbow to the dorsal MCP joints *(O, P)*. The wrist should be in neutral position with regard to both flexion-extension and supination-pronation in most cases.
3. The patient should sit with the elbow on a table and fingers upward, with the fingers held either by an assistant or by finger traps.
4. After reduction of a Colles'-type fracture, slight wrist flexion and ulnar deviation are often used. This position can be reserved for the definitive cast, however, because it is difficult to achieve with a splint alone. After reduction of a Colles'-type fracture, constant dorsal pressure should be held on the fracture fragment, before and after splint application, to prevent displacement.
5. An arm sling may be helpful to prevent shoulder strain. Shoulder range of motion maneuvers should be taught (Codman's exercises) to prevent adhesive capsulitis.

FINGER SPLINT
1. The finger splint is useful for stable phalangeal fractures, mallet finger injuries *(Q)*, and boutonniere deformities *(R)*.
2. A paper clip or commercially available metal splint may be placed over the affected joint, with tape applied to the finger on either side of the joint. For mallet finger injuries the splint should be placed on the dorsal surface of the DIP joint in extension *(S)*. For boutonniere deformities the splint should be placed on the volar surface of the PIP joint in extension *(T)*.
3. For stable phalangeal fractures (not intraarticular, spiral, or displaced), "buddy taping" to the adjacent finger is usually adequate. Alternatively, a metal splint may be placed on the volar surface of the injured finger (extending beyond the fingertip) to protect against bumping the finger and causing pain.

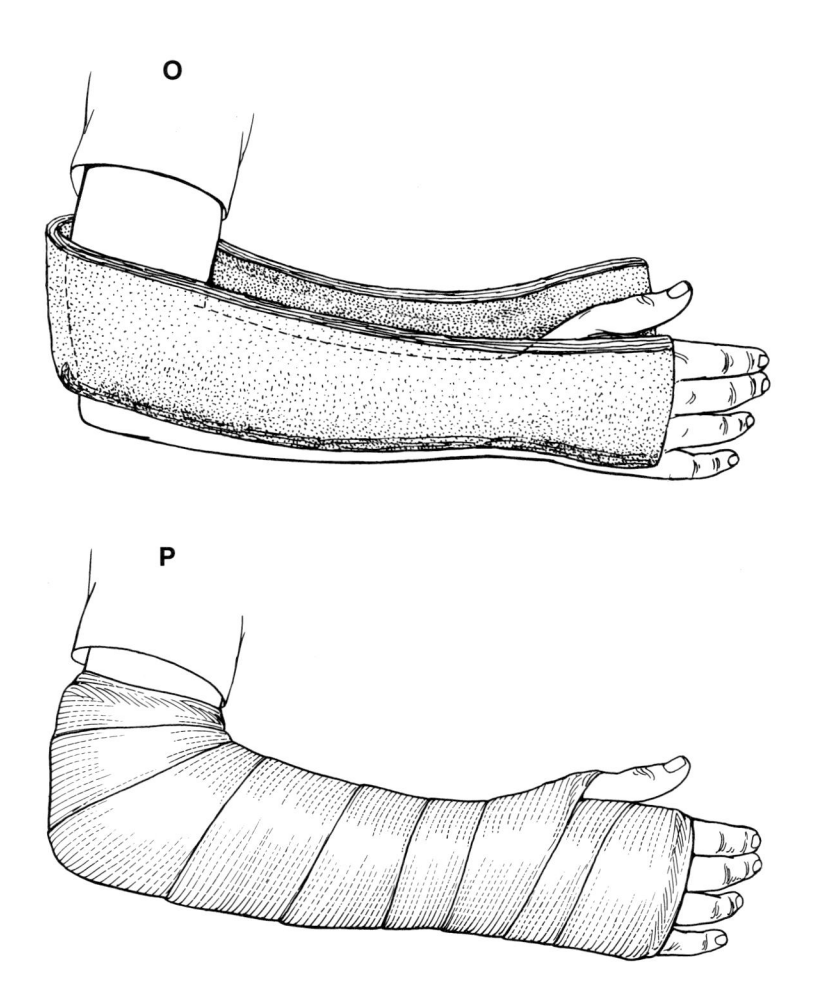

Q

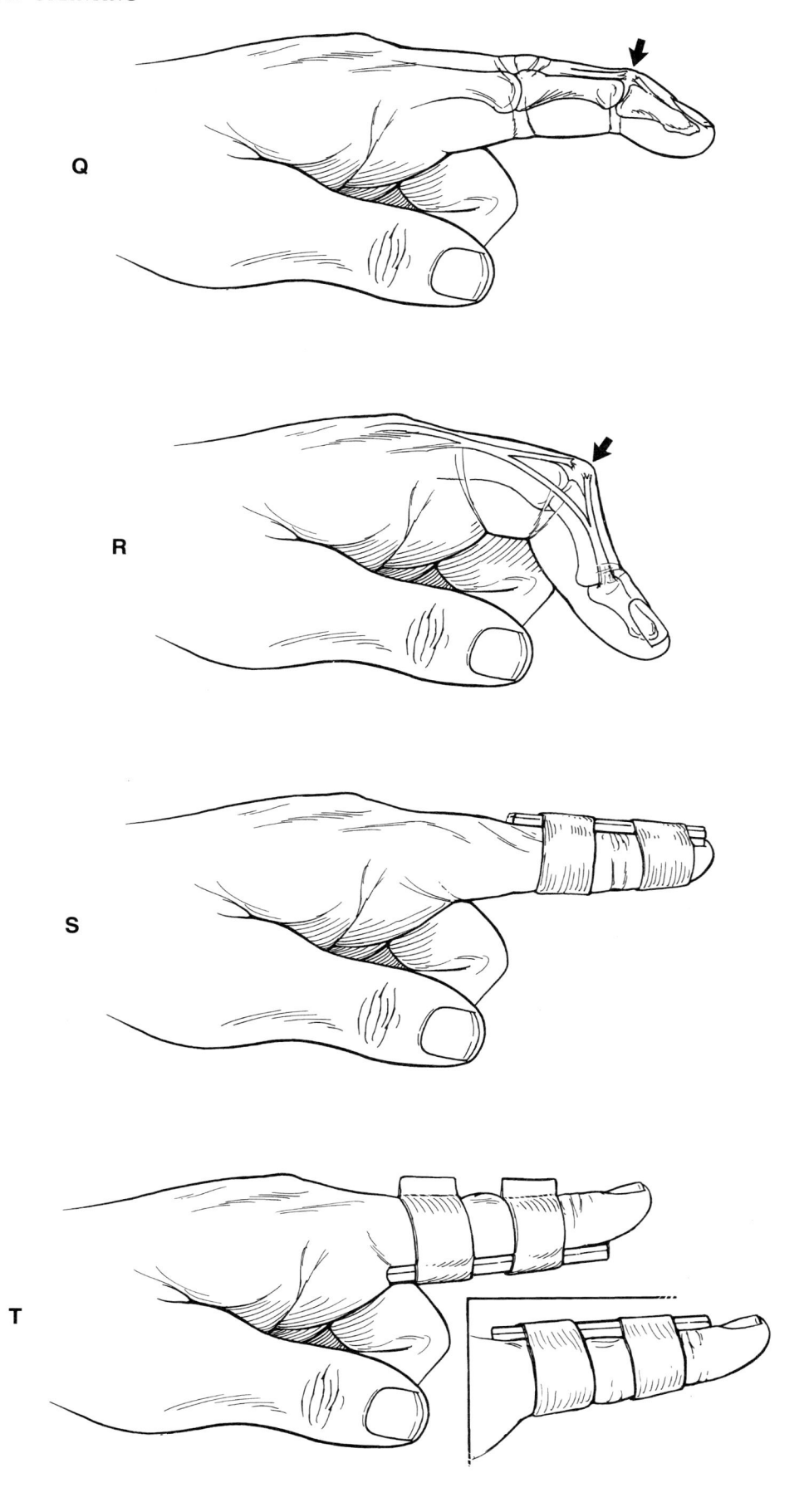

R

S

T

Lower extremity

Posterior splint (U, V)

1. The posterior splint is useful as an adjunct to the coaptation splint or for Achilles' tendon injuries, calcaneus fractures, or metatarsal fractures. This splint alone is inadequate for ankle injuries because it does not provide enough strength to prevent plantar flexion and does not prevent inversion and eversion.
2. The splint should extend from the toes to the upper calf. Care should be taken to avoid placing the splint edge against the posterior knee, which could cause abrasions or compression of the popliteal fossa. For Achilles' tendon injuries the ankle should be placed in plantar flexion; otherwise, the ankle should be placed at 90° to 110°.
3. The patient should be placed prone with the knee bent to allow the practitioner access to the foot and ankle.
4. A bulky Jones dressing (see below) may be placed first when swelling is significant.
5. For tibia injuries (other than the distal tibia) the splint may be extended up to the midthigh with the knee in slight flexion.
6. For isolated knee injuries the splint may extend from the midcalf to the midthigh, excluding the ankle. Lateral knee splints ("struts") may be added for additional valgus-varus stability.

U

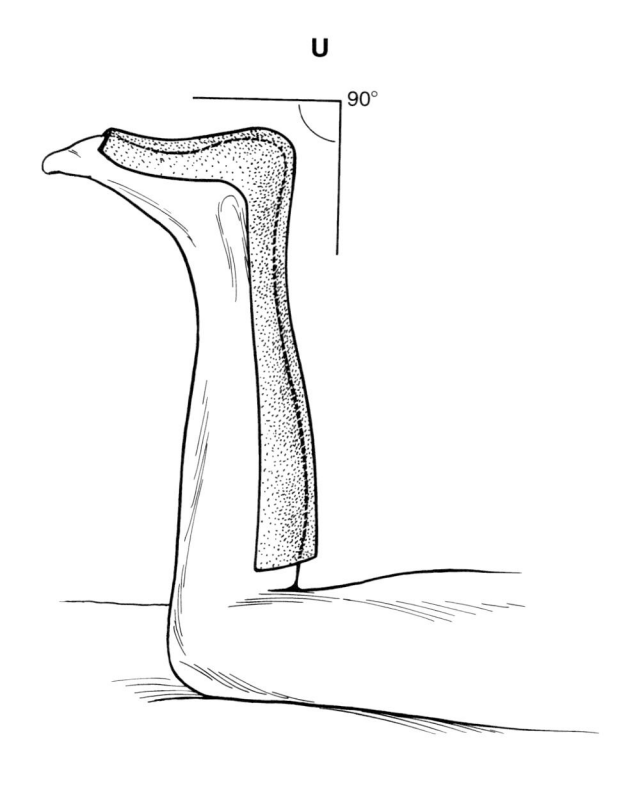

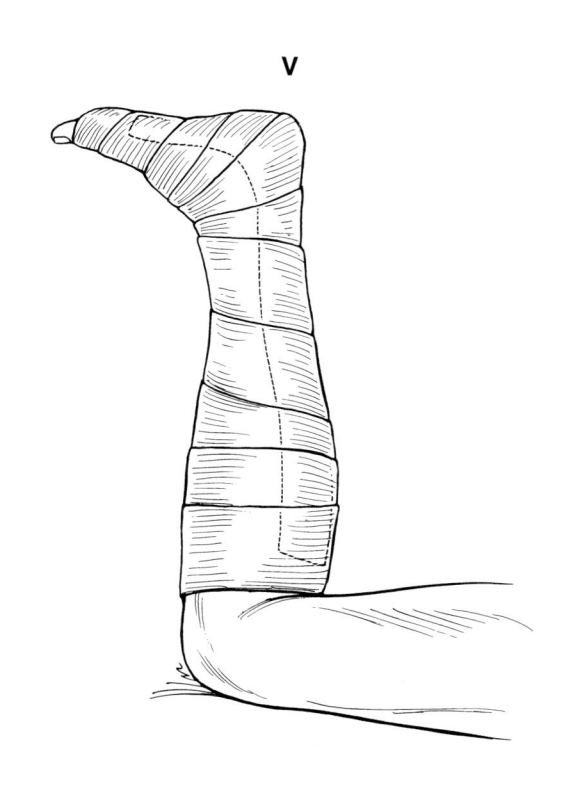

90°

V

BULKY JONES DRESSING
1. The bulky Jones dressing is useful for any lower leg, ankle, or foot injury with significant swelling.
2. The cotton roll should first be completely unrolled and split in half (with regard to thickness rather than length or width). It is then rerolled loosely to make application easier.
3. A stockinette is applied to the affected extremity. The extremity is then wrapped loosely from toes to knee (distal to proximal) with the split cotton roll *(W)*.
4. A layer of Webril is applied to compress the cotton roll. As much tension as Webril will allow should be used to produce the proper amount of compression (elastic bandage should not be used for this step). Each Webril layer is overlaid by half its width *(X)*. If the Webril tears (as it often will if proper tension is being applied), layering should start again with a complete overlap of the last layer.
5. No tape or clips are necessary to seal this layer. The splint is applied over the top of the bulky Jones dressing (Y_1-Y_3). Most commonly a posterior splint is placed in combination with a coaptation splint.

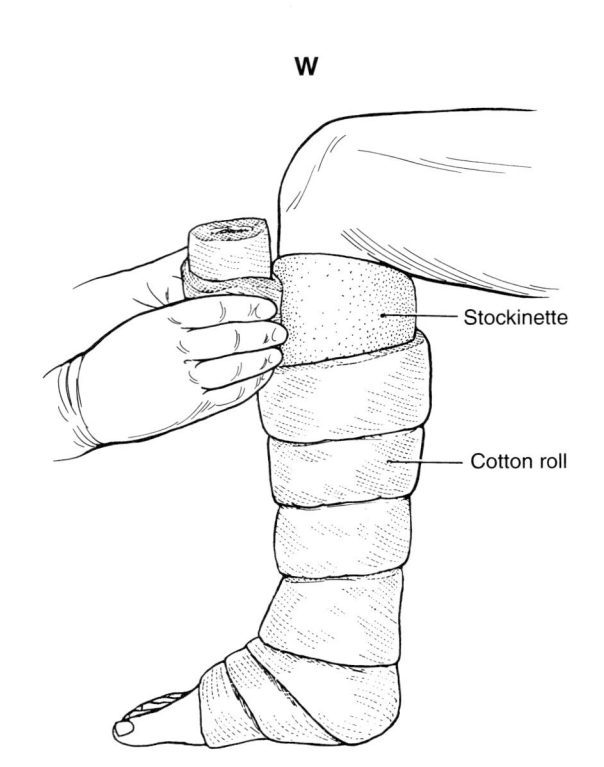

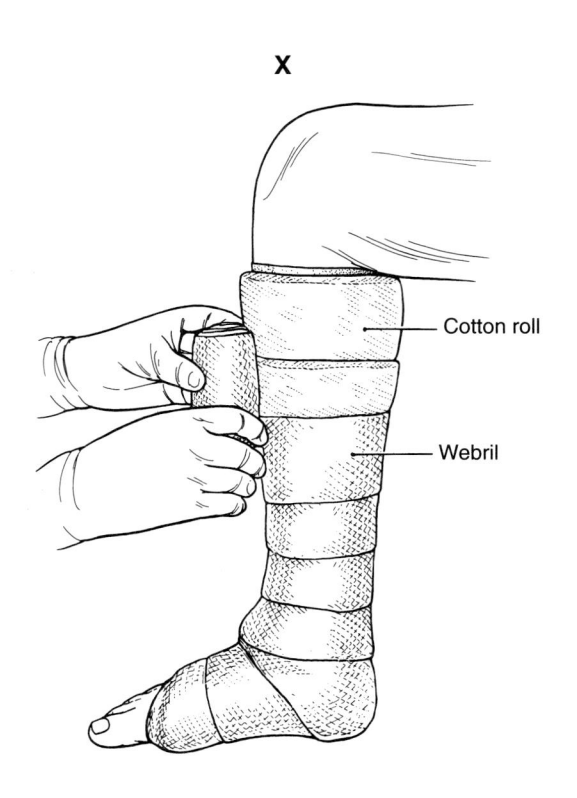

W

Stockinette
Cotton roll

X

Cotton roll
Webril

REDUCTION AND SPLINTING 283

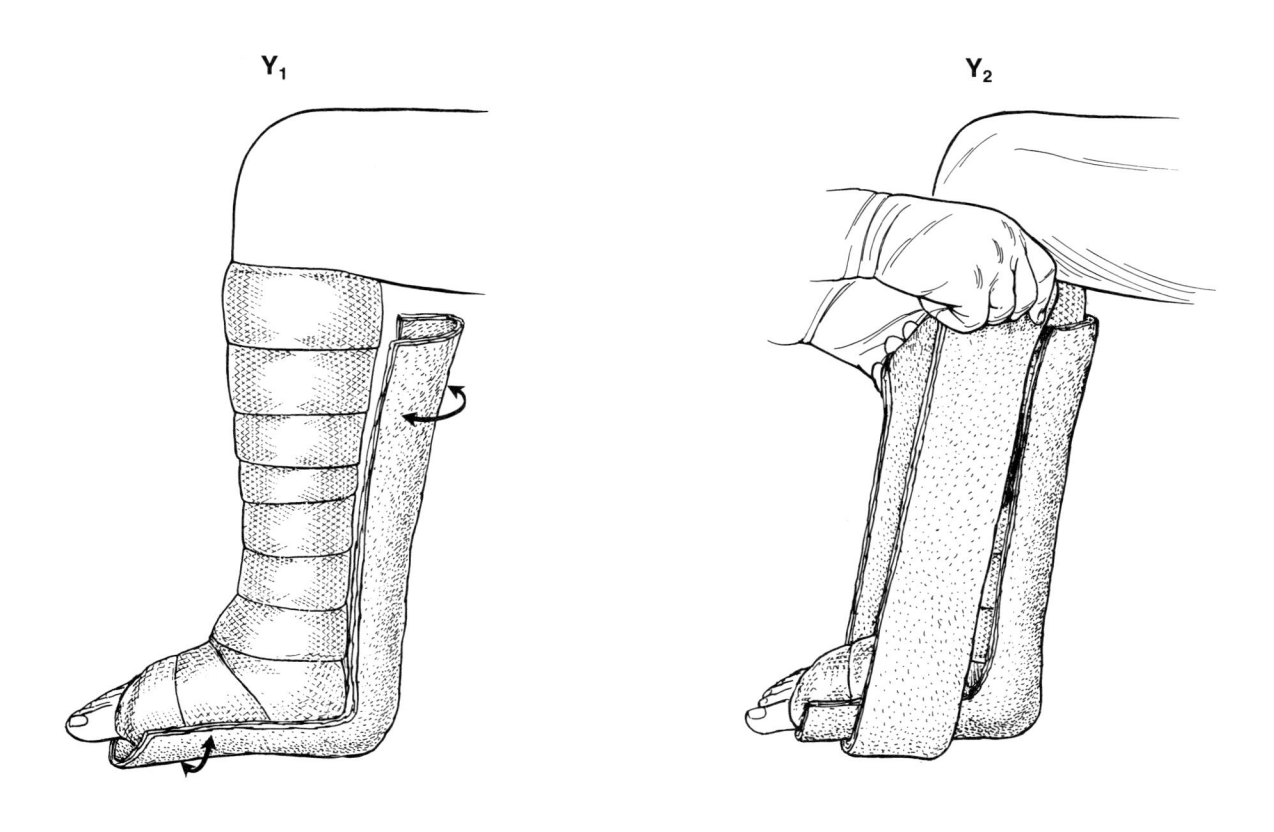

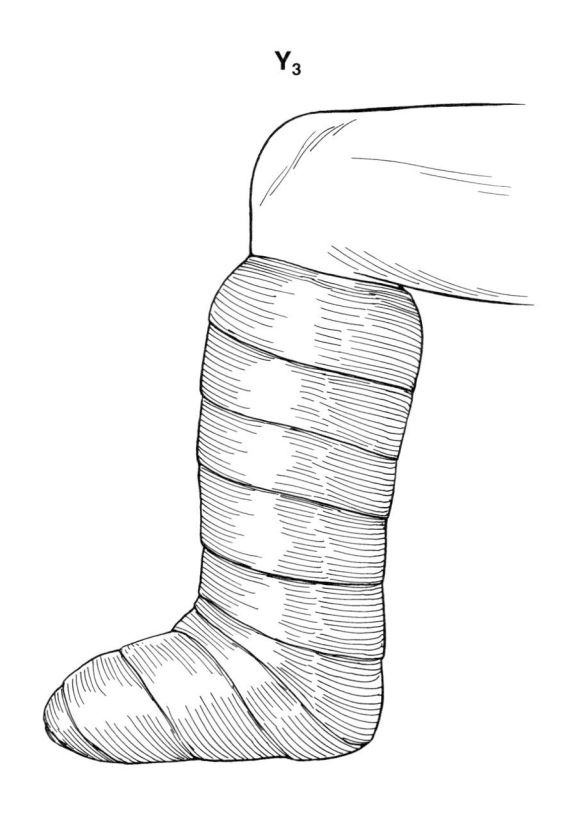

Y_1

Y_2

Y_3

Complications

- Compartment syndrome resulting from edema or excessive pressure from the splint and Ace wrap
- Skin breakdown from pressure over bony prominences
- Skin breakdown and maceration in areas of excessive pressure
- Paresthesias caused by nerve compression
- Inadequate immobilization of unstable fractures
- Joint stiffness or adhesions caused by prolonged immobilization

Discussion

- Care should be taken to avoid allowing the opposite sides of a splint to touch each other and create a circumferential "cast." If necessary, the plaster can be folded over or a narrower size can be used.
- Although a temporary splint is useful while preparations are being made for operative intervention, a splint should never be considered an appropriate alternative when immediate intervention is needed, as in cases of open fracture, extreme instability, or dislocation before reduction.
- The most common preparation mistakes involve inadequate planning, such as running out of Ace wraps or failing to enlist the help of an assistant to help hold the position.
- The most common technical mistakes involve movement while the splint is setting, rendering it useless. This can be avoided by warning the patient in advance and by holding the patient in proper position for at least 10 minutes after splint application.
- The patient should be instructed to elevate the limb. In the presence of paresthesias or numbness, the Ace wrap may be carefully loosened, but if the paresthesias or numbness does not subside, the patient should return immediately for reevaluation.
- When multiple splints are being placed (coaptation and posterior splints for ankle injuries or posterior splints with medial-lateral struts for knee injuries), the initial splint may be held in place with a layer of Webril before the final Ace wrap to prevent excessive compression and compartment syndrome.

Bibliography

Connolly JF: *Fractures and dislocations,* vol 2, Philadelphia, 1995, WB Saunders.

McRae R: *Practical fracture treatment,* ed 3, Edinburgh, 1994, Churchill Livingstone.

Simon RR, Koenigsknecht SJ: *Emergency orthopedics: the extremities,* ed 2, Norwalk, Conn, 1987, Appleton & Lange.

Index

A

Abdomen, 103-121
  anoscopy, 114-115
  excision of thrombosed external hemorrhoid, 116-117
  nasogastric intubation, 104-107
  paracentesis, 112-113
  perianal abscess drainage, 120-121
  pilonidal abscess drainage, 118-119
  semiopen diagnostic peritoneal lavage, 108-111
Abscess
  Bartholin's, incision and drainage of, 152-153
  incision and drainage of, 222-225
  perianal, drainage of, 120-121
  peritonsillar, drainage of, 202-203
  pilonidal, drainage of, 118-119
Adults, bladder aspiration in, 130
Airway, 1-29
  assisted neck ventilation, 2-3
  cricothyrotomy, 24-29
  digital intubation, 12-13
  endotracheal intubation
    pediatric, 18-19
    standard, 4-7
    using lighted stylet, 14-15
  fiberoptic intubation, 8-9
  nasotracheal intubation, 16-17
  needle cricothyrotomy, 22-23
  retrograde intubation, 10-11
  tracheal suctioning, 20-21
Allis method, posterior hip reduction by, 268-269
Alternative venous access, 90-101
Alveolar block
  anterosuperior, 163
  posterosuperior, 163
Ankle, arthrocentesis of, 234-235
Anoscopy, 114-115
Anterior approach to internal jugular central venous access, 84
Anterior fascial compartment pressure measurement, 228-231
Anterior packing, 190-191
Anterior shoulder dislocations, closed reduction of, 258-261
Anterosuperior alveolar block, 163
Aortic cross-clamping, 58-60
Arm venipuncture, 68-70
Arthrocentesis
  of ankle, 234-235
  of elbow, 240-241
  of knee, 232-233
  of metatarsophalangeal joint, 236-237
  of wrist, 242-243
Aspiration
  bladder, 130-131
  before injections, 163

Aspiration—cont'd
  needle, peritonsillar abscess drainage and, 202
  of shoulder, 238-239
Assisted mask ventilation, 2-3
Auricular hematoma drainage, 200-201

B

Baby; *see* Infants
Bag-valve-mask (BVM) resuscitator, 2-3
Bartholin's abscess, incision and drainage of, 152-153
Basilic vein cutdown, 96
Bier block, 168-169
Bladder aspiration, 130-131
Block; *see* Nerve block
Breech vaginal delivery, 142-143
Bulky Jones dressing, 282-283
Buried suture, 212-213
BVM resuscitator; *see* Bag-valve-mask resuscitator

C

Cannulation, radial artery, 62-63
Cardiac massage, 50-53
Cardiorrhaphy, 54-55
Cardiovascular system, 61-101
  alternative venous access, 90-101
    greater saphenous venous cutdown, 90-93
    intraosseous infusion, 98-99
    saphenous venous cutdown, 94-95
    umbilical venous catheter, 100-101
    upper extremity venous cutdown, 96-97
  central venous access, 74-89
    femoral, 86-89
    internal jugular, 82-85
    Seldinger guidewire technique of, 74-77
    subclavian, 78-81
  pericardiocentesis, 66-67
  peripheral venipuncture, 68-73
  peripheral venous access, 68-73
  radial artery cannulation, 62-65
Catheter, umbilical venous, 100-101
Catheterization, urethral; *see* Urethral catheterization
Central venous access, 74-89
  femoral, 86-89
  general approach to, 74-77
  internal jugular, 82-85
  Seldinger guidewire technique of, 74-77
  subclavian, 78-81
Cephalic vein cutdown, 96
Cesarean section, perimortem, 146-149
Children; *see* Infants; Pediatric patients
Closed reduction of anterior shoulder dislocations, 258-261
Coaptation splint, 278-279

Compression dressing, auricular hematoma drainage and, 200
Contact lens removal, 184-185
Corneal foreign body removal, 180-181
Corner stitch suture, 216-217
Cricothyroid membrane (CTM), retrograde intubation and, 10
Cricothyrotomy, 24-29
　needle, 22-23
Cross-clamping, aortic, 58-60
CTM; see Cricothyroid membrane
Culdocentesis, 140-141
Cutdown
　basilic vein, 96
　cephalic vein, 96
　venous; see Venous cutdown
Cystostomy, 128-129

D

Deep peroneal nerve block, 176-177
Deep posterior fascial compartment pressure measurement, 230-232
Defibrillation
　external, 32-33
　internal, 56-57
Delivery, vaginal; see Vaginal delivery
Diagnostic peritoneal lavage, semiopen, 108-111
Digital intubation, 12-13
Digital nerve block, 174-175
Directional tip endotracheal tubes, nasotracheal intubation and, 16-17
Dislocation
　anterior shoulder, closed reduction of, 258-261
　finger, 266-267
Dislocation reduction, 258-271
　closed reduction of anterior shoulder dislocations, 258-261
　finger dislocations, 266-267
　patellar, 270-271
　posterior elbow, with puller technique, 262-263
　posterior hip reduction by standard supine (Allis) method, 268-269
　radial head subluxation reduction by flexion-supination method, 264-265
Distal interphalangeal joint reduction, 266-267
Dog ear repair, 218-219
Dorsal slit in phimosis, 132-133
Drainage
　of abscess, 222-225
　auricular hematoma, 200-201
　of Bartholin's abscess, 152-153
　felon, 244-245
　paronychia, 245-246
　perianal abscess, 120-121
　peritonsillar abscess, 202-203
　pilonidal abscess, 118-119
　septal hematoma, 198-199

E

Ear, nose, and throat, 191-205
　anterior packing, 192-193
　auricular hematoma drainage, 200-201
　mandibular reduction, 204-205
　peritonsillar abscess drainage, 202-203
　posterior packing, 194-197
　septal hematoma drainage, 198-199
Elbow
　arthrocentesis of, 240-241
　posterior, dislocation reduction of, with puller technique, 262-263

Emergency procedures
　abdomen, 103-121
　airway, 1-29
　cardiovascular system, 61-101
　ear, nose, and throat, 189-205
　extremities, 227-255
　eye, 179-187
　genitourinary system, 123-137
　nervous system, 155-177
　obstetrics and gynecology, 139-153
　reduction and splinting, 257-284
　skin and subcutaneous tissue, 205-223
　thorax, 31-60
Endotracheal intubation
　pediatric, 18-19
　standard, 4-7
　using lighted stylet, 14-15
Endotrol, nasotracheal intubation and, 16-17
Episiotomy and repair, 150-151
Eversion of upper eyelid, 182-183
Excision of thrombosed external hemorrhoid, 116-117
External defibrillation, 32-33
External hemorrhoid, thrombosed, excision of, 116-117
External jugular vein venipuncture, 70-71
External rotation technique, closed reduction of anterior shoulder dislocations and, 258-261
Extremities, 227-255
　arthrocentesis
　　of ankle, 234-235
　　of elbow, 240-241
　　of knee, 232-233
　　of metatarsophalangeal joint, 236-237
　　of wrist, 242-243
　aspiration of shoulder, 238-239
　fascial compartment pressure measurement (anterior compartment, lower leg), 228-231
　hand, 244-257
　　felon drainage, 244-245
　　fish hook removal, 252-255
　　paronychia drainage, 246-247
　　ring removal, 248-251
　　nail removal, 252-253
Extremity blocks, 168-177
　Bier block, 168-169
　digital nerve block, 174-175
　foot, 176-177
　wrist blocks, 170-173
Eye, 179-187
　contact lens removal, 184-185
　corneal foreign body removal, 180-181
　eversion of upper eyelid, 182-183
　measurement of intraocular pressure–Schiøtz tonometry, 186-187
Eyelid, eversion of, 182-183

F

Facial and oral blocks, 158-167
　infraorbital nerve block, 160-161
　internal maxillary–superior alveolar nerve block, 162-163
　mandibular and inferior alveolar nerve block, 164-165
　mental nerve block, 166-167
　supraorbital nerve block, 158-159
Fascial compartment pressure measurement, 228-231
Felon drainage, 244-245
Female patient, urethral catheterization for, 124-125
Femoral central venous access, 86-89
Fiberoptic intubation, 8-9

Index

Finger dislocations, 266-267
Finger splint, 278-279
Fish hook removal, 252-255
Flexion-supination method, radial head subluxation reduction by, 264-265
Foley posterior pack, 194
Foot blocks, 176-177
Foreign body, corneal, removal of, 180-181

G

Genitourinary system, 123-137
    bladder aspiration, 130-131
    cystostomy, 128-129
    dorsal slit in phimosis, 132-133
    manual phimosis reduction, 134-135
    urethral catheterization, 124-127
        for female patient, 124-125
        for male patient, 126-127
    zipper removal, 136-137
Greater saphenous venous cutdown, 90-93
Gynecology; see Obstetrics and gynecology

H

Half-buried horizontal mattress suture, 216-217
Hand, 244-255
    felon drainage, 244-245
    fish hook removal, 252-255
    paronychia drainage, 246-247
    ring removal, 247-251
    venipuncture and, 68-70
Hard contact lens, removal of, 184-185
Hematoma
    auricular, drainage of, 200-201
    septal, drainage of, 198-199
Hemorrhoid, thrombosed external, excision of, 116-117
Hip, posterior, reduction of, by standard supine (Allis) method, 268-269
Horizontal mattress suture, 210-211
    half-buried, 216-217

I

Incision
    of abscess, 222-225
    and drainage of Bartholin's abscess, 152-153
Infants; see also Pediatric patients
    care after delivery of, 144-145
    scalp vein for, venipuncture using, 72
Inferior alveolar nerve block, 164-165
Infraclavicular approach to subclavian central venous access, 78
Infraorbital nerve block, 160-161
Infusion, intraosseous, 98-99
Intercostal nerve block, 34-35
Internal defibrillation, 56-57
Internal jugular central venous access, 82-85
Internal maxillary–superior alveolar nerve block, 162-163
Interphalangeal joint reduction, distal, 266-267
Interphalangeal joint reduction, proximal, 266-267
Interrupted suture, 208-209
Intradermal suture, 212-213
Intraocular pressure, measurement of, 186-187
Intraosseous infusion, 98-99
Intubation
    digital, 12-13
    endotracheal; see Endotracheal intubation
    fiberoptic, 8-9
    nasogastric, 104-107

Intubation—cont'd
    nasotracheal, 16-17
    retrograde, 10-11

J

Joint
    distal interphalangeal, reduction of, 266-267
    proximal interphalangeal, reduction of, 266-267
Jones dressing, bulky, 282-283
Jugular vein, external, venipuncture using, 70-71

K

Knee, arthrocentesis of, 232-233

L

Laceration, scalp, repair of, 214-215
Lateral fascial compartment pressure measurement, 230-231
Lavage, semiopen diagnostic peritoneal, 108-111
Lens, contact, removal of, 184-185
Lighted stylet, endotracheal intubation using, 14-15
Lower extremity splints, 280-284
Lumbar puncture, 156-157

M

Male patient, urethral catheterization for, 126-127
Mandibular and inferior alveolar nerve block, 164-165
Mandibular reduction, 204-205
Manual paraphimosis reduction, 134-135
Mask ventilation, assisted, 2-3
Massage, cardiac, 50-53
Mastoid dressing, auricular hematoma drainage and, 200
Mattress suture, 210-211
    half-buried horizontal, 216-217
    horizontal, 210-211
    vertical, 210-211
Measurement
    fascial compartment pressure, 228-231
    of intraocular pressure, 186-187
Median nerve block, 172-173
Mental nerve block, 166-167
Metacarpophalangeal reduction, 266-267
Metatarsophalangeal joint, arthrocentesis of, 234-235
Middle approach to internal jugular central venous access, 82

N

Nail removal, 252-253
Nasogastric intubation, 104-107
Nasotracheal intubation, 16-17
Needle aspiration, peritonsillar abscess drainage and, 202
Needle cricothyrotomy, 22-23
Needle thoracostomy, 38-39
Nerve block
    anterosuperior alveolar, 163
    Bier, 168-169
    deep peroneal, 176-177
    digital, 174-175
    extremity; see Extremity blocks
    facial and oral; see Facial and oral blocks
    foot, 176-177
    infraorbital, 160-161
    intercostal, 34-35
    internal maxillary–superior alveolar, 162-163
    mandibular and inferior alveolar, 164-165
    median, 172-173
    mental, 166-167
    posterior tibial, 176-177

Nerve block—cont'd
　　posterosuperior alveolar, 163
　　radial, 170-171
　　superficial peroneal, 176-177
　　supraorbital, 158-159
　　sural, 176-177
　　ulnar, 172
　　wrist; see Wrist blocks
Nervous system, 155-177
　　extremity blocks, 168-177
　　　　Bier block, 168-169
　　　　digital nerve block, 174-175
　　　　foot blocks, 176-177
　　　　wrist blocks, 170-173
　　facial and oral blocks, 158-167
　　　　infraorbital nerve block, 160-161
　　　　internal maxillary–superior alveolar nerve block, 162-163
　　　　mandibular and inferior alveolar nerve block, 164-165
　　　　mental nerve block, 166-167
　　　　supraorbital nerve block, 158-159
　　lumbar puncture, 156-157
Nose; see Ear, nose, and throat

O

Obstetrics and gynecology, 139-153
　　culdocentesis, 140-141
　　episiotomy and repair, 150-151
　　incision and drainage of Bartholin's abscess, 152-153
　　perimortem cesarean section, 146-149
　　vaginal delivery, 142-145
Oral blocks; see Facial and oral blocks

P

Packing
　　anterior, 190-193
　　posterior, 194-197
Paracentesis, 112-113
Paraphimosis reduction, manual, 134-135
Paronychia drainage, 246-247
Patellar dislocation reduction, 270-271
Pediatric patients; see also Infants
　　bladder aspiration in, 130
　　endotracheal intubation in, 18-19
Perianal abscess drainage, 120-121
Pericardiocentesis, 66-67
Perimortem cesarean section, 146-149
Peripheral venipuncture, 68-73
　　external jugular vein, 70-71
　　hand and arm venipuncture, 68-70
　　scalp vein for infants, 72
Peripheral venous access, 68-73
　　external jugular vein, 70-71
　　hand and arm venipuncture, 68-70
　　scalp vein for infants, 72
Peritoneal lavage, semiopen diagnostic, 108-111
Peritonsillar abscess drainage, 202-203
Phimosis, dorsal slit in, 132-133
Pilonidal abscess drainage, 118-119
PIP joint; see Proximal interphalangeal joint
Posterior approach to internal jugular central venous access, 82
Posterior elbow dislocation reduction with puller technique, 262-263
Posterior fascial compartment pressure measurement, 230-231
Posterior hip reduction by standard supine (Allis) method, 268-269
Posterior packing, 194-197
Posterior splint, 280-281
Posterior tibial nerve block, 176-177

Posterosuperior alveolar block, 163
Proximal interphalangeal (PIP) joint reduction, 266-267
Puller technique, posterior elbow dislocation reduction with, 262-263

R

Radial artery cannulation, 62-63
Radial head subluxation reduction by flexion-supination method, 264-265
Radial nerve block, 170-171
Reduction
　　closed, of anterior shoulder dislocations, 258-261
　　dislocation; see Dislocation reduction
　　distal interphalangeal joint, 266-267
　　mandibular, 204-205
　　manual paraphimosis, 134-135
　　metacarpophalangeal, 266-267
　　posterior hip, by standard supine (Allis) method, 268-269
　　proximal interphalangeal joint, 266-267
　　and splinting, 257-284
　　　　dislocation reduction, 258-271
　　　　　　closed reduction of anterior shoulder dislocations, 258-261
　　　　　　posterior elbow dislocation reduction with puller technique, 262-263
　　　　　　radial head subluxation reduction by flexion-supination method, 264-265
　　　　　　finger dislocations, 266-267
　　　　　　lower extremity, 280-284
　　　　　　patellar dislocation reduction, 270-271
　　　　　　posterior hip reduction by standard supine (Allis) method, 268-269
　　　　　　upper extremity, 274-279
　　subluxation, radial head, by flexion-supination method, 264-265
Resuscitator, bag-valve-mask, 2-3
Retrograde intubation, 10-11
Ring removal, 248-251
Running suture, 208-209

S

Saphenofemoral venous cutdown, 94-95
Scalp laceration repair, 214-215
Scalp vein for infants, venipuncture using, 72
Scapular rotation modification, Stimson's technique with, closed reduction of anterior shoulder dislocations and, 258-259
Schiøtz tonometry, 186-187
Seldinger guidewire technique of central venous access, 74-77
Semiopen diagnostic peritoneal lavage, 108-111
Septal hematoma drainage, 198-199
Shoulder
　　anterior, dislocations of, closed reduction of, 258-261
　　aspiration of, 238-239
Skin and subcutaneous drainage, 207-225
　　abscess incision and drainage, 222-225
　　buried suture, 211-213
　　corner stitch, 216-217
　　dog ear repair, 218-219
　　half-buried horizontal mattress suture, 216-217
　　interrupted and running suture, 208-209
　　intradermal suture, 212-213
　　mattress suture, 210-211
　　scalp laceration repair, 214-215
　　V-Y closure, 220-221
Slit, dorsal, in phimosis, 132-133
Soft contact lens, removal of, 184-185
Splints, 272-284
　　bulky Jones, 282-283
　　coaptation, 278

Index

Splints—cont'd
 finger, 278-279
 posterior, 280-281
 reduction and; see Reduction and splinting
 thumb spica, 276-277
 ulnar gutter, 274-275
 upper extremity, 274-279, 280-281
 volar, 274-275
Standard endotracheal intubation, 4-7
Standard supine (Allis) method, posterior hip reduction by, 268-269
Stimson's technique with scapular rotation modification, closed reduction of anterior shoulder dislocations and, 258-259
Stylet, lighted, endotracheal intubation using, 14-15
Subclavian central venous access, 78-81
Subcutaneous drainage; see Skin and subcutaneous drainage
Subluxation reduction, radial head, by flexion-supination method, 264-265
Suctioning, tracheal, 20-21
Sugar tong splint, 278-279
Superficial peroneal nerve block, 176-177
Superficial posterior fascial compartment pressure measurement, 230-231
Supine method, standard, posterior hip reduction by, 268-269
Supraclavicular approach to subclavian central venous access, 78-81
Supraorbital nerve block, 158-159
Sural nerve block, 176-177
Suture
 buried, 212-213
 half-buried horizontal mattress, 216-217
 horizontal mattress, 210-211
 interrupted, 208-209
 intradermal, 212-213
 mattress, 210-211
 running, 208-209
 vertical mattress, 210-211

T

Thoracentesis, 36-37
Thoracostomy
 needle, 38-39
 tube, 40-45
Thoracotomy, 46-49
Thorax, 31-60
 aortic cross-clamping, 58-60
 cardiac massage, 50-53
 cardiorrhaphy, 54-55
 external defibrillation, 32-33
 intercostal nerve block, 34-35
 internal defibrillation, 56-57
 needle thoracostomy, 38-39
 thoracentesis, 36-37
 thoracotomy, 46-49
 tube thoracostomy, 40-45
Throat; see Ear, nose, and throat
Thrombosed external hemorrhoid, excision of, 116-117
Thumb spica splint, 276-277
Tonometry, Schiøtz, 186-187
Tracheal suctioning, 20-21
Traction-countertraction technique, closed reduction of anterior shoulder dislocations and, 260-261
Tube thoracostomy, 40-45

U

Ulnar gutter splint, 274-275
Ulnar nerve block, 172
Umbilical venous catheter, 100-101
Upper extremity splints, 274-279
Upper extremity venous cutdown, 96-97
Upper eyelid, eversion of, 182-183
Urethral catheterization, 124-127
 for female patient, 124-125
 for male patient, 126-127

V

Vaginal delivery, 142-145
 after delivery of baby, 144-145
 breech, 142
 vertex, 142-143
Venipuncture
 hand and arm, 68-70
 peripheral; see Peripheral venipuncture
Venous access
 alternative, 90-101
 central; see Central venous access
 greater saphenous venous cutdown, 90-93
 intraosseous infusion, 98-99
 peripheral; see Peripheral venous access
 saphenofemoral venous cutdown, 94-95
 umbilical venous catheter, 100-101
 upper extremity venous cutdown, 96-97
Venous catheter, umbilical, 100-101
Venous cutdown
 greater saphenous, 90-93
 saphenofemoral, 94-95
 upper extremity, 96-97
Ventilation, assisted mask, 2-3
Vertex vaginal delivery, 142-143
Vertical mattress suture, 210-211
Volar splint, 274-275
V-Y closure, 220-221

W

Wrist, arthrocentesis of, 242-243
Wrist blocks, 170-173
 median nerve block, 172-173
 radial nerve block, 170-171
 ulnar nerve block, 172

Z

Zipper removal, 136-137